EMT - Basic
Review

A CASE-BASED APPROACH

EMT-Basic Review

Review

A CASE-BASED APPROACH

KAYE NAGELL, BSN, RN, CEN
Sevierville, Tennessee

NEIL COKER, BS, EMT-P
Director of Simulation Teaching, Assessment, and Research Programs
Division of Health Sciences
Temple College
Temple, Texas

*with **48** illustrations*

MOSBY
ELSEVIER

MOSBY JEMS
ELSEVIER

11830 Westline Industrial Drive
St. Louis, Missouri 63146

EMT-BASIC REVIEW: A CASE-BASED APPROACH, REVISED EDITION

NOTICE

ISBN-13: 978-0-323-04776-0
ISBN-10: 0-323-04776-9

Executive Editor: Linda Honeycutt
Developmental Editor: Laura Bayless
Publishing Services Manager: Pat Joiner
Project Manager: David Stein
Design Manager: Gail Morey Hudson

Printed in the United States

Last digit is the print number: 9   8   7   6   5   4   3

To

Rosalie Ward, MSED, MSRN

You are truly an asset to your profession,
a fantastic instructor, and an inspiration to all.
Thank you for being such a great friend over the years.

I would also like to dedicate this to
my co-author
Neil
Thank you for all your help and advice.

KAYE NAGELL

To

my parents.

NEIL COKER

Preface

Yes, it is time to study for your EMT certification examination. You may be taking an original EMT-Basic course or you may be reviewing for the State or the National Registry examination. In either case, this book is designed to help you.

Being an EMT is one of the most rewarding professions in the world, but it also is one of the most demanding. Whether you volunteer or are paid, an EMT's responsibilities require your best efforts 24 hours a day, 7 days a week. When you join the EMS world, you embark on a career of helping others. You will gather a multitude of memories. As you meet and overcome obstacles along the way, you will continue to build your own character. Many of your patients will remain in your heart forever.

Along with the rest of the world, medicine changes constantly. Fifty years ago EMS was almost unheard of. Forty years ago many ambulances were "load and go horizontal taxicabs." Thirty years ago paramedics were just coming into being. And 20 years ago standing orders were being introduced into prehospital medicine for the first time. Skills have changed, equipment has changed, and even our thinking about how and where to treat patients has changed. Now, try to imagine what EMS will be like 20 or 30 years in the future! For the sake of your patients, you must remain abreast of these changes. Keep reviewing, keep studying, and keep learning. Your knowledge, skills, performance, common sense, and abilities always will be under the greatest scrutiny. You must give every patient 100% of your expertise.

This book is not intended to replace your EMT-Basic textbook. It is a review manual designed to help you focus on the most important ideas and identify areas in which you need additional study. Each chapter begins with an outline that reviews essential concepts. In most of the chapters the outline is followed by several patient care scenarios, many of which are based on actual calls. Accompanying each scenario is a space for you to write your treatment plan for the patient and a series of multiple-choice, completion, matching, or true-false questions to test your understanding of the patient's disease process and its treatment. At the end of each chapter, an appropriate treatment plan for each scenario and its rationale are provided along with answers to the questions.

Scenarios involving responses to acts of terrorism are presented in several chapters. Additionally, we have included a complete chapter on chemical and biological terrorism. In today's world, we never know if terror will strike in a large city or a small town. EMTs, paramedics, firefighters, and law enforcement officers must understand the tools terrorists use so they can protect themselves and the public. The only way to survive is to be prepared.

We have provided a CD with several practice examinations so you can test your overall understanding of the material presented in the EMT-Basic course. In some areas, EMT-Basics now are taking their examinations on computers, and the National Registry may move to this format in the near future. The CD will help you feel better prepared to take a comprehensive final examination and allow you to become more comfortable with computer-administered tests.

We are proud to have been involved with the emergency services for most of our lives and very proud of the EMTs and paramedics we have worked with and had the opportunity to teach. Kaye volunteered for 23 years with the Four Town Ambulance Squad. Many of the cases and scenarios in this book are based on responses to actual calls while working as a paramedic with Eastern Ambulance and as a volunteer paramedic with the Four Town Ambulance Squad. Neil has had the privilege of teaching EMS personnel in settings ranging from metropolitan Dallas to rural communities in the Texas Panhandle and South Plains, where EMTs and paramedics often are the only healthcare providers in an area of thousands of square miles. His experiences with these dedicated professionals, who are too numerous to even begin to name, have shaped his contributions to this book. All of you have our thanks and our admiration. Please, please be careful out there.

Acknowledgments

AUTHOR ACKNOWLEDGMENTS

To Claire Merrick: With your support this project grew into reality. Thank you for your support and help.
To Laura Bayless: I really appreciate all your support, help, and guidance. Thank you for being there through all those phone calls. You are the best in your profession.
To David Stein: A very special thank you for your terrific guidance and support as an editor, and for always listening with an open mind. You are a great addition to the Mosby publishing staff.

Kaye Nagell

PUBLISHER ACKNOWLEDGMENTS

The editors wish to acknowledge the following reviewers for their invaluable help in developing and fine-tuning this book:

Robert D. Cook, NREMT-P, PS, EMS-I, EMD
Iowa Central Community College
Ft. Dodge, Iowa

Julie Crawshaw, BSN, MICN
University of California, Los Angeles (UCLA), Westwood, California;
Long Beach Community College (LBCC), Long Beach, California;
St. Mary's Medical Center, Long Beach, California

Marti Driscoll, AS EMS, AA, NREMT-P
Clinical Coordinator, Instructor Emergency Medical Services Education
Daytona Beach, Florida

Dennis Edgerly, EMT-P
HealthOne EMS
Englewood, Colorado

Mike Loreg, MICT, EMT-B I/C
Director, Harper County EMS
Anthony, Kansas

David S. Pecora, PA-C, NREMT-P, RN
Department of Emergency Medicine, West Virginia University
Morgantown, West Virginia

Eric Powell, PhD(c)
EMS Curriculum Area Coordinator
Health Sciences Division, Carteret Community College
Morehead City, North Carolina

Anne Robenstein, DO
Cortland Memorial Hospital for Emergency Medicine Physicians
Cortland, New York

Janet L. Schulte BS, AS, NR-CCEMT-P
Training Center Coordinator
IHM Health Studies Center
St. Louis, Missouri

Study and Test-Taking Skills for EMT Students

BEFORE THE TEST

1. If you have a history of not doing well on written examinations, you may suffer from a reading or learning disability. Professionals at the counseling center of a college or university can help you determine if this is the case. If you have a diagnosed learning disability, they can help you identify strategies to help compensate for it. Also, in some cases, certifying agencies will allow reasonable accommodations such as increased time to take a test if you have a documented learning disability.

2. Keep up with the course material. Try to schedule time to study every day. As part of your schedule allow some time each week to review all course content presented up to that point.

3. Try to identify and learn the major concepts before you learn the details. Understanding the major concepts gives you a structure to associate the details with.

4. Do *not* simply memorize the material. Take the time to understand why patients with specific problems present with specific signs and symptoms or why you manage particular problems in a specific way. If you understand the material and try to make it meaningful to yourself, you will be able to remember and apply it more effectively and efficiently.

5. Schedule time for both personal and group study. When you study alone, you have a chance to go over material you are unsure of. When you study in a group, you can learn from your partners and help others.

6. Do *not* study and review with the goal of passing the test. Study and review to prepare yourself to be the best EMT you possibly can be. If you remain focused on this goal, you also will be able to pass the tests.

7. Get plenty of rest. Do not pull an "all nighter" just before a test.

8. Do *not* cram. Cramming tends to clutter your mind and lead to confusion. Also, material you study during a "cram" session will not be stored in your long-term memory where you can use it later. Study regularly and learn the material in small steps.

9. On the day of the test, dress comfortably. Wear layered clothing so you can add or remove clothing if the testing room is too hot or too cold.

10. Eat a low-fat, complex carbohydrate meal before coming to a test. Avoid overeating or eating foods that may be hard to digest.

11. Avoid too much caffeine, which can affect your attention and concentration. Do *not* drink alcohol before a test. While you should *not* self-medicate, there are a number of medications your doctor can prescribe if you suffer from severe test anxiety that hampers your performance.

12. Try to arrive at the test site early. Running late will raise your anxiety. Also, by arriving early, you may have an opportunity to choose a seat in an area that is as free from distractions as possible. Avoid last minute reviewing or quizzing with others. They can confuse you.

13. Use the restroom immediately before you go to the testing room. You do not want to be distracted or have to stop during the test if at all possible.

14. Try to relax. Sitting up straight, closing your eyes, and taking five slow, deep breaths are a simple, nondisruptive way of relaxing yourself.

DURING THE TEST

1. Read all the directions carefully before starting the test.

2. Read every question completely before attempting to answer it. Important background information may be contained in the sentences leading up to the actual question.

3. After reading the entire question, try to answer it without looking at the choices. Then look at the choices to see if your answer is the same as, or close to, one of the choices.

4. Read *all* of the choices. Even if the first choice seems to be the correct answer, read the other choices so you do not overlook a better choice.

5. Read carefully. Give all the words in the question and answer choices equal attention. A missed or misread word can mean the difference between a correct answer and an incorrect answer.

6. Look for key words or phrases in the question such as "first," "most important," "next," or "least."

7. Skip questions you do not know the answer to and come back to them later. If you first answer all questions to which you know the answer, you will be reviewing the course material and forming associations that may help you answer questions whose answer you do not immediately remember. Also, a question further on in the test may contain information that will help you answer a question you are having difficulty with.

8. Be sure the number on the answer sheet corresponds to the number of the question you are answering. Check periodically to ensure the question number and answer number correspond.

9. Do *not* change an answer to a question unless you realize you marked the wrong spot on the answer sheet or misread the question. Your first choice will almost always be correct.

10. If you are having difficulty with a question, read the question using each of the answer choices given. Reading the question and each answer choice together in their entirety allows you to focus on choices that make sense logically and grammatically.

11. Remember the fundamentals. In most cases, confirming scene safety, ensuring an open airway, ensuring adequate oxygenation and ventilation, and correcting life-threatening problems take precedence. Look for answers that deal with these aspects of patient management.

12. If you do not immediately know the correct answer, eliminate any choice you are sure is incorrect before you make a guess.

13. Be wary of answers that contain words or information you have never heard of before, even if they seem to be plausible choices. If it was not mentioned in lecture or in your textbook, it is probably *not* correct.

14. Base your answers on the material presented in lecture or in your textbook. Do *not* rely on personal experience or the experiences of EMS personnel you may know.

15. Know how the test will be scored. If no penalty is applied for guessing, answer *every* question. However, to discourage guessing, some tests are scored with a system that applies a penalty for each incorrect response. For example, a correct response is worth 1 point, an unanswered

question is worth 0 points, and an incorrect response is worth –0.25 points. On this type of test it is better to leave questions unanswered unless you are very sure of the correct response.

16. Use all of the allotted time. You are being tested on your knowledge, *not* on the speed with which you can take a test.

17. Use any time remaining near the end of the examination to be sure you marked the correct spots on your answer sheet. However, do *not* change an answer unless you know you marked the answer sheet incorrectly or you discover you misread a question. Your first choice will almost always be correct.

CHOOSING THE "BEST" ANSWER FOR A QUESTION

Multiple choice test items usually consist of a "stem" (a question or incomplete statement) followed by three to five "responses." One of these responses, the "keyed response," is the correct answer. The other responses are called "distractors" because they are designed to distract you from selecting the keyed response as your answer. Distractors are designed to seem right without being the best answer to the question. The following tips may help you eliminate distractors and identify the best response to a question.

1. The best response to a question may not be the perfect response. It is just the best choice among those presented for the question.

2. If the responses to a question consist of a series of steps in a procedure, the correct answer will be the series that is most complete and in the correct order.

3. If two or more responses seem to be correct, be sure all of them relate directly to the question. A common strategy used by test writers to develop distractors is to include statements that are correct but that are not related to the question. For example, a question related to management of airway and breathing might include a true statement about management of circulation as a distractor. Although the statement might be true, it does not relate to the question, so it is not the best choice.

4. If two or more responses seem correct, look for one that is more specific. For example, a medical-legal question might present a scenario in which you knowingly write information in a patient care report that is not true and that damages the patient's reputation. You might then be asked what you could be sued for and presented with choices that include "slander," "libel," "defamation of character," and "an intentional tort." The best choice is libel. Although both slander and libel are legally classified as defamation of character, which in turn is an intentional tort, libel is the most specific response to this question.

5. If three responses seem correct, look for one that includes the other two. For example, you might be asked what kinds of ingestions administration of activated charcoal is inappropriate for. The answers might include "aspirin," "alkalis," "acids," and "corrosive substances." Aspirin clearly is *not* a correct response. Alkalis and acids both appear to be correct. However, the choice "corrosive substances" includes both acids and alkalis. Therefore, it is the best response.

Contents

1 The EMS System and the Role of the EMT-Basic, 1

2 Medical Terminology, 9

3 The Well-Being of the EMT-Basic, 22

4 Medical-Legal Issues, 36

5 Anatomy and Physiology, 46

6 Moving and Lifting Patients, 73

7 Scene Size-Up, Initial Assessment, and SAMPLE, 96

8 Airway Management, 119

9 Trauma Assessment, 137

10 Musculoskeletal Injuries, 155

11 Head and Spinal Injuries, 177

12 Soft Tissue Injuries and Bleeding Control, 201

13 Shock Management, 229

14 Medical Assessment, 258

15 Respiratory Diseases, 284

16 Cardiovascular Emergencies, 314

17 Altered Mental Status, 349

18 Poisons and Overdoses, 369

19 Environmental Problems, 391

20 Behavioral Emergencies, 421

21 Obstetric and Gynecologic Emergencies, 438

22 Pediatric Emergencies, 457

23 Geriatric Emergencies, 478

24 Communications and Documentation, 499

25 Ambulance Operations, 510

26 Extrication and Rescue, 520

27 Biological and Chemical Terrorism, 529

28 Advanced Airway Management, 545

Appendix: National Registry Skills Sheets, 560

EMT-Basic Review

A CASE-BASED APPROACH

1

The EMS System and the Role of the EMT-Basic

RESPONSIBILITIES OF THE EMT

- Personal safety, crew safety, patient safety, and bystander safety
- Proper recognition of need for and use of body substance isolation and other personal protective equipment
- Proper maintenance and handling of emergency vehicles
- Rapid scene size-up
- Rapid recognition of patients needing immediate intervention (initial assessment)
- Recognition of "load-and-go" situations
- Complete and thorough head-to-toe assessment, including reevaluation of any change in patient status
- Efficient, effective communication with partner, other responders, patient, family, and receiving facilities
- Appropriate, safe patient lifting, moving, and transport
- Complete, accurate, and legible documentation
- Proper transfer of care to personnel of equal or greater training, including verbal report
- Acting as patient advocate
- Safeguarding patient rights

TRAITS OF THE EMT-BASIC

- Be pleasant—Inspire confidence, calm the patient
- Be resourceful—Adapt ideas, tools, and techniques for unusual situations
- Be a self-starter—Show initiative, accomplish tasks that need to be done
- Be a leader—Take charge when necessary, control the scene, and organize bystanders
- Be neat and clean—Promote a good impression of yourself, your organization, and your profession
- Have good moral character—The patient has to be able to trust you
- Be able to control personal habits—Smoking, alcohol
- Be compassionate, patient, and nonjudgmental
- Be cooperative—For efficient care, better coordination with crew members
- Be sincere
- Be in good health—To be able to meet the mental, emotional, and physical challenges of the job
- Be flexible—You cannot control everything that happens during an emergency response
- Take pride in your profession
- Keep a sense of humor

LEVELS OF EMS TRAINING

- First responder—Personnel trained and equipped to provide immediate patient care before EMS arrives on scene
- EMT-Basic—Personnel trained according to the U.S. Department of Transportation (DOT) National Standard EMT-Basic Curriculum to:
  - Control life-threatening injuries, including maintaining an open airway, performing cardiopulmonary resuscitation, controlling bleeding, treating shock, and caring for poisoning
  - Stabilizing non–life-threatening injuries, including dressing and bandaging wounds, splinting injured extremities, delivering and caring for infants, and dealing with psychological stress

- Using nonmedical operational skills such as driving emergency vehicles, maintaining supplies and equipment, using good communication and record-keeping skills, performing extrication and rescue, and coping with legal and ethical issues
- EMT-Intermediate—EMT-Basic personnel who have completed additional training according to the DOT National Standard EMT-Intermediate Curriculum in roles and responsibilities, EMS systems, medical and legal considerations, medical terminology, EMS communications, patient assessment, airway management, and assessment and management of shock. Additional skills include IV therapy and advanced airway management skills.
- Paramedic—Personnel trained in all aspects of prehospital emergency care, equal to or exceeding the DOT National Standard Paramedic Curriculum. Additional skills include administration of medications, chest decompression, interpretation of electrocardiograms, and use of manual defibrillators.

MEDICAL DIRECTION

- Medical director—The physician who assumes responsibility for patient care provided by the EMS system in his or her community or region
- Medical control—The process used by physicians to ensure quality and accountability in delivery of out-of-hospital care
  - On-line medical control—Direct communication by telephone or radio with physicians at receiving facilities providing further direction and support for EMS personnel actively caring for patients in the field
  - Off-line medical control—Physician development of EMS system procedures, standards, guidelines, protocols, and standing orders and review of patient care to ensure quality and accountability
- Designated agent—EMS personnel are an extension of their medical director. This allows them to provide care and give medications under the medical director's license.
- Protocols—Written step-by step instructions for EMS personnel to use for assessment and treatment in the field
- Standing orders—Protocols issued by the medical director that authorize EMS personnel to perform certain skills and give certain medications without having to ask for permission by radio or telephone
- Quality improvement—A system for continuously reviewing the performance of an EMS system, identifying areas that can be improved, developing strategies for improvement, and implementing these strategies

REVIEW QUESTIONS

Multiple Choice

1.1. To practice effectively as an EMT-Basic, you need all of the following *except:*
   a. knowledge of patient care protocols.
   b. a positive attitude.
   c. ability to ensure your safety and the safety of your crew and patients.
   d. national licensure.

1.2. All of the following are nationally recognized EMS certification levels *except:*
   a. EMT-Basic.
   b. EMT-Critical Care.
   c. paramedic.
   d. first responder.

1.3. The EMT-Basic's role in quality improvement includes all of the following *except:*
   a. maintaining a clean, neat appearance.
   b. attending run reviews and other quality assurance activities.
   c. ensuring equipment is functioning properly by doing regular maintenance checks.
   d. participating in continuing education.

1.4. All of the following are responsibilities of an EMT-Basic *except:*
   a. maintaining a neat, clean appearance.
   b. having knowledge of state and national EMS issues.
   c. documenting patient care completely and legibly.
   d. placing patient needs before personal safety.

1.5. Which of the following is an example of off-line medical control?
   a. Receiving a radio order to give activated charcoal
   b. Following directions from an on-scene physician to check a blood glucose level and give oral glucose
   c. Defibrillating a patient according to the local protocol
   d. Calling the ER on a cell phone for an order to give albuterol to an asthmatic patient

1.6. Standing orders are issued by the:
   a. state EMS director.
   b. nurse manager of the regional level I trauma center.
   c. local or regional EMS medical director.
   d. National Registry.

1.7. Keeping accurate written records, obtaining feedback from patients and hospital, maintaining equipment, and participating in continuing education activities are elements of:
   a. quality assurance and improvement.
   b. quality standing protocols.
   c. quality service.
   d. quality assessment.

1.8. Medical direction is:
   a. all operational policies and procedures issued by the local EMS director.
   b. the process used for physician oversight of the EMS system.
   c. the physician who assumes responsibility for out-of-hospital patient care.
   d. any person authorized by the medical director to give on-line orders for administration of medications to patients.

1.9. The National Registry does all of the following *except:*
   a. develop standardized written and practical examinations for EMS personnel.
   b. maintain records of personnel who have met requirements for registration.
   c. assist in evaluating training programs.
   d. provide national authorization to practice as an EMT-Basic.

1.10. All of the following are responsibilities of the EMS medical director *except:*
   a. overseeing the clinical practice of EMTs working under his or her license.
   b. establishing protocols for out-of-hospital patient care.
   c. providing on-line orders for patient care by EMTs working under his or her license during every patient contact.
   d. evaluating and approving patient care equipment used by EMTs under his or her supervision.

1.11. Which of the following is one of the *most important* goals of quality improvement?
   a. Maintaining a clean ambulance and functioning patient care equipment
   b. Ensuring appropriate supplies are always available
   c. Ensuring patient satisfaction with services provided
   d. Providing a billing system fair to all patients regardless of financial status

1.12. The person ultimately responsible for patient care and the clinical aspects of a local or regional EMS system is the:
   a. state EMS director.
   b. chief or director of EMS operations.
   c. regional EMS coordinator.
   d. EMS medical director.

Matching

1.13. _____ C _____ Certification/registration
1.14. _____ B _____ Licensure
1.15. _____ A _____ Reciprocity

a. Granting an individual licensure or certification based on licensure or certification by another agency or association
b. The process by which a government agency grants permission to an individual to engage in and practice a profession or occupation
c. The process under which an agency or association recognizes that an individual meets specific knowledge and skill requirements

Multiple Choice

1.16. Which agency develops and maintains national standards for EMS training?
   a. The U.S. Department of Health and Human Services
   b. The Office of the U.S. Surgeon General
   c. The Federal Emergency Management Agency
   d. The U.S. Department of Transportation

1.17. A tiered system:
   a. includes some units staffed only by EMT-Basic personnel and other units staffed by personnel with more advanced training.
   b. ensures that state and federal funding is available to emergency response systems based on the level of care they provide.
   c. matches personnel continuing education requirements to levels of certification or licensure.
   d. consists of ambulances staffed by crews consisting of an EMT-Basic and a paramedic.

1.18. Positioning ambulances to reduce response times based on projected call volume and location is:
   a. strategic unit deployment.
   b. tiered response.
   c. priority dispatching.
   d. system status management.

1.19. You have just delivered a patient to the emergency department when you hear another unit dispatched to a full arrest. The other unit's ETA is 10 minutes. You are 2 minutes from the scene. However, the ER is busy, and the nurse who is to take your patient is not available. She is assisting with the care of a critical trauma patient and will be with you in about 5 minutes. You should:

   a. go to the room where the nurse is, give report, and leave for the full arrest.

   b. leave your run report on the cot with the patient, tell the nurse it is there, and advise the dispatcher you are available to respond to the full arrest.

   c. give report to a nursing student who is not busy and go to the full arrest.

   d. wait until the nurse is free, give her a report, and advise the dispatcher you are available to respond to the full arrest.

1.20. A system for reviewing and auditing calls, patient care, and run records is known as:

   a. constant quality assessment.

   b. system status improvement.

   c. program assurance and evaluation.

   d. quality improvement.

1.21. Federal ambulance specifications developed by the General Services Administration (GSA) are known as:

   a. Type I and II specifications.

   b. KKK-1822 standards.

   c. GSA-FAS.

   d. Type III specifications.

1.22. All of the following skills may be performed by an EMT-Basic without additional training *except*:

   a. using an automated external defibrillator (AED).

   b. giving epinephrine using an autoinjector.

   c. inserting an endotracheal tube to ensure an open airway.

   d. using a metered dose inhaler to give albuterol.

Matching

1.23. _____ 1966

1.24. _____ Standing orders

1.25. _____ EMT-Basic

1.26. _____ 1970

1.27. _____ 1973

1.28. _____ Tiered response system

1.29. _____ On-line medical control

a. Direct supervision of prehospital patient care by a physician; this occurs when a physician gives direct radio or telephone orders to EMS personnel.

b. The year the National Registry of Emergency Medical Technicians was founded

c. Steps or actions that can be taken without contacting a physician when the EMT-Basic determines them necessary

d. An EMS system that includes some units with basic patient capability and some units with advanced patient care capability

e. The year the National Highway Safety Act gave the job of developing EMS standards to the U.S. Department of Transportation

f. An emergency responder trained to provide patient care that includes oxygen administration, spinal immobilization, emergency childbirth assistance, splinting and hemorrhage control, and automated defibrillation

g. The year Congress passed the Emergency Medical Services Systems (EMSS) Act and specifically identified standardized prehospital personnel training as an essential goal

Answer Key—Chapter 1

66% −10/29

1.1. **D,** Knowledge of patient care protocols, a positive attitude, and the ability to ensure crew and patient safety are all abilities needed to practice as an EMT-Basic. Authorization to practice as an EMT-Basic is received from the state. There is no national licensure of EMS personnel.

1.2. **B,** EMT-Critical Care technician is not a nationally recognized level. The nationally recognized levels of EMS certification are first responder, EMT-Basic, EMT-Intermediate, and paramedic.

1.3. **A,** The EMT-Basic's role in quality improvement includes attending continuing education classes, maintaining skill levels with refresher courses, preparing neat and legible documentation, attending run reviews, performing preventive maintenance on vehicles and equipment, and gathering feedback from patients, other EMS personnel, and hospital staff. Although maintaining a neat, clean appearance is an important characteristic of EMS personnel, it is not part of the quality improvement process.

1.4. **D,** Your safety and the safety of your crew ALWAYS come first. You do not do the patient any good if you become injured or incapacitated.

1.5. **C,** An EMT performing defibrillation according to the local protocols would be an example of off-line medical control. In all of the other situations described, the EMT is performing a procedure under a direct order received from a physician.

1.6. **C,** The local or regional EMS medical director issues standing orders.

1.7. **A,** Quality improvement includes keeping accurate, complete records; obtaining feedback on patient care; maintaining equipment and vehicles; and participating in continuing education.

1.8. **B,** Medical direction is the process used by a physician to oversee all aspects of the EMS system related to patient care.

1.9. **D,** The National Registry does NOT provide national licensure. Licensure or certification to practice is provided by the states. The National Registry promotes a national standard for EMS personnel knowledge and skill and maintains records of personnel who have met this standard. The performance of students on the National Registry's written and practical examinations is a useful tool to evaluate and improve training programs.

1.10. **C,** The medical control physician sometimes is involved with on-line communications but not every time. He or she establishes protocol and procedures followed by other physicians who provide direct on-line supervision of patient care.

1.11. **C,** Ensuring patient (customer) satisfaction is always the most important goal of quality improvement.

1.12. **D,** Because the care provided by EMTs and paramedics is carried out under the medical director's license, he or she ultimately is responsible for the clinical aspects of an EMS system.

1.13. **C,** Certification—the process by which an agency or association grants recognition to an individual who meets specific knowledge and skill requirements.

1.14. **B,** Licensure—the process by which a government agency grants permission to an individual to engage in and practice a profession or occupation.

1.15. A, Reciprocity—granting an individual licensure or certification based on licensure or certification by another agency or association.

1.16. D, The U.S. Department of Transportation is the agency that develops and is responsible for maintaining the national standards for EMS personnel education and training.

1.17. A, The tiered response system includes some units staffed by basic personnel and other units staffed by advanced personnel. Dispatchers using medically approved protocols match unit patient care capabilities to patient needs.

1.18. D, In systems status management, dispatchers use projections of call volume and locations to strategically place ambulances near locations where calls are expected to occur, reducing response times.

1.19. D, The patient you currently have is your top priority. You must give report and turn the care of the patient over to a nurse or another health care professional with equal or higher training. If you leave your patient without doing this, you are placing yourself and your organization at risk for a lawsuit.

1.20. D, Quality assurance, quality improvement, or continuous quality improvement should include clear, accurate documentation; quality improvement committees that focus on improving specific aspects of the system; feedback from hospital personnel, other EMS agencies, patients, or their families regarding the quality of care given; maintenance of knowledge and skills so the same level of care is given every time; continuing education; and run reviews and audits.

1.21. B, Federal ambulance design specifications are known as the KKK or KKK-1822 standards. The ambulances are classified as Type I, Type II, and Type III according to their design and style, but all fall under the federal KKK specifications.

1.22. C, Endotracheal intubation is not part of the core curriculum for EMT-Basic training. However, with additional training and appropriate legal and medical authorization, EMT-Basic personnel in some areas perform this skill.

1.23. E, 1966—The National Highway Safety Act gave the job of developing EMS standards to the U.S. Department of Transportation.

1.24. C, Standing orders are lists of actions or steps that can be taken by the EMT-Basic without contacting the physician directly.

1.25. F, The EMT-Basic has the level of training to allow him or her to perform basic airway skills, cardiopulmonary resuscitation (CPR), oxygen administration, splinting, spinal immobilization, emergency childbirth assistance, hemorrhage control, and automated defibrillation.

1.26. B, The National Registry of EMTs was organized in 1970.

1.27. G, In 1973, Congress passed the Emergency Medical Services Systems (EMSS) Act and specifically identified standardized training for prehospital personnel as an essential goal.

1.28. D, A tiered response system includes some units with basic patient care capability and some units with advanced capabilities. Dispatchers use medically approved protocols to match units with appropriate capabilities with patient needs.

1.29. A, On-line medical control is direct supervision of the prehospital care by a physician on the radio or via telephone.

2

Medical Terminology

DEFINITIONS
Anatomical Definitions

Anatomical position—The standard position in which the body is always visualized when describing anatomical positions and movements: standing upright, facing forward, arms to the side, and palms forward (Figure 2-1)

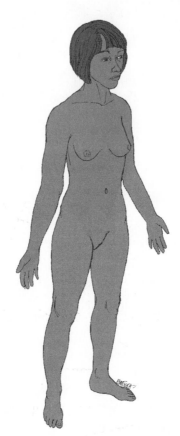

Figure 2-1   The anatomical position. (From Shade B, Rithenburg MA, Wertz E, et al: *Mosby's EMT-intermediate textbook*, ed 2, St Louis, 2002, Mosby.)

Midline—A vertical plane passed through the body from front to back dividing it into right and left halves

Anterior—Closer to the front surface of the body; opposite of posterior

Posterior—Closer to the back surface of the body; opposite of anterior

Ventral—Closer to the front surface of the body; opposite of dorsal

Dorsal—Closer to the back surface of the body; opposite of ventral

Superior—Closer to the head; opposite of inferior

Inferior—Closer to the feet; opposite of superior

Cephalad—Closer to the head; opposite of caudad

Caudad—Closer to the feet (or tail); opposite of cephalad

Lateral—Away from the midline; opposite of medial

Medial—Closer to the midline; opposite of lateral

Proximal—Closer to the point of origin of a structure; opposite of distal. The elbow is proximal to the wrist.

Distal—Farther away from the point of origin of a structure; opposite of proximal. The foot is distal to the knee.

Superficial—Near the body's surface; opposite of deep

Deep—Farther away from the body's surface; opposite of superficial

External—Outside of the body or involving the body's surface; opposite of internal

Internal—Inside the body; opposite of external

Palmar—The anterior surface of the hand (the palm)

Plantar—The inferior surface of the foot (the sole)

Midaxillary line—An imaginary vertical line extending from the middle of the axilla (armpit) down the patient's lateral surface

Midclavicular line—An imaginary vertical line extending from the middle of the clavicle (collarbone) down the patient's anterior surface parallel to the midline

Movements

Abduction—Movement away from the midline; opposite of adduction

Adduction—Movement toward the midline; opposite of abduction

Flexion—Bending or moving jointed parts closer together; opposite of extension

Extension—Straightening or moving jointed parts further apart; opposite of flexion

Lateral rotation—Turning an extremity away from the midline; opposite of medial rotation

Medial rotation—Turning an extremity toward the midline; opposite of lateral rotation

Pronation—Turning the palm of the hand downward; opposite of supination

Supination—Turning the palm of the hand upward; opposite of pronation

Positions

Supine—Lying in a face-up position; opposite of prone

Prone—Lying in a face-down position; opposite of supine

Left lateral recumbent—Lying on the left side; opposite of right lateral recumbent

Right lateral recumbent—Lying on the right side; opposite of left lateral recumbent

Shock—Lying supine with the lower extremities elevated approximately 12 inches

Trendelenburg—Lying on an inclined plane with the head down and the body and legs elevated. Sometimes used interchangeably with "shock position"; however, it does not have precisely the same meaning.

Fowler's—Lying on the back with the upper body elevated at a 45- to 60-degree angle

PREFIXES AND SUFFIXES

AN = absence of, without, lack of; *an*uria—absence of urine production

BI = double or two of; *bi*lateral—both sides

BRADY = slow; *brady*cardia—abnormally slow heart rate

BRONCH/O = pertaining to the bronchi (large lower airways); *broncho*scopy—a procedure in which the lower airways are visualized

CARDI/O = pertaining to the heart; *cardio*genic shock—shock caused by failure of the heart as a pump

DYS = difficult, abnormal; *dys*pnea—difficulty breathing

ECTOMY = surgical removal of an organ; append*ectomy*—surgical removal of the appendix

EMIA = pertaining to a condition of the blood; hypovol*emia*—low (inadequate) blood volume

GASTR/O = pertaining to the stomach; *gastr*itis—inflammation of the stomach

HEMAT/O = pertaining to blood; *hemat*emesis—vomiting blood

HEMI = half; *hemi*plegia—paralysis of one side of the body

HEPAT/O = pertaining to the liver; *hepat*itis—inflammation of the liver

HYPER = excessive or high; *hyper*tension—high blood pressure

HYPO = low or below, abnormally low condition; *hypo*tension—low blood pressure

INTER = between; *inter*costal—between the ribs

INTRA = within; *intra*muscular—within a muscle

ITIS = inflammation of; append*icitis*—inflammation of the appendix

LARYNG/O = pertaining to the larynx; *laryng*ectomy—surgical removal of the larynx

MY/O = pertaining to muscle; *my*ocardium—the heart muscle

NAS/O = pertaining to the nose; *nas*opharynx—the portion of the pharynx (throat) posterior to the nasal cavity

NEPHR/O = pertaining to the kidney; *nephr*itis—inflammation of the kidney

NEUR/O = pertains to the nerves; *neur*ologist—a physician who specializes in disorders of the nervous system

OMA = a swelling or tumor; hemat*oma*—local swelling caused by accumulation of blood under the skin

ORTH/O = straight or correct; *orth*opedist—a physician who corrects or straightens deformities of the skeletal system

OSTOMY = creating a surgical opening in; trache*ostomy*—creating a surgical opening in the trachea

PERI = around; *peri*cardium—the sac that surrounds the heart

PHARYNG/O = pertaining to the throat; *pharyng*itis—inflammation of the throat

PHOT/O = pertaining to light; *phot*osensitivity—sensitivity to light

PLEGIA = paralysis; quadri*plegia*—paralysis involving all four extremities

PNEA = pertaining to breathing; dys*pnea*—difficulty breathing

PSYCH/O = the mind, soul; *psych*iatrist—a physician who specializes in disorders of the mind

PULMON/O = refers to the lungs; *pulmon*ologist—a physician who specializes in disorders of the lungs

SUPRA = over or above; *supra*pubic—the area of the abdomen just above the pubic bone

TACHY = fast; *tachy*pnea—fast breathing

THORAC/O = pertaining to the chest or chest cavity; *thorac*ostomy—surgically opening the chest cavity

PATIENT ASSESSMENT ACRONYMS, MNEMONICS, AND ABBREVIATIONS

AVPU—*A*lert, Responds to *V*erbal Stimulus, Responds to *P*ainful Stimulus, *U*nresponsive. Used to describe levels of responsiveness

DCAP-BTLS—*D*eformities, *C*ontusions, *A*brasions, *P*unctures and *P*enetrations, *B*urns, *T*enderness, *L*acerations, and *S*welling. Used to remember problems sought during the rapid trauma examination

HPI—*H*istory of *P*resent *I*llness

LOC—*L*evel *O*f *C*onsciousness or *L*oss *O*f *C*onsciousness

MOI—*M*echanism *O*f *I*njury. Factors involved in producing injury to a patient, including nature, strength, and directions of forces causing the injury

NOI—*Nature Of Illness*. Type of medical condition or complaint a patient is suffering from

OPQRST—*Onset, Provocation, Quality, Radiation, Severity, Time*. Used to remember questions to ask when assessing patient's chief complaint

PEARL—*Pupils Equal And Reactive to Light*

PERRLA—*Pupils Equal, Round, Reactive to Light and Accommodation*

Rx or Tx—Treatment

SAMPLE—*Signs and Symptoms, Allergies, Medications, Pertinent Past Medical History, Last Oral Intake, Events Leading to Injury or Illness*. Used to recall categories of information necessary to the patient's history

REVIEW QUESTIONS

Scenario One

On your way to work you find a car that has gone off the road and down a 15-foot embankment. An 18-y.o. (2.1) female has been ejected from the vehicle. She is lying on the ground in a **supine** (2.2) position with the **inferior** (2.3) part of her body partly in a small pond. The patient is conscious and tells you she thinks there was no **LOC** (2.4). However, she is only alert × 3 to **PPT** (2.5). There is a 2-inch laceration on her left thigh **c̄** (2.6) minimal bleeding. However, considerable **edema** (2.7) and a large contusion also are present. The **distal** (2.8) portion of the left lower extremity is **laterally** (2.9) rotated. You know the patient's airway is adequate because she is able to talk to you **s̄** (2.10) difficulty. Her pupils are **PERRLA** (2.11). She **c/o** (2.12) of pain in the **RUQ** (2.13) and rates it as a 4 on the 1 to 10 scale. You do not have the equipment to take a **BP** (2.14). However, the patient has a radial pulse, so you know the systolic pressure is more than 80 **mm Hg** (2.15). At this point an ambulance arrives, and its crew takes over patient care. You give a quick report on the **pt.** (2.16) and the **treatment** (2.17) you have given.

Fill in the Blank

2.1. The abbreviation y.o. means _____ years old _____.

Multiple Choice

2.2. Supine means the patient is:
   a. lying face up.
   b. lying face down.
   c. lying with her palms turned up.
   d. lying on her right side.

A

2.3. Inferior means:
   a. closer to the feet.
   b. toward the back.
   c. closer to the head.
   d. toward the front.

A

Fill in the Blank

2.4. In this case, the abbreviation LOC means _____ level of Consciousness _____.

2.5. The abbreviation PPT means the patient is oriented to _____ person _____, _____ place _____, and _____ time _____, but not to _____.

2.6. The abbreviation c̄ means _____ with _____.

Multiple Choice

2.7. Edema refers to:
   a. thickening.
   b. discoloration.
   c. enlargement.
   d. swelling. *(d circled)*

2.8. Distal means:
   a. closer to the point of origin.
   b. closer to the head.
   c. closer to the feet. *(c circled)*
   d. farther from the point of origin.

2.9. Lateral means:
   a. toward the front.
   b. closer to the midline.
   c. away from the midline. *(c circled)*
   d. toward the back.

Fill in the Blank

2.10. The abbreviation s̄ means _____ without _____.

2.11. The abbreviation PERRLA means that the patient's pupils are _____, _____, and _____ to _____ and _____.

2.12. The abbreviation c/o means _____ complains of _____.

2.13. The abbreviation RUQ refers to the _____ right upper quadrant _____.

2.14. When referring to a BP, you are referring to _____ blood pressure _____.

2.15. The abbreviation mm Hg means _____ levels _____ of _____ mercury _____.

2.16. The abbreviation pt. means _____ patient _____.

2.17. When you write your report, the abbreviation you could use for treatment is _____ Tx _____.

Scenario Two

You are dispatched to a report of a man with "difficulty breathing." On arrival you find a 72-y.o. male c̄ moderate **dyspnea** (2.18). He is alert and oriented × 4. His family tells you the difficulty breathing began 2 days ago and has steadily worsened. The patient has a past medical **hx** (2.19) of **COPD** (2.20) for 15 years and of an **MI** (2.21) 4 years ago that led to his developing **CHF** (2.22). He has a **DNR** (2.23) order in place. On examination you note **wheezes** (2.24) in the **posterior** (2.25) lung fields and some **cyanosis** (2.26 and 2.27). There is a considerable amount of secretions in his **oropharynx** (2.28). The patient is using his diaphragm and **intercostal muscles** (2.29) with the **active phase** (2.30) of each breath. His respirations are **rapid** (2.31 and 2.32) at a rate of 28 per minute. To obtain a complete hx, you use the mnemonic **SAMPLE** (2.33, 2.34, 2.35, 2.36, 2.37, and 2.38). While you obtain the history, your partner takes the patient's **VS** (2.39).

Fill in the Blank

2.18. Dyspnea means _____ trouble breathing _____.

2.19. The abbreviation hx means _____ history _____.

2.20. The abbreviation COPD means _____.

2.21. MI is the abbreviation for ___myocardial infarction___, commonly
called a ___heart attack___.

2.22. CHF is the abbreviation for ___coronary heart failure___.

2.23. DNR is the abbreviation for ___do not resuscitate___.

Multiple Choice

2.24. Wheezes are:
  a. low-pitched sounds caused by fluid in the lower airways.
  b. high-pitched sounds produced by narrowing of the lower airways.
  c. low-pitched sounds caused by fluid in the upper airway.
  d. high-pitched sounds produced by narrowing of the upper airways.

B

2.25. Posterior means toward the:
  a. back.
  b. head.
  c. front.
  d. feet.

A

2.26. A patient who is cyanotic has:
  a. decreased blood flow to the skin.
  b. blue-gray skin color.
  c. skin that is cold to touch.
  d. pale, moist skin.

B

2.27. Cyanosis is:
  a. an early sign of inadequate oxygenation.
  b. a late sign of increased blood pressure.
  c. an early sign of decreased blood pressure.
  d. a late sign of inadequate oxygenation.

D

2.28. The oropharynx is the:
  a. mouth.
  b. part of the throat just posterior to the oral cavity.
  c. area between the nasal cavity and the larynx.
  d. complete ring of cartilage at the inferior boundary of the larynx.

B

2.29. Intercostal muscles are the muscles:
  a. of the anterior abdominal wall.
  b. that connect the clavicles to the upper ribs.
  c. located between the ribs.
  d. that run from the neck to the clavicles and upper ribs.

C

2.30. Which phase of respiration is active?
  a. Inhalation
  b. Exhalation
  c. Both inhalation and exhalation
  d. Inhalation, but only if a chronic respiratory problem is present

A

2.31. The term for a rapid respiratory rate is:
  a. apnea.
  b. bradypnea.
  c. tachypnea.
  d. dyspnea.

C

2.32. If the patient was breathing at a rate of 6 per minute you would describe this as:
   a. apneic.
   b. bradypneic.
   c. tachypneic.
   d. dyspneic.

B

Fill in the Blank
2.33. In the mnemonic SAMPLE, "S" stands for _Sms (Symptoms)_.
2.34. In the mnemonic SAMPLE, "A" stands for _Allergies_.
2.35. The "M" of SAMPLE history stands for _Medications_.
2.36. The "P" in SAMPLE history stands for _Past Hx_.
2.37. In the SAMPLE history, "L" stands for _Last oral Intake_.
2.38. In the SAMPLE history, "E" stands for _Events Prior_.

Scenario Three

While you are responding to an **MVC** (2.39), the dispatcher calls and ask what your **ETA** (2.40) is. On arrival you are told a car went off the road and rolled over. The fire-rescue department has secured the scene. Patient #1 is a 64-y.o. female who was not wearing a seatbelt and was ejected from the vehicle. She is awake and alert × 4, lying in a **prone** (2.41) position, and c/o of **midaxillary** (2.42) pain on the right side. Her left ankle is **laterally** (2.43) rotated. She has a past history of **CAD** (2.44) and angina pectoris and had a **TIA** (2.45) 2 years ago. The **ROM** (2.46) of her left foot is very limited. Patient #2 is a 69-y.o. male who was wearing a seat belt and is still in the vehicle. He is c/o mild chest pain and has a 3-inch laceration on the **medial** (2.47) aspect of his left arm, a large bruise on the **dorsal** (2.48) aspect of his right hand, and a laceration on the **ventral** (2.48) portion of his left hand. His skin is slightly **jaundiced** (2.50). He tells you his past medical hx includes cirrhosis of the liver and a **CVA** (2.51) 3 years ago. Your partner performs a rapid trauma assessment on Patient #2 by quickly examining him from head-to-toe for **DCAP-BTLS** (2.52 to 2.59).

Fill in the Blank
2.39. The abbreviation MVC stands for _Motor Vehicle Crash_.
2.40. The abbreviation ETA stands for _estimated time of arrival_.

Multiple Choice
2.41. Prone means that the patient is:
   a. lying on her back.
   b. lying on her left side.
   c. lying face down.
   d. lying on her right side.

C

2.42. Midaxillary refers to an imaginary:
   a. vertical line drawn from either clavicle down to the lower chest margin.
   b. vertical line drawn from the middle of the armpit to the ankle.
   c. vertical line drawn down the body's center dividing it into right and left halves.
   d. horizontal line drawn from the middle of the armpit to the ankle.

B

2.43. Lateral means:
  a. away from the midline.
  b. away from the point of origin of a structure.
  c. toward the midline.
  d. toward the point of origin of a structure.

A

Fill in the Blank

2.44. The abbreviation CAD stands for ___coronary artery disease___.
2.45. The abbreviation TIA stands for ___transient ischemic attack___.
2.46. The abbreviation ROM stands for ___range of motion___.

Multiple Choice

2.47. Medial means:
  a. toward the midline.
  b. away from the midline.
  c. toward the front.
  d. away from the front.

A

2.48. When you use the term "dorsal," you mean:
  a. closer to the torso, the opposite of distal.
  b. away from the torso, the opposite of proximal.
  c. located on or closer to the back, a synonym for posterior.
  d. located on or closer to the front, a synonym for anterior.

C

2.49. When you use the term "ventral," you mean:
  a. closer to the torso, the opposite of distal.
  b. away from the torso, the opposite of proximal.
  c. located on or closer to the back, a synonym for posterior.
  d. located on or closer to the front, a synonym for anterior.

D

2.50. "Jaundiced" means the patient has a:
  a. bluish-gray skin color caused by liver disease.
  b. yellowish skin color caused by liver disease.
  c. bluish-gray skin color usually seen in older patients who have had a CVA.
  d. yellowish skin color usually seen in older patients who have had a CVA.

B

Fill in the Blank

2.51. The abbreviation CVA stands for ___cerebral vascular accident___, commonly known as a ___stroke___.
2.52. The "D" in DCAP-BTLS stands for ___Deformities___.
2.53. The "C" in DCAP-BTLS stands for ___Contusions___.
2.54. The "A" in DCAP-BTLS stands for ___Abrasions___.
2.55. The "P" in DCAP-BTLS stands for ___Punctures___.
2.56. The "B" in DCAP-BTLS stands for ___Burns___.
2.57. The "T" in DCAP-BTLS stands for ___tenderness___.
2.58. The "L" in DCAP-BTLS stands for ___lacerations___.
2.59. The "S" in DCAP-BTLS stands for ___Swelling___.

Multiple Choice

2.60. Which end of the femur connects to the tibia?

    a. Proximal
    b. Distal
    c. Lateral
    d. Medial

Matching

Match the following terms to the definitions below:

Abduction   ~~Medial~~
~~Adduction~~   ~~Palmar~~
~~Anterior~~   ~~Plantar~~
~~Caudal~~   ~~Posterior~~
~~Cephalic~~   ~~Prone~~
~~Distal~~   ~~Proximal~~
~~Dorsal~~   ~~Recumbent~~
~~Inferior~~   ~~Superior~~
~~Lateral~~   ~~Supine~~

2.61. _Superior_ Situated above another structure
2.62. _Caudal_ Toward spine's lower end
2.63. _Dorsal_ The back of the body *Posterior*
2.64. _Abduction_ Movement away from the body's midline
2.65. _Lateral_ Located or situated away from the midline of the body
2.66. _Recumbent_ Lying in a horizontal position
2.67. _Prone_ Lying flat, face down
2.68. _Posterior_ Pertaining to the back surface of the body *Dorsal*
2.69. _Inferior_ Situated below
2.70. _Anterior_ The front surface of the body
2.71. _Supine_ Lying flat, face up
2.72. _Palmar_ Regarding the palm of the hand
2.73. _~~Bottom~~ Adduction_ Movement toward the body's midline
2.74. _Plantar_ Regarding the sole of the foot
2.75. _Medial_ Situated toward the body midline
2.76. _Proximal_ Situated nearest the point of origin
2.77. _Distal_ Situated farthest from the point of origin
2.78. _Cephalic_ Toward the head

81%

2.1. The abbreviation "y.o." stands for *year old* or *years old*.

2.2. **A,** Supine means lying flat on the back with your face up. Prone is lying face down. Lying on the right side is right laterally recumbent.

2.3. **A,** Inferior means closer to the feet.

2.4. In this case, the abbreviation "LOC" stands for *loss of consciousness*.

2.5. The abbreviation "PPT" means the patient is oriented to *person*, *place*, and *time*. In other words, she knows who she is, where she is, and what day it is, but she cannot remember the events that led up to the current incident.

2.6. **A,** A "c̄" refers to the term *with*; a "q̄" means *every*; and "s̄" means *without*.

2.7. **D,** Edema refers to an abnormal accumulation of fluid in the tissues of the body, causing swelling.

2.8. **D,** Distal means farther from a structure's point of origin. In the case of an arm or leg, it means further from the trunk.

2.9. **C,** Lateral means away from the midline. For example, the outer surface of the thigh could be referred to as the lateral surface or lateral aspect.

2.10. The "s̄" symbol means *without*.

2.11. The abbreviation "PERRLA" means that the *p*upils are *e*qual in size, *r*ound, and *r*eact to *l*ight and *a*ccommodation.

2.12. "c/o" stands for *complaining of* or *complains of*.

2.13. "RUQ" refers to the *right upper quadrant* of the abdomen.

2.14. "BP" refers to the *blood pressure*.

2.15. "mm Hg" is the abbreviation for *millimeters* of *mercury*.

2.16. "pt" stands for *patient*.

2.17. To shorten or abbreviate treatment, use *Rx* or *Tx*.

2.18. Dyspnea means difficulty breathing (*dys* = difficult or labored; *pnea* = breathing).

2.19. "hx" is an abbreviation for *history*.

2.20. "COPD" stands for *chronic obstructive pulmonary disease*.

2.21. The abbreviation "MI" refers to *myocardial infarction*, commonly called a *heart attack*. You may also see this condition referred to as an "AMI," *acute myocardial infarction*.

2.22. "CHF" stands for *congestive heart failure*.

2.23. "DNR" is the abbreviation for *do not resuscitate*.

2.24. **B,** Wheezes are a high-pitched musical sound caused by a high-velocity airflow trying to go through narrowed portions of the lower airways. Wheezes are found in patients with various conditions, including asthma, COPD, bronchitis, chronic bronchitis, and others.

2.25. **A,** Posterior means in toward the back.

2.26. **B,** Cyanosis is a bluish-gray skin color.

2.27. **D,** Cyanosis is a blue-gray skin color that appears as a late sign of hypoxia. Other significant changes that may occur in skin color include pallor—paleness from blood loss, shock, or fright; flushing—redness from exertion or sometimes exposure to sun or heat; and jaundice—yellowish colored skin or yellow cast to the skin from liver disease.

2.28. **B,** The oropharynx is the area directly posterior to the mouth or oral cavity.

2.29. **C,** The intercostal muscles are the muscles between the ribs. During inhalation, the intercostal muscles contract. The ribs move upward and outward, increasing the volume of the chest cavity and decreasing the pressure in the lower airways, which allows the lungs to expand. With exhalation the intercostal muscles relax. The ribs move down and inward, causing the chest to decrease in size and the pressure in the lower airways to increase. This increase in pressure makes air flow out of the lungs.

2.30. **A,** Inhalation is the active phase of respirations whether or not pulmonary disease is present.

2.31. **C,** Tachypnea means rapid respirations (*tachy* = rapid; *pnea* = breathing); apnea means without respirations; bradypnea refers to slow respirations; and dyspnea means difficulty breathing.

2.32. **B,** A respiratory rate less than 12 per minute is slow and would be called bradypneic (*brady* = slow; *pnea* = breathing).

2.33. The "S" in SAMPLE stands for *signs and symptoms*.

2.34. The "A" in SAMPLE stands for *allergies* the patient may have to medications or foods.

2.35. The "M" stands for the *medications* the patient takes daily.

2.36. The "P" stands for the patient's pertinent *past medical history*.

2.37. The "L" stands for the patient's *last oral intake*. Last intake of food or liquids will be particularly significant if the patient must undergo surgery.

2.38. The "E" stands for the *events* leading up to the patient's illness or injury.

2.39. The abbreviation "MVC" stands for *motor vehicle collision* or *motor vehicle crash*.

2.40. The abbreviation "ETA" stands for *estimated time of arrival*.

2.41. **C,** Prone means to be lying face down.

2.42. **B,** The midaxillary line is an imaginary line drawn from the middle of the armpit down to the ankle.

2.43. **A,** Lateral means to the side or away from the body's midline.

2.44. The abbreviation "CAD" stands for *coronary artery disease*.

2.45. "TIA" stands for *transient ischemic attack*.

2.46. "ROM" stands for *range of motion*.

2.47. **A,** Medial is the opposite of lateral, meaning toward the midline of the body.

2.48. **C,** Dorsal is a synonym for posterior, referring to the back, for example, the back of the head, the back of the hand or foot, or the back of the body.

2.49. **D,** The term ventral is a synonym for anterior, referring to the front of the body.

2.50. **B,** Jaundiced means the skin has a yellowish color. Jaundice is produced by liver disease. It also can develop in patients with kidney and gallbladder disease.

2.51. The abbreviation "CVA" stands for *cerebrovascular accident*, commonly known as a *stroke*.

2.52. "D" stands for *deformities*.

2.53. "C" stands for *contusions*.

2.54. "A" stands for *abrasions*.

2.55. "P" stands for *punctures* or *penetrating wounds*.

2.56. "B" stands for *burns*.

2.57. "T" stands for *tenderness*.

2.58. "L" stands for *lacerations*.

2.59. "S" stands for *swelling*.

2.60. B, The end of the femur that is connected to the knee would be the "distal" part of the femur. The end that is connected to the hip is the "proximal" part of the femur.

2.61. "Superior"—situated above another structure.

2.62. "Caudal"—toward the distal end of the spine, toward the inferior in humans, and toward the tail in animals.

2.63. "Posterior"—the back of the body.

2.64. "Abduction"—movement away from the body's midline.

2.65. "Lateral"—located or situated away from the midline of the body.

2.66. "Recumbent"—lying in a horizontal position.

2.67. "Prone"—lying flat, face down.

2.68. "Dorsal"—pertaining to the back surface of the body.

2.69. "Inferior"—situated below.

2.70. "Interior"—the front surface of the body.

2.71. "Supine"—lying flat, face up.

2.72. "Palmar"—the inner surface of the hand, the palm.

2.73. "Adduction"—movement toward the body's midline.

2.74. "Plantar"—regarding the sole of the foot.

2.75. "Medial"—toward the body's midline.

2.76. "Proximal"—nearest the point of origin.

2.77. "Distal"—farthest from the point of origin.

2.78. "Cephalic"—toward the head.

3

The Well-Being of the EMT-Basic

EMOTIONAL ASPECTS OF EMERGENCY CARE

Definitions

Stress—The body's nonspecific response to events that are threatening or challenging

Burnout—A state of exhaustion and irritability brought on by chronic stress

Death and Dying

Stages of Grief

- Denial
- Anger
- Bargaining
- Depression
- Acceptance

Dealing with Dying Patients

- Do everything possible to maintain patient's dignity
- Show greatest possible respect for patient
- Communicate
- Allow family members to express themselves
- Listen empathetically
- Do not give false assurances
- Use a gentle, reassuring tone of voice
- Let patient know everything that can be done to help will be done
- Use reassuring touch, if appropriate
- Do what you can to comfort the family

Other Stressful Situations

- Mass casualty incidents
- Infant and child trauma
- Traumatic amputation
- Child, elder, or spouse abuse
- Response to injury or illness of a friend or family member
- Injury of a co-worker or other public safety personnel
- Death of a co-worker or other public safety personnel

Stress Warning Signs

- Irritability with co-workers, family, friends, or patients
- Inability to concentrate
- Difficulty sleeping or nightmares
- Anxiety
- Indecisiveness
- Guilt
- Loss of appetite
- Loss of interest in sexual activities
- Isolation
- Loss of interest in work
- Increased substance use or abuse

Stress Management

- Change your diet
  - Cut down on sugar, alcohol, and caffeine
  - Avoid fatty foods
  - Increase carbohydrate intake
- Stop smoking
- Exercise more often
- Learn to relax
- Keep balance between work, family, and recreation
- Make changes in your work environment
  - Develop a "buddy" system with a co-worker
  - Encourage and support your co-workers
  - Periodically take a break
  - Request work shifts that allow more time to relax
  - Request a rotation of duty assignment
- Get professional help

Critical Incident Stress

- Critical incident—Any situation that causes you to experience unusually strong emotions that may interfere with your ability to function
  - Line-of-duty death or serious injury
  - Suicide of emergency team member
  - Injury or death of friend or family member
  - Death of patient under especially tragic circumstances or after prolonged or intense rescue procedures
  - Sudden death of infant or child
  - Injuries caused by child abuse
  - Civilian injuries or deaths caused by EMS personnel
  - Events that threaten your life
  - Events that attract unusual media attention
  - Events with distressing sights, sounds, or smells
  - Multiple-casualty incidents
- Critical incident stress debriefing (CISD)
  - Formal process that allows personnel to work through emotional responses to a critical incident and to release stress
  - Conducted by team of peer counselors and mental health professionals
  - Ideally held within 24 to 72 hours of critical incident

Comprehensive Critical Incident Stress Management

- Preincident stress education
- On-scene peer support
- One-on-one support
- Disaster support services
- Defusing
- CISD

- Follow-up services
- Spouse and family support
- Community outreach programs
- Other health and welfare programs, such as wellness programs

COMMUNICABLE DISEASE

Definitions

Pathogens—Microorganisms such as bacteria, viruses, or fungi that can cause disease

Infectious disease—A disease caused by the presence of a pathogenic organism in the body

Communicable disease—An infectious disease that can be transmitted from one infected person to another

How Diseases Spread

- Direct contact
- Indirect contact
- Airborne transmission
- Vehicle transmission (food, water, needles, or clothing)
- Vector transmission (mosquitoes, ticks, fleas, or lice)

Communicable Disease Prevention

- Maintain good personal health status
- Immunizations for:
  - Tetanus/diphtheria
  - Hepatitis A
  - Hepatitis B
  - Measles, mumps, and rubella
  - Influenza
  - Chicken pox
- Tuberculosis skin test at least annually
- Wash hands after patient contact—10 to 15 seconds with plain soap
- Personal protective equipment
  - Gloves when any contact with body fluids is anticipated
  - Face mask if patient has airborne disease or splashing of body fluids is anticipated
  - High-efficiency particulate air (HEPA) respirator if tuberculosis is suspected
  - Eye protection if splashing of body fluids is anticipated
  - Gown if significant contact with body fluids is anticipated
- Avoid needle stick; do NOT recap needles
- Dispose of needles and other sharp instruments in rigid, puncture-proof container
- Clean up blood and body fluid spills as soon as possible
- Use disposable equipment whenever possible
- Disinfect or sterilize nondisposable equipment as soon as possible
- Document any contact with blood or body fluids and any cleaning done as a result
- Report any suspected exposures according to local protocol

Common Communicable Diseases
Tuberculosis

- Bacterial infection (*Mycobacterium tuberculosis*)
- Transmitted by droplets

Signs and Symptoms

- Cough
- Fever
- Infected sputum
- Hemoptysis (coughing up blood)
- Night sweats
- Weight loss
- Pleuritic chest pain

Precautions

- Wear disposable gloves
- Wear HEPA mask
- Mask patient to reduce contamination of ambulance
- Clean exposed surfaces and nondisposable equipment
- Routine skin tests; follow up on positive reactors

Viral Hepatitis
Hepatitis A

- Fecal-oral transmission
- Most infections very mild
- Does not cause chronic liver disease or carrier state
- Vaccine available

Hepatitis B

- Transmitted by blood exposure or sexual contact
- Can cause liver failure
- Carrier state possible
- Vaccine available

Hepatitis C

- Transmitted by blood exposure or sexual contact
- Can cause liver failure
- Carrier state possible
- No vaccine available

Hepatitis D

- Occurs as coinfection with hepatitis B
- Increases severity of hepatitis B infection

Hepatitis E

- Fecal-oral transmission
- Rare in United States, occurs mostly after international travel

Signs and Symptoms

- Fatigue
- Nausea
- Loss of appetite
- Abdominal pain
- Headache
- Fever
- Yellowish color of skin and whites of eyes
- Joint pain
- Dark urine

Precautions

- Wear disposable gloves
- Wash hands thoroughly
- Obtain vaccination for hepatitis B and consider being vaccinated for hepatitis A
- Clean up blood spills as soon as possible using bleach solution
- If exposed, obtain immune serum globulin as soon as possible

Meningococcal Meningitis

- Inflammation of membranes covering brain and spinal cord
- Caused by *Neisseria meningitidis*
- Transmitted by droplets created when patient coughs or sneezes

Signs and Symptoms

- Headache
- Nausea
- Fever
- Stiff neck
- Rash consisting of tiny hemorrhages under skin (petechiae)
- Ecchymosis
- Septic shock

Precautions

- Wear disposable gloves
- Wear face mask
- Avoid contact with patient's oral and nasal secretions
- Clean all exposed surfaces in patient compartment
- Obtain appropriate antibiotic prophylaxis

Acquired Immunodeficiency Syndrome (AIDS)

- Caused by human immunodeficiency virus (HIV)
- Virus damages helper T cells and suppresses immune system
- Patient develops recurring infections with organisms that normally are not pathogenic (opportunistic infections)
- Virus transmitted through:
  - Sexual contact
  - Infected needles

- ○ Infected blood or blood products
- ○ Mother-fetus transmission
- *Cannot* be transmitted by casual contact

Signs and Symptoms
- Persistent low-grade fever
- Night sweats
- Swollen lymph glands
- Loss of appetite
- Nausea
- Persistent diarrhea
- Headache
- Sore throat
- Fatigue
- Weight loss
- Shortness of breath
- Muscle and joint pain
- Rash
- Various opportunistic infections

Precautions
- Wear disposable gloves
- Wash hands thoroughly
- Clean up blood spills as soon as possible
- Report exposures immediately so appropriate prophylaxis can be started
- Consider use of face mask to protect patient from possible infection by EMT
- Consider use of HEPA mask if patient has shortness of breath or cough. A significant portion of patients with AIDS acquire tuberculosis infections.

REVIEW QUESTIONS
Scenario One

You are dispatched to a report of a "child with a fever." The patient is an 8-y.o. female who has had a "cold" for 2 days. Today she began complaining of headache, nausea, and vomiting. When you try to sit her up to listen to her lungs, she says, "my neck hurts." She is unable to touch her chin to her chest, and her neck feels stiff when you try to move it. She has been taking an over-the-counter decongestant but is on no other medications. She has no known allergies. Vital signs are blood pressure (BP)—106/78; pulse (P)—116, strong, regular; and respiration (R)—24, regular, unlabored.

Multiple Choice

3.1. This patient probably has:
   a. measles.
   b. hepatitis.
   c. meningitis.
   d. mumps.

3.2. Which of the following statements *best* describes precautions to be taken with this disease?

   a. You should wear gloves and a mask to avoid transmission.

   b. The disease is communicable but is not easily transmitted, so only gloves and hand washing are necessary.

   c. No special precautions are needed because this disease is not communicable.

   d. The disease is spread by blood contact only, so only gloves and hand washing are necessary.

3.3. All of the following diseases are airborne *except:*

   a. mumps.

   b. measles.

   c. tuberculosis.

   d. hepatitis A. — blood + body fluid

3.4. Which form of communication with the hospital would be *most appropriate* in this situation?

   a. Report only the chief complaint and vital signs so persons listening with scanners will not know what the patient's problem is.

   b. Let the emergency department know what problem you suspect so they can prepare.

   c. Relay all radio transmissions through the dispatcher.

   d. Document the problem you suspect in your patient care report but do not call in a radio report.

Scenario Two

Your patient is a 59-y.o. male c/o RUQ pain and nausea that have been recurring intermittently for approximately 2 weeks. He says he feels weak and has no appetite. He normally smokes two packs of cigarettes a day but has not smoked for almost a week because his cigarettes "don't taste right." The patient's skin has a yellowish color. He is not on any medications, and he had a reaction to penicillin 20 years ago. Vital signs are BP—130/77; P—104, weak, regular; R—18, regular, nonlabored; and SaO_2—96%.

Multiple Choice

 3.5. The patient probably has:

   a. meningitis.

   b. measles.

   c. hepatitis. — liver failure + Jaundice

   d. anemia.

 3.6. Precautions you should take would include all of the following *except:*

   a. wearing gloves.

   b. wearing a mask if there are any body secretions, i.e., vomit or blood.

   c. using a respirator-type mask.

   d. wearing eye protection if any body fluids are present.

 3.7. Which blood component fights infection?

   a. Red blood cells

   b. White blood cells

   c. Platelets

   d. Plasma

3.8. Organisms that cause disease are also known as:
  a. pathogens.
  b. T cells.
  c. fungi.
  d. phagocytes.

True/False

3.9. Some forms of hepatitis can be fatal.
  a. True
  b. False

3.10. A person can carry hepatitis without ever experiencing the disease.
  a. True
  b. False

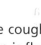

Scenario Three

Your patient is a 38-y.o. female who has had shortness of breath and a productive cough for 4 days. She is very weak, and she experiences chest pain when she breathes deeply. Her skin is flushed, warm, and moist. Rhonchi are present in both lung fields. She has a history of AIDS contracted while she was in the hospital for surgery 2 years ago. She takes AZT and has no allergies. Vital signs are BP—98/62; P—110, weak, regular; R—22, regular, labored; and SaO$_2$—94%.

Multiple Choice

3.11. The incubation period for AIDS is:
  a. 10 to 14 days.
  b. 14 to 21 days.
  c. 2 to 4 weeks.
  d. several months to years.

3.12. All of the following diseases are airborne *except:*
  a. tuberculosis.
  b. meningitis.
  c. AIDS.
  d. chicken pox.

3.13. Appropriate infection control procedures would include:
  a. hand washing with bleach solution.
  b. gloves and a respirator-type mask.
  c. isolating the patient in the ambulance patient compartment while both crewmembers sit in the driver's compartment.
  d. gloves, mask, eye protection, a gown, a hair cover, and shoe covers.

3.14. After the call is completed, what steps would be *most appropriate?*
  a. Change clothing.
  b. Sterilize all equipment that was present on the ambulance.
  c. Empty the ambulance, and clean all exposed surfaces with bleach solution.
  d. Wash your hands, and disinfect any equipment the patient came in contact with.

3.15. The *most* common route for transmission of HIV is:

  a. needle sticks.

  b. sexual contact with an infected person.

  c. exposure to droplets produced by coughing and sneezing.

  d. vomitus from an infected person.

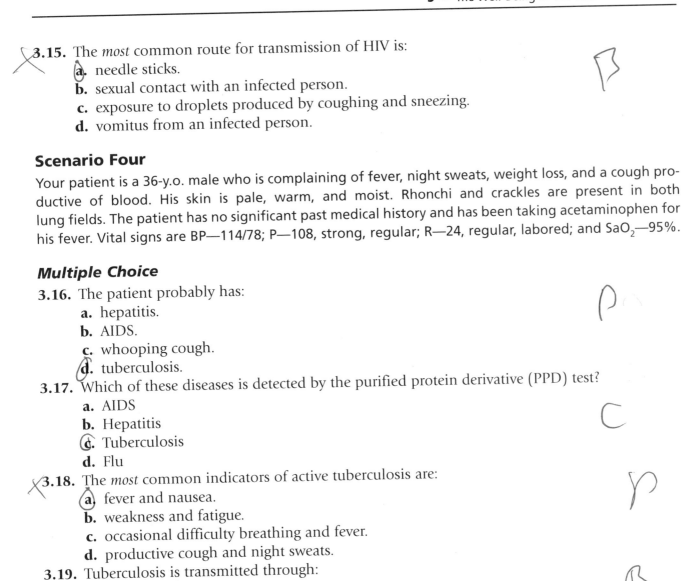

Scenario Four

Your patient is a 36-y.o. male who is complaining of fever, night sweats, weight loss, and a cough productive of blood. His skin is pale, warm, and moist. Rhonchi and crackles are present in both lung fields. The patient has no significant past medical history and has been taking acetaminophen for his fever. Vital signs are BP—114/78; P—108, strong, regular; R—24, regular, labored; and SaO$_2$—95%.

Multiple Choice

3.16. The patient probably has:

  a. hepatitis.

  b. AIDS.

  c. whooping cough.

  d. tuberculosis.

3.17. Which of these diseases is detected by the purified protein derivative (PPD) test?

  a. AIDS

  b. Hepatitis

  c. Tuberculosis

  d. Flu

3.18. The *most* common indicators of active tuberculosis are:

  a. fever and nausea.

  b. weakness and fatigue.

  c. occasional difficulty breathing and fever.

  d. productive cough and night sweats.

3.19. Tuberculosis is transmitted through:

  a. sexual contact.

  b. droplets from coughing.

  c. emesis from vomiting.

  d. contact with blood.

3.20. Which of the following is the *most* common serious infectious disease?

  a. Herpes

  b. Tuberculosis

  c. Hepatitis

  d. Syphilis

Scenario Five

You are dispatched to a motor vehicle collision. On arrival you find a 28-y.o. female lying in the roadway. She has a major open skull fracture and is in cardiac arrest. An 8-y.o. female is pinned in the front seat with part of the steering wheel embedded in her chest. She is pulseless and apneic. The fire department has removed a 5-y.o. male and a 6-m.o. (month-old) female from the back seat. Both were properly restrained, but the 5-y.o. male is unconscious and has crushing injuries to both legs. The 6-m.o. female is awake with no signs of injury but is unusually quiet. The fire captain tells you the victims are the family of the local fire chief.

Multiple Choice

3.21. The stage of grief characterized by refusal to accept the possibility something bad has happened is:

    a. depression.

    b. denial.

    c. anger.

    d. bargaining.

3.22. Critical incident debriefings should be held within:

    a. 6 to 12 hours.

    b. 24 to 72 hours.

    c. 5 to 7 days.

    d. 7 to 14 days.

3.23. All of the following statements about stress in prehospital care personnel are correct *except*:

    a. job-related stress is characterized by irritability, fatigue, and insomnia.

    b. cumulative effects of stress take years to reach dangerous levels.

    c. burnout is a common problem among prehospital care providers.

    d. job-related stress exists to some degree in most prehospital providers.

3.24. Which of the following would be appropriate techniques for stress management?

    a. Maintaining a healthy lifestyle and using sedatives for sleep when needed

    b. Getting regular counseling after each call

    c. Maintaining a balance between work and leisure activities

    d. Taking sick leave when necessary and avoiding discussion of bad calls

3.25. Chronic job stress may cause a state of constant fatigue and irritability known as:

    a. depression.

    b. denial.

    c. burnout.

    d. acceptance.

3.26. The purpose of a critical incident stress debriefing session is to:

    a. allow EMTs to pass through the depression stage of grief.

    b. give EMTs a chance to talk with an expert in critical stress.

    c. assure the EMTs they did nothing wrong.

    d. allow the EMTs to work through emotional reactions they have had to a disturbing call.

3.27. Hand washing should be done for a minimum of:

    a. 10 to 15 seconds.

    b. 15 to 30 seconds.

    c. 30 to 60 seconds.

    d. 1 to 2 minutes.

3.28. A face mask and eye protection should be worn when you are:

    a. applying a traction splint.

    b. splinting a closed fracture.

    c. suctioning the airway.

    d. giving oxygen to an asthma patient.

3.29. Salmonella is transmitted by:

    a. infected persons who do not wash their hands adequately.

    b. mosquitoes.

    c. exposure to droplets when an infected person coughs.

    d. ticks.

3.30. Biohazard waste disposal bags are:
   a. black with red letters.
   b. yellow with black letters.
   c. red with black letters.
   d. orange with black letters.

3.31. Lyme disease is characterized by:
   a. flulike symptoms, joint pain, stiff neck, chest pain, and cardiac arrhythmias.
   b. painful muscle spasms in the throat, difficulty swallowing, dehydration, and death.
   c. a cough productive of blood, weight loss, night sweats, and fever.
   d. fever, rash, vomiting, headache, and stiff neck.

3.32. The Ryan White Act requires hospitals to notify emergency personnel of possible infectious disease exposure within:
   a. 6 hours.
   b. 12 hours.
   c. 24 hours.
   d. 48 hours.

Answer Key—Chapter 3

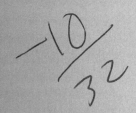

69%

3.1. **C,** The patient's complaints of a stiff neck and headache indicate the patient probably has meningitis. Hepatitis would be characterized by jaundice (yellow skin), dark urine, loss of appetite, and right upper quadrant pain. A patient with measles would have a rash consisting of red, slightly raised spots accompanied by symptoms of a respiratory infection. Mumps would produce tenderness and swelling of one or more of the salivary glands.

3.2. **A,** A mask and gloves should be worn for protection against meningitis. Droplets produced when the patient sneezes or coughs transmit meningitis.

3.3. **D,** Hepatitis A is not an airborne disease. It is transmitted via the fecal-oral route. Mumps, measles, and tuberculosis are airborne diseases.

3.4. **B,** You should let the emergency department know you suspect the patient has meningitis so they can prepare for your arrival and minimize the potential number of exposures. Calling by cell phone would be best if you have one available.

3.5. **C,** The patient's yellowish skin, abdominal pain, loss of appetite, and nausea suggest he has hepatitis. Meningitis would cause headache and a stiff neck. Measles would produce a distinctive rash and symptoms of a respiratory infection. Anemia would cause pale skin.

3.6. **C,** You would not need to wear a respirator-type mask because hepatitis is not spread by sneezing or coughing. In most cases gloves would be sufficient. However, if the patient is vomiting or if there are other body secretions present, gloves, a mask, and eye protection should be worn.

3.7. **B,** White blood cells (leukocytes) fight infection. Red blood cells (erythrocytes) contain hemoglobin and transport oxygen to the tissues. Plasma, the liquid portion of blood, contains electrolytes, lipids, enzymes, clotting factors, and glucose. Platelets (thrombocytes) take part in the blood's clotting process.

3.8. **A,** Pathogens are organisms that cause disease. T cells are lymphocytes that aid in the immune response. Fungi are organisms such as mushrooms, molds, and yeasts. Some fungi are pathogens. Phagocytes are cells that ingest microorganisms.

3.9. **A,** Severe hepatitis can cause liver failure, leading to death.

3.10. **A,** A person can carry and spread hepatitis without actually developing signs and symptoms of the disease.

3.11. **D,** The incubation period for AIDS is several months to years.

3.12. **C,** AIDS is spread through contact with infected blood or body fluids.

3.13. **B,** Appropriate infection control for a patient with AIDS would be gloves and respirator-type mask. AIDS is spread through contact with body fluids, particularly blood, semen, and vaginal secretions. Although AIDS is not an airborne disease, AIDS patients are susceptible to infection by airborne viruses transmitted by their caregivers. Additionally, a significant number of AIDS patients become infected by tuberculosis.

3.14. **D,** You should wash your hands and clean any equipment the patient may have come into contact with. Changing clothing is unnecessary unless your uniform has become contaminated with blood and body fluid. There is no need to clean or sterilize equipment that did not come into contact with the patient or the patient's body fluids.

3.15. B, The most common route for transmission of the HIV virus is sexual contact with an infected person.

3.16. D, Fatigue, fever, night sweats, weight loss, productive cough, and hemoptysis (coughing up blood) are signs and symptoms of tuberculosis.

3.17. C, The PPD test detects exposure to the bacterium that causes tuberculosis.

3.18. D, Active tuberculosis most commonly causes night sweats and coughing of blood or blood sputum.

3.19. B, Tuberculosis is spread through droplets produced by coughing.

3.20. C, Hepatitis is the most common serious infectious disease in the United States.

3.21. B, Denial is characterized by refusal to accept that something bad has happened.

3.22. B, A debriefing should be held within 24 to 72 hours of a critical incident.

3.23. B, Cumulative effects of stress do NOT take years to reach dangerous levels.

3.24. C, Maintaining a balance between work and leisure activities is an appropriate, effective way to manage stress. Using sedatives for sleep is not a good idea because of the risks of addiction. Counseling after each call is unnecessary because most EMS calls will not result in significant stress. Discussing bad calls or other stressful experiences is a way of relieving stress.

3.25. C, Burnout is a state of constant fatigue and irritability that results from chronic stress.

3.26. D, The purpose of a CISD is to allow EMTs to work through the emotional responses they have had to a disturbing call.

3.27. A, The minimum time for good hand washing is 10 to 15 seconds.

3.28. C, A face mask and eye protection should be worn when you are suctioning the airway because there is an increased risk of contacting secretions from the mucous membranes.

3.29. A, Salmonella, a bacterium that lives in the intestines, is transmitted by infected persons who do not wash their hands adequately after using the restroom.

3.30. C, Biohazard bags are red with black letters and markings.

3.31. A, Lyme disease is characterized by flulike symptoms, joint pain, stiff neck, chest pain, and cardiac arrhythmias.

3.32. D, The Ryan White Act requires hospitals to notify EMS personnel of possible infectious disease exposure within 48 hours.

4

Medical-Legal Issues

DEFINITIONS

Abandonment—Discontinuing care of a patient either without the patient's consent or before the patient has been transferred to another healthcare provider with equal or greater training

Assault—Acting in a manner that places another person in immediate fear of being harmed

Battery—Touching another person without his or her consent or other just cause

Confidentiality—A patient's right to expect that information about himself or herself and his or her present or past medical problems will not be revealed except to healthcare professionals involved in his or her care, under subpoena, in a court of law, or when a release of confidentiality has been signed

Duty to act—An obligation to provide care to a patient

Emancipated minor—A person who is still legally a minor but whose parents have relinquished authority and control over him or her. Legal definitions vary from state-to-state, but typically emancipated minors must be living apart from their parents and managing their own financial affairs. Be sure to check the definition in your state's laws.

Expressed consent—Permission to provide care given by a person who is an adult and possesses the mental competence and capacity to make rational decisions in regard to their health and well-being

False imprisonment—Intentionally detaining a person without his or her consent or other just cause

Implied consent—A legal doctrine that assumes that in a situation that reasonably appears to be life threatening a person who is unable to provide consent would do so. Implied consent is assumed with adults when the patient is unconscious or unable to communicate and has what reasonably appears to be a life-threatening injury or illness. Implied consent is assumed with minors or adults who have been declared mentally incompetent by a court of law if the patient has what reasonably appears to be a life-threatening injury or illness and a person who can legally consent to the patient's care is not present.

Informed consent—Permission to provide care given by a person who understands the nature of his or her illness or injury and risks of the care about to be provided

Libel—Making a false statement in *writing* or through some other *graphic representation* (such as drawing a picture) that will injure a person's name or character or hold him or her up to ridicule in the community

Negligence—To cause harm or injury to a patient by failing to meet or perform the expected standard of care. Normally four elements must be demonstrated to prove negligence has occurred:
- Duty to act
- Breach of duty
- Damages
- Proximate cause (a link between the breach of duty and the damages)

Negligence per se—Failing to perform a duty or meet an obligation imposed by law or by an administrative regulation adopted under law. An EMT-Basic who fails to follow all relevant federal, state, and local laws or regulations has, by definition, failed to meet the standard of care.

Res ipsa loquitur—Literally, "the thing speaks for itself." A legal doctrine that allows a plaintiff to demonstrate the defendant in a civil suit was negligent by showing that:
- The damages could not have occurred unless someone had been negligent.
- The defendant was in control of the instrument or thing that caused the damages.
  Invoking the doctrine of *res ipsa loquitur* during a lawsuit for negligence shifts the burden of proof from the plaintiff to the defendant.

Slander—Making a false statement using *spoken* words that will injure a person's name or character or hold him or her up to ridicule in the community

Standard of care—The actions a reasonable person with the same or similar training would have taken under the same or similar circumstances. To prove that an EMT-Basic was negligent, the person bringing a lawsuit must demonstrate that the EMT-Basic's actions differed from those that another EMT-Basic would have taken under the same or similar circumstances.

Tort—A violation of civil law other than a breach of contract for which the law provides a remedy. Negligence, abandonment, false imprisonment, assault, battery, slander, and libel are torts.

REVIEW QUESTIONS

Scenario One

You have been called to transfer a 78-y.o. male from the local hospital to a nursing home. The patient is very upset about leaving the hospital. After you have explained several times where he is going, he says, "I won't go with you." The patient was in the hospital for treatment of diverticulitis. He has a history of angina pectoris and peptic ulcer disease. He does not have any history of psychiatric disease and has not been declared incompetent.

Multiple Choice

4.1. What should you do *next*?
  a. Transport the patient because you have an order from a physician.
  b. Take the patient to the emergency department for a psychiatric evaluation.
  c. Return to your station and try again later.
  d. Tell the nurse what has happened and ask her to call the patient's doctor.

4.2. If you transport the patient, which statement would be *most* correct?
  a. You would have implied consent because the patient's family wants him to go to the nursing home.
  b. You would have expressed consent from the nurse who arranged the transfer.
  c. You would have committed assault, battery, and kidnapping by treating and transporting the patient against his will.
  d. You would not have consent to transport, but you would be protected from legal action by the Good Samaritan Law.

Scenario Two

A 16-y.o. female is experiencing cramping lower abdominal pain accompanied by moderate vaginal bleeding. Her last normal menstrual period was approximately 8 weeks ago. Her skin is pale and cool. She has no significant past medical history and is taking no medications. Vital signs are blood pressure (BP)—104/76; pulse (P)—114, weak, regular; and respiration (R)—18, regular, nonlabored. The patient left home 6 months ago and has been supporting herself.

Multiple Choice

4.3. You can treat this patient because you have:
  a. implied consent.
  b. involuntary consent.
  c. expressed consent.
  d. a duty to act.

4.4. This patient would be considered:
   a. an adult.
   b. an emancipated minor.
   c. a minor without consent.
   d. a minor using implied consent.

Scenario Three

A 49-y.o. male with a history of chronic alcohol abuse complains of weakness and mild chest pain. He denies any other symptoms. The patient is unshaven, and his clothing is filthy and wrinkled. Empty whisky bottles are strewn about his apartment; he smells of whisky; and his speech is slurred. Vital signs are BP—188/98; P—106, weak, regular; and R—24, regular, nonlabored. This patient calls EMS frequently for a variety of trivial problems. Although local protocol requires you to call for an advanced life support (ALS) ambulance when a patient complains of chest pain, you decide to transport him in your basic life support (BLS) unit. At the emergency department, the patient is found to be suffering from an acute myocardial infarction.

Multiple Choice

4.5. The patient would be *most* likely to sue you for:
   a. assault and battery.
   b. negligence.
   c. libel.
   d. implied standard of care.

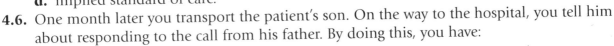

4.6. One month later you transport the patient's son. On the way to the hospital, you tell him about responding to the call from his father. By doing this, you have:
   a. libeled his father.
   b. breached confidentiality.
   c. slandered his father.
   d. been negligent.

Scenario Four

You have been dispatched to the home of a retired federal judge for an "unknown medical emergency." The patient is confused, has slurred speech, and staggers when he attempts to walk. His skin is pale, cool, and moist. Vital signs are BP—136/88; P—122, strong, regular; and R—22, shallow, regular. You are unable to obtain a history because of the patient's confusion. As you are moving him to the ambulance, a neighbor asks what is wrong. You reply, "Oh, he's just drunk." At the hospital, it is determined that the patient is diabetic and has hypoglycemia (low blood sugar) caused by taking insulin and then not eating.

Multiple Choice

4.7. Your comment about the patient's being "just drunk" would be:
   a. negligence.
   b. slander.
   c. libel.
   d. an intentional tort.

Scenario Five

The patient is a 5-y.o. male who was struck by a car while he was riding his bicycle. He does not respond to verbal or painful stimuli. He has an abrasion on his forehead, and his pupils are dilated and sluggish. His abdomen is distended, and his left thigh is swollen and deformed. Vital signs are BP—66/42; P—138, weak, regular; and R—28, shallow, regular.

Multiple Choice

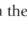

4.8. What should you do?
- a. Remain on the scene until the patient's parents are notified.
- b. Transport immediately and let the hospital notify the parents.
- c. Treat the patient under implied consent, call for ALS, and remain on the scene until the paramedics arrive.
- d. Ask a police officer for permission to treat and transport the patient.

4.9. If the patient was conscious and alert, he could be treated using:
- a. implied consent.
- b. expressed consent.
- c. informed consent.
- d. the Good Samaritan Law.

Scenario Six

An 8-y.o. male fell down an escalator at a mall. He has a deep laceration on the left leg that is bleeding profusely and a contusion on his forehead. He is screaming, "Don't touch me!"

Multiple Choice

4.10. What should you do?
- a. Withhold treatment until the parents are found because you could be sued for assault if you touch the patient without his permission
- b. Treat the child, and take the chance of being sued for battery and assault
- c. Treat the child under implied consent
- d. Control the bleeding with direct pressure, and then wait for the parents before transporting

4.11. You have expressed consent when:
- a. the patient gives you his or her permission to treat.
- b. a patient is unconscious or unable to communicate and has what reasonably appears to be a life-threatening injury or illness.
- c. the patient is aware of the nature of his or her illness and risks associated with the care about to be given.
- d. a duty or obligation to act exists.

Scenario Seven

You respond to a motor vehicle collision (MVC) in which one vehicle rear-ended another vehicle at a traffic light. On arrival you find two females talking with a police officer. They say they are not hurt and refuse treatment or transportation. They both were wearing seat belts, and the speed of impact was only 5 miles per hour.

Multiple Choice

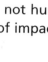

4.12. Which of the following would be *most* appropriate?
- a. Transport them to the hospital.
- b. Tell them to follow up with their doctors and clear from the scene.
- c. Obtain a refusal of service from each patient and document the situation thoroughly.
- d. Perform a detailed physical examination on both patients.

4.13. When several patients at the scene of an MVC refuse treatment, you should:
  a. have the police officer sign each refusal as a witness.
  b. have all of the patients sign the same refusal form.
  c. document that you told the patients the risks of not being examined, treated, and transported.
  d. document that you told every patient to follow up with his or her doctor.

Scenario Eight

You are called for "a child injured by a fall." The patient is a 7-y.o. female with a painful, swollen, and deformed right elbow. She says she tripped over the dog while running, but you don't see any animals in the house. The patient's father says he wants her "checked out" but does not want her taken to the hospital. You can smell beer on his breath and see a large number of empty beer cans scattered around the house. He is belligerent and keeps insisting that his daughter not be taken to the hospital.

Multiple Choice

4.14. Which of the following would be *most* appropriate?
  a. Have the father sign a refusal form after you have examined the child and splinted the deformed elbow.
  b. Return to the ambulance, call the police, and stand by until they arrive.
  c. Examine the child, leave the scene, notify the police, and document the call thoroughly.
  d. Contact on-line medical control to see if the doctor can convince the patient's father to allow her to be transported.

True/False

4.15. Leaving the house but remaining on scene until the police arrive would be abandonment.
  a. True
  b. False

Multiple Choice

4.16. Laws that protect healthcare personnel from liability when they provide care at the scene of an emergency are:
  a. implied consent laws.
  b. Duty to Act laws.
  c. delegation of authority laws.
  d. Good Samaritan laws.
4.17. The expectation that an EMT treat patients in the same way as another EMT would in the same situation is called:
  a. the standard of reciprocity.
  b. the standard of care.
  c. *res ipsa loquitur*.
  d. the duty to act.
4.18. An EMT-Basic may release patient information in all of these situations *except:*
  a. when a police officer asks for the information.
  b. when an insurance company requires the information to pay a claim.
  c. when hospital personnel need the information to provide patient care.
  d. when a subpoena is presented ordering its release.

4.19. What is slander?
   a. Damaging a person's reputation by saying things that are untrue
   b. Touching a patient without his or her consent
   c. Damaging a person's reputation by written statements that are untrue
   d. Placing another person in immediate fear of bodily harm

4.20. What is battery?
   a. Damaging a person's reputation by saying things that are untrue
   b. Restricting a person's freedom of movement without consent or just cause
   c. Touching a patient without his or her consent
   d. Placing another person in immediate fear of bodily harm

4.21. What is assault?
   a. Restricting a person's freedom of movement without consent or just cause
   b. Damaging a person's reputation by saying things that are untrue
   c. Touching a patient without his or her consent
   d. Placing another person in immediate fear of bodily harm

4.22. You would have consent to treat all of the following patients *except:*
   a. a 48-y.o. male who has paralysis of one side of his body and is unable to speak.
   b. a 3-y.o. child struck by a car whose parents cannot be located.
   c. a 14-y.o. child with a painful, swollen, and deformed left knee whose mother tells you to go away.
   d. a 16-y.o. adolescent involved in a car accident who is awake but oriented only to person.

4.23. Your *best* defense in the event of a lawsuit is:
   a. statements from other EMS personnel who were working with you.
   b. the physician who was in the ER when you brought in the patient.
   c. how well you performed patient care techniques during the call.
   d. the documentation on your patient care report.

4.24. Which of the following would be battery?
   a. A 30-y.o. female who suffers a broken tooth during placement of an airway adjunct
   b. Examining an 18-y.o. female's chest without asking permission
   c. A patient's head moving because the EMS did not apply an appropriately sized cervical collar
   d. An EMT's writing in a run report that a patient was drunk because his speech was slurred and he was having difficulty walking

67% 8/24

4.1. **D,** You should speak to the nurse in charge and ask the nurse to call the patient's doctor. A patient who has not been declared incompetent by a court of law has the right to refuse treatment and transport. Transporting a patient without his or her consent is kidnapping. In this situation, the patient's physician should be notified so he or she can evaluate the patient for a possible underlying medical problem that is affecting his ability to reason.

4.2. **C,** If you transport the patient without his consent, you will have committed assault, battery, and kidnapping. The patient's family does not have the right to make medical decisions for him or to consent to his transport. Because the patient refuses transport, you do not have his expressed consent. Good Samaritan Laws provide a defense in lawsuits for negligence. They do not apply to suits for intentional torts such as assault, battery, or kidnapping.

4.3. **C,** You have this patient's expressed consent to treat her. Involuntary consent exists when a court or a law enforcement officer who has a patient in custody directs treatment. You have implied consent when an individual who is unable to provide expressed consent has what reasonably appears to be a life-threatening injury or illness. The duty to act that arises from you being on duty as an EMT does not automatically give you the right to examine or treat a patient. You must have the patient's consent.

4.4. **B,** Although this patient is only 16 y.o., she is living apart from her parents and managing her own financial affairs. In most states she would be an *emancipated minor* and would have the right to consent to her own medical care. Additionally, most states give a minor who may be pregnant the right to consent to her own medical care in matters related to the pregnancy.

4.5. **B,** The patient probably will sue you for negligence, which is failure to follow the accepted standard of care that results in damages or injury. Assault is placing a patient in fear of immediate bodily harm. Battery is touching a patient without his or her consent. Libel is making untrue statements in writing that damage another person's reputation.

4.6. **B,** Telling the patient's son about his father's medical problems is a breach of confidentiality. Slander and libel involve making untrue verbal or written statements about another person that damage his or her reputation. Negligence is a breach of the standard of care that leads to damages to a patient.

4.7. **B,** Slander is something untrue about another person that damages his or her reputation. If the untrue statement is made in writing, you have committed libel. Slander and libel fall into the category of civil wrongs known as intentional torts. Negligence, which is failure to follow the standard of care, is an unintentional tort. In other words, whether you meant to breach the standard of care is not relevant. It only matters that the standard of care was breached and damages resulted.

4.8. **B,** This patient is a minor and is suffering from life-threatening injuries. You should transport immediately to the closest facility that can take him to the operating room immediately. When a minor has what reasonably appears to be an immediately life-threatening injury or illness and a parent is not present, you have the parent's implied consent to treat and transport. Because this child probably has a head injury and internal bleeding, waiting on the scene for an ALS unit would not be a good choice. He needs to be transported as quickly as possible.

4.9. **A,** The patient's being conscious does not change the fact he is a minor. A minor is treated using *implied consent* when a parent or guardian is not present and the patient has a life-threatening injury or illness.

4.10. **C,** The patient is a minor; therefore, he cannot make his own medical decisions. You can treat and transport him because his parent's implied consent is assumed.

4.11. **C,** You have *expressed consent* when a patient gives you verbal or written permission to treat. Obtaining informed consent involves telling the patient the nature of his or her illness and all risks associated with the care you are about to provide. True informed consent usually is not practical in emergency care settings. If a patient with a life-threatening problem is unconscious or otherwise unable to communicate, you have implied consent.

4.12. **C,** Because the patients do not appear to be hurt and the mechanism is unlikely to have caused serious injuries, you should have them sign refusal forms. You then should document the nature of the accident, the patients' appearance, their refusal of care, and your instructions to them to follow up with their physicians if necessary.

4.13. **C,** When patients refuse treatment, you should document that they were informed of the risks of not being examined, treated, and transported. Each patient should sign a separate form refusing service. Although the police officer does not need to sign each refusal, you should document the name and badge numbers of any police officers on the scene who witnessed the refusals.

4.14. **B,** You should return to the ambulance, call for the police, and stand by until they arrive. The inconsistent history and the father's belligerence suggest that the patient is a victim of child abuse. Confronting the patient's father could result in you being attacked or in the father's fleeing with the patient before the police arrive. You should wait near the ambulance until the police have secured the scene, and then you can return to care for the patient.

4.15. **B,** Because you notified the police and waited nearby until they could secure the scene, you did not abandon the patient. Temporarily leaving an unsafe scene until law enforcement officers could respond was a prudent action on your part necessary to prevent a possible attack on yourself or further injury to the patient.

4.16. **D,** Good Samaritan Laws provide a defense against civil liability for individuals who provide care at the scene of an emergency as long as they were not grossly negligent.

4.17. **B,** The standard of care expected of an EMT is that he or she will treat a patient the way another EMT would in the same situation. An EMT's quality of care is judged by comparing it with the quality of care that would be delivered in the same situation by another EMT.

4.18. **A,** Police officers do not have any special privilege or status that requires you to release medical information to them. You may assist the police to identify a patient and provide general information about the seriousness of the patient's condition, but you may not provide law enforcement officers with information about the specific nature of a patient's problem. Insurance companies have a right to obtain patient information needed to pay claims. Hospital personnel may be given information needed to provide patient care. Otherwise, you should release or discuss patient information only when a court of law orders you to do so by issuing a subpoena.

4.19. **A,** Slander is damaging someone's reputation by making false verbal statements about him or her. Making a false written statement that damages another person's reputation is libel.

4.20. **C,** Battery is touching another person without his or her consent.

4.21. **D,** Assault is saying or doing anything that places another person in immediate fear of bodily harm, regardless of whether actual contact occurs.

4.22. **C,** Because this patient is a minor and her mother has told you to go away, you do not have consent to treat. In this situation, you will have to obtain involuntary consent to treat the patient by either obtaining a court order or having the police or child protective service place the patient in protective custody. The 48-y.o. male with hemiplegia who is unable to speak has given you his implied consent. You also have implied parental consent to treat the 3-y.o. child who was struck by a car and the 16-y.o. adolescent who was involved in an MVC.

4.23. **D,** Your best defense in the event of a lawsuit is the documentation on your patient care report.

4.24. **B,** Examining a patient without first obtaining his or her consent would be battery. Breaking a tooth during placement of an airway adjunct and improperly sizing a cervical collar causing excessive movement of an injured neck are examples of negligence. Writing untrue statements about a patient in a run report could constitute libel.

5

Anatomy and Physiology

Study Set Body Structure

— Body Function

DEFINITIONS

Anatomy—Study of body structure
Homeostasis—Ability of organism to maintain stable internal environmental balance compatible
    with life and harmonious function
Physiology—Study of body function

LEVELS OF ANATOMICAL STRUCTURE

- Cell—Basic unit of life; smallest structural element of the body. Example: cardiac muscle cell
  (Figure 5-1)

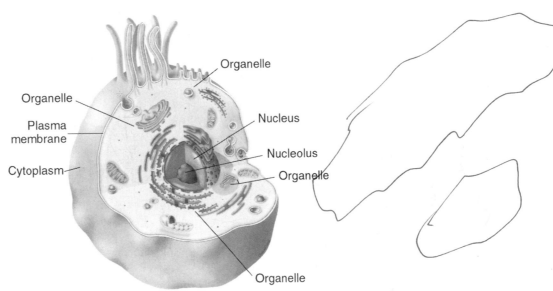

Figure 5-1   A typical cell in the human body. (Christine Oleksyk
from Seely R: *Essentials of anatomy and physiology*, ed 2, St Louis,
1996, Mosby.)

- Tissue—A group of cells that performs a similar function. Example: the myocardium
- Organ—A group of tissues that functions together to perform a function. Example: the heart
- Organ system—A group of organs that works together to perform a function. Example: the
  cardiovascular system
- Organism—The sum of all of the organ systems functioning together; the individual. Example:
  you

TYPES OF TISSUES

- Epithelial tissue—Lines body surfaces; provides protection, specialized functions such as
  secretion, absorption, diffusion, and filtration. Examples: skin surface, lining of gastrointestinal
  tract, and lining of respiratory tract
- Muscle tissue—Has ability to contract on stimulation. Examples: skeletal muscle, smooth
  muscle, and cardiac muscle
- Nervous tissue—Conducts motor, sensory impulses throughout the body. Examples: brain,
  spinal cord, and peripheral motor and sensory nerves
- Connective tissue—Most abundant tissue in body; provides support, connection insulation.
  Examples: bone, cartilage, tendons (connect muscles to bones), and ligaments (connect bones to
  bones)

MAJOR ORGAN SYSTEMS
Skeletal System
- Supports body against gravity, gives it shape; produces red blood cells, protects vital organs, and works with muscles to allow movement (Figure 5-2)

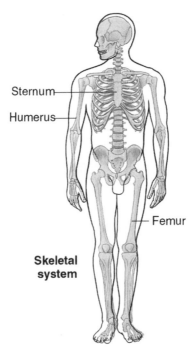

Figure 5-2   Skeletal system. (Joan M. Beck from Thibideau GA, Patton KT: *Anatomy and physiology*, ed 3, St Louis, 1996, Mosby.)

- ○ Skull
    - ■ Cranium—Frontal, parietal, temporal, and occipital bones
    - ■ Face—Maxilla (upper jaw), mandible (lower jaw), zygoma (cheek), and nasal bones
- ○ Spine—Cervical (7 vertebrae), thoracic (12 vertebrae), lumbar (5 vertebrae), sacral (5 fused vertebrae), and coccyx (3 to 5 fused vertebrae)
- ○ Rib cage—Sternum, 12 pairs of ribs
- ○ Pelvis—Ilium, ischium, and pubis
- ○ Lower extremities—Femur, patella (kneecap), tibia, fibula, tarsals, metatarsals, and phalanges
- ○ Upper extremities—Clavicle, scapula, humerus, radius, ulna, carpals, metacarpals, and phalanges

Muscular System
- Provides for movement, posture, and production of heat (Figure 5-3)
    - ○ Voluntary muscle—Also called skeletal or striated muscle; major muscle mass of body; forms body walls; generally attached to bones by tendons; and under conscious control
    - ○ Involuntary muscle—Also called smooth muscle; under control of autonomic nervous system; and found in walls of blood vessels, respiratory tract, and hollow organs
    - ○ Cardiac muscle—Possesses automaticity, ability to stimulate own contractions; found only in heart

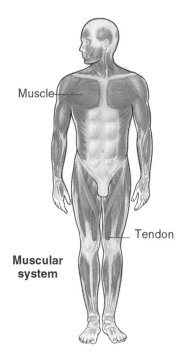

Figure 5-3   Muscular system. (Joan M. Beck from Thibideau GA, Patton KT: *Anatomy and physiology*, ed 3, St Louis, 1996, Mosby.)

Respiratory System

- Provides for exchange of oxygen and carbon dioxide between the bloodstream and the atmosphere (Figure 5-4)

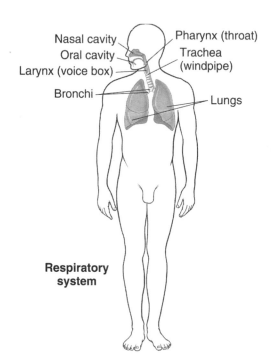

Figure 5-4   Respiratory system. (Joan M. Beck from Thibideau GA, Patton KT: *Anatomy and physiology*, ed 3, St Louis, 1996, Mosby.)

○ Nose and mouth—Nose normally warms, moistens, and filters air
○ Pharynx—Throat; shared passage for air and food; divided into nasopharynx and oropharynx
○ Epiglottis—Leaf-shaped valve; protects entrance to lower airway during swallowing
○ Larynx—Voice box; contains vocal cords; ring-shaped cricoid cartilage forms lower edge
○ Trachea—Windpipe
○ Bronchi—Carry air between trachea and lungs; two mainstem bronchi branch into smaller bronchi, which branch into bronchioles leading to the alveoli
○ Alveoli—Thin-walled air sacs in lungs where gas exchange with bloodstream takes place
○ Diaphragm—Dome-shaped muscle that separates thoracic cavity from abdominal cavity; contraction increases height of thoracic cavity, leading to inhalation
○ Intercostal muscles—Muscles located between ribs; contraction pulls ribs up and out, increasing width of thoracic cavity, leading to inhalation

Circulatory (Cardiovascular) System

- Transports oxygen, nutrients, carbon dioxide, waste, hormones, heat, and antibodies (Figure 5-5)

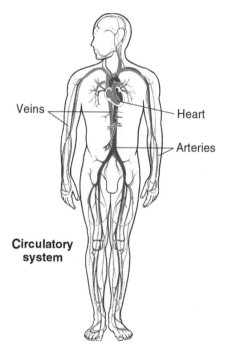

Figure 5-5   Circulatory system. (Joan M. Beck from Thibideau GA, Patton KT: *Anatomy and physiology*, ed 3, St Louis, 1996, Mosby.)

○ Heart—Two atria (upper chambers); two ventricles (lower chambers)
○ Blood vessels—Arteries (carry blood away from heart); veins (return blood to heart); and capillaries (connect arteries and veins, allow for exchange of gases, nutrients, and waste with tissues)
  ▪ Aorta—Largest artery; carries oxygenated blood from left side of heart to body
  ▪ Venae cavae—Superior and inferior; two largest veins; return unoxygenated blood from body to right side of heart
  ▪ Pulmonary artery—Carries unoxygenated blood from heart to lungs; the only artery that carries unoxygenated blood

■ Pulmonary veins—Carry oxygenated blood from lungs to heart; the only veins that carry oxygenated blood
○ Blood—Plasma (liquid portion of blood); erythrocytes (red blood cells); leukocytes (white blood cells); and thrombocytes (platelets)

Gastrointestinal (Digestive) System

● Takes in and digests food, absorbs nutrients, eliminates waste products (Figure 5-6)

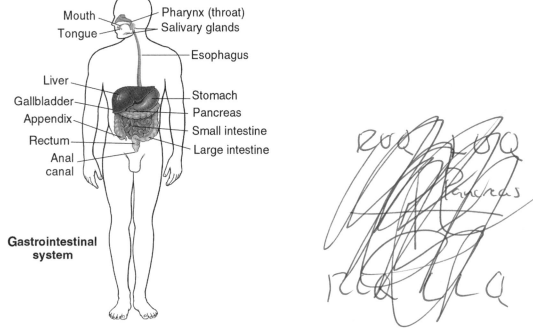

Figure 5-6   Gastrointestinal system. (Joan M. Beck from Thibideau GA, Patton KT: *Anatomy and physiology*, ed 3, St Louis, 1996, Mosby.)

○ Esophagus—Hollow organ; connects pharynx with stomach
○ Stomach—Hollow organ; left upper quadrant; secretes gastric juices to break down food
○ Pancreas—Solid organ; primarily in left upper quadrant; secretes pancreatic juices to aid in digestion of proteins, starches, and fats
○ Liver—Solid organ; right upper quadrant; produces bile, stores sugar, makes proteins needed for blood clotting and plasma production, and breaks down toxins
○ Gallbladder—Right upper quadrant; stores bile, which assists in fat digestion
○ Small intestine—Hollow organ; made up of duodenum, jejunum, and ileum; absorbs nutrients into bloodstream
○ Large intestine—Hollow organ; consists of cecum, ascending colon, transverse colon, descending colon, sigmoid colon, and rectum; reabsorbs water from digestive tract into body; and stores feces until removed from body

Nervous System

● Controls all activities of the body, voluntary and involuntary; allows individual to be aware of and react to environment (Figure 5-7)

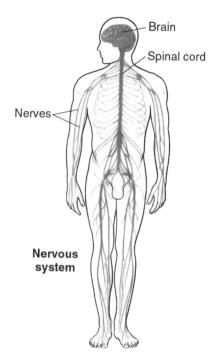

Figure 5-7 Nervous system. (Joan M. Beck from Thibideau GA, Patton KT: *Anatomy and physiology*, ed 3, St Louis, 1996, Mosby.)

○ Central nervous system
  ▪ Brain—Cerebrum, cerebellum, brain stem
  ▪ Spinal cord
○ Peripheral nervous system—All nerves outside brain and spinal cord
  ▪ 31 pairs of spinal nerves
  ▪ 12 pairs of cranial nerves

Endocrine System

- Secretes hormones directly into blood stream; hormones affect growth, metabolic rate, blood sugar levels, blood electrolytes, and reproduction (Figure 5-8)
  ○ Pituitary gland—Located at base of brain; "master gland"; regulates growth; and controls function of thyroid, parathyroid, adrenals, and gonads
  ○ Thyroid gland—Located in neck; regulates metabolism
  ○ Parathyroid glands—Behind thyroid; regulates blood calcium and phosphorus levels
  ○ Adrenal glands—On top of kidneys; release adrenalin in response to stress; and help regulate body's sugar, salt, and water balance
  ○ Pancreas—Islets of Langerhans produce insulin; causes uptake of sugar from blood into body tissues
  ○ Gonads (ovaries and testes)—Produce hormones that govern reproduction, sexual characteristics

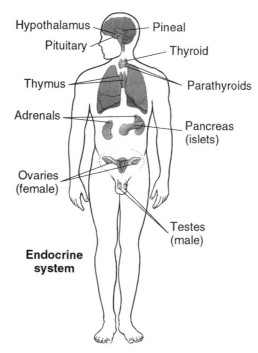

Figure 5-8   Endocrine system. (Joan M. Beck from Thibideau GA, Patton KT: *Anatomy and physiology*, ed 3, St Louis, 1996, Mosby.)

Integumentary System

- The skin; largest organ; protects body from pathogens; prevents excessive loss of body water; helps regulate body temperature; and senses heat, cold, touch, pressure, and pain (Figure 5-9)

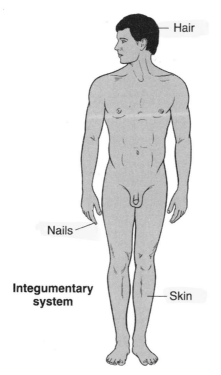

Figure 5-9   Integumentary system. (Joan M. Beck from Thibideau GA, Patton KT: *Anatomy and physiology*, ed 3, St Louis, 1996, Mosby.)

○ Epidermis—Outermost layer; top consists of dead, hardened cells that form protective barrier
○ Dermis—Contains blood vessels, nerves, hair follicles, and oil glands
○ Subcutaneous layer—Made of fat; helps insulate body

Urinary System

• Helps regulate water and electrolyte balance; eliminates waste products (Figure 5-10)

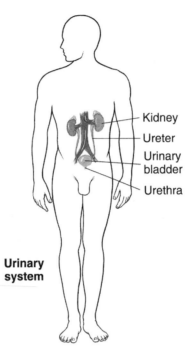

Kidney
Ureter
Urinary bladder
Urethra

Urinary system

Figure 5-10 Urinary system. (Joan M. Beck from Thibideau GA, Patton KT: *Anatomy and physiology*, ed 3, St Louis, 1996, Mosby.)

○ Kidneys—Filter waste from bloodstream; control fluid balance
○ Ureters—Carry urine from kidney to urinary bladder
○ Urinary bladder—Stores urine before excretion
○ Urethra—Carries urine out of body

Reproductive System

- Responsible for reproduction (Figure 5-11)

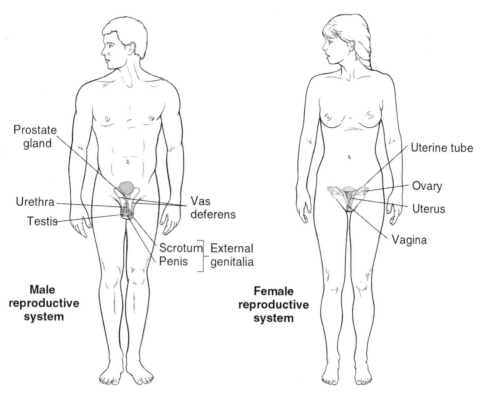

Figure 5-11   Reproductive system. (Joan M. Beck from Thibideau GA, Patton KT: *Anatomy and physiology*, ed 3, St Louis, 1996, Mosby.)

- Male—Testes, epididymis, vas deferens, prostate, seminal vesicles, penis, and urethra
- Female—Ovaries, fallopian tubes, uterus, cervix, vagina, and external genitalia

REVIEW QUESTIONS

Scenario One

You have been dispatched to a "motor vehicle collision (MVC) with injuries." On arrival you see a car that has left the roadway, struck a utility pole, and rolled onto its side. The fire department is extricating the patient, who is an 18-y.o. male c/o LUQ abdominal pain and left shoulder pain. He was wearing a seat belt. He does not appear to have any other injuries. He has no significant past medical history, and NKA. Vital signs are blood pressure (BP)—100/72; pulse (P)—112, regular, strong; and respiration (R)—22, regular, unlabored. You immediately request a response by an advance life support (ALS) unit, but they are 5 to 10 minutes away.

Your Plan of Action

Fill in the blank lines with your treatment plan for this patient. Then compare your plan with the questions, answers, and rationale.

1. _____
2. _____
3. _____
4. _____
5. _____
6. _____
7. _____
8. _____
9. _____

Multiple Choice

5.1. The left upper quadrant (LUQ) of the abdomen contains which major organs?
   a. Left kidney, spleen, pancreas, and stomach
   b. Left kidney, stomach, appendix, and gallbladder
   c. Left kidney, spleen, stomach, and appendix
   d. Left kidney, pancreas, liver, and gallbladder

5.2. Which of this patient's organs are most likely injured?
   a. Pancreas or spleen
   b. Stomach or gallbladder
   c. Spleen or gallbladder
   d. Left kidney or liver

5.3. If the patient were having left flank pain rather than left shoulder pain, you might suspect an injury of what organ?
   a. Liver
   b. Kidney
   c. Stomach
   d. Spleen

5.4. Which of the following organs are located in the right upper quadrant (RUQ)?
   a. Right kidney, spleen, pancreas, and stomach
   b. Right kidney, stomach, appendix, and gallbladder
   c. Right kidney, spleen, stomach, and appendix
   d. Right kidney, part of pancreas, liver, and gallbladder

5.5. Which of the following are solid organs?
   a. Gallbladder, stomach
   b. Liver, urinary bladder
   c. Spleen, liver
   d. Spleen, descending colon

5.6. Which of the following are "hollow organs"?
   a. Gallbladder, stomach
   b. Liver, urinary bladder
   c. Spleen, liver
   d. Spleen, descending colon

5.7. How much blood may be lost into the abdomen without noticeable distension?
   a. 250 to 500 mL
   b. 500 to 1000 mL
   c. 1000 to 1500 mL
   d. greater than 2000 mL

5.8. One of the major functions of the pancreas is to produce:
   a. red blood cells.
   b. bile.
   c. insulin.
   d. gastric juices.

Scenario Two

You are dispatched to a collision between a car and a motorcycle. The motorcyclist is a 20-y.o. male who struck the car at approximately 35 mph. He was wearing a helmet. He is conscious and oriented × 4, c/o pain in the right lateral chest wall. A superficial laceration is present over the 4th rib in the midaxillary line. He denies any past medical hx and has NKA. Vital signs are BP—122/74; P—88, strong, regular; R—22, shallow, regular, unlabored; and SaO_2—96%.

> **Your Plan of Action**
>
> *Fill in the blank lines with your treatment plan for this patient. Then compare your plan with the questions, answers, and rationale.*
>
> 1. _____
> 2. _____
> 3. _____
> 4. _____
> 5. _____
> 6. _____
> 7. _____
> 8. _____
> 9. _____

Multiple Choice

5.9. All of the following are immediate concerns with thoracic trauma *except:*
   a. bruising of the myocardium may cause effects similar to a heart attack.
   b. tearing of one of the great vessels could result in massive blood loss.
   c. a blood clot may form, resulting in a pulmonary embolism.
   d. bruising of the lungs or the presence of blood in the pleural space may interfere with gas exchange.

5.10. All of the following are arteries in the chest *except*:
a. aorta.
b. pulmonary.
c. axillary.
d. left subclavian.

5.11. During your examination you find a "flail segment" on the right side. This means:
a. the affected chest wall section will move out on inspiration.
b. the diaphragm is torn.
c. there will be air or blood in the pleural space.
d. three or more ribs in a row on the same side of the chest are fractured in two places.

5.12. The sternum is:
a. the double-walled membrane that surrounds the lung.
b. the sac that surrounds the heart.
c. the breastbone.
d. a flat, elongated bone located in the shoulder.

5.13. The *primary* concern with this patient is the possibility of:
a. fractured ribs causing significant pain and resulting in inadequate breathing.
b. bruising of the lung causing inadequate gas exchange with the blood.
c. an impending heart attack caused by the inadequate oxygenation of the blood.
d. internal bleeding in the abdominal cavity from an injury to the spleen.

Scenario Three

You are dispatched to a report of an explosion at a coffee shop. On arrival you find multiple victims from what appears to have been a pipe bomb explosion. A police sergeant and two other officers are on the scene. Additional police are en route. A fire department engine company with a lieutenant, a driver-engineer, and two firefighters is pulling onto the scene at the same time you arrive. A second engine company, a truck company, and a district fire chief also are responding. Their ETA is 5 to 7 minutes.

Your Plan of Action

Fill in the blank lines with your treatment plan for this patient. Then compare your plan with the questions, answers, and rationale.

1. _____
2. _____
3. _____
4. _____
5. _____
6. _____
7. _____
8. _____
9. _____

Your partner establishes initial EMS command and starts setting up a command post with the police sergeant and fire department lieutenant. You are designated triage officer. After donning appropriate protective equipment, you enter the damage area with the firefighters to begin triage.

Multiple Choice

5.14. Patient #1 is a 16-y.o. female who has a fracture of her right femur. This bone is located in the:

   a. upper arm.
   b. lower leg.
   c. thigh.
   d. ankle.

5.15. The head of the femur sits in an indentation in the pelvis is known as the:

   a. ischium.
   b. acetabulum.
   c. greater trochanter.
   d. ilium.

5.16. Patient #2 is a 41-y.o. male with massive facial trauma. The bones involved could include the:

   a. maxilla, zygoma, and mandible.
   b. mandible, maxilla, and scapula.
   c. zygoma, mandible, and occipital.
   d. mandible, maxilla, and manubrium.

5.17. Patient #3 is a 12-y.o. male who has a large bruise on the posterior surface of the skull just superior to the cervical spine. Which bone is *most* likely to be injured?

   a. Frontal
   b. Occipital
   c. Parietal
   d. Temporal

5.18. Patient #4 is a 24-y.o. male who has a 2-inch laceration on the right lateral chest and is experiencing difficulty breathing. Your *principal* concern should be that he might have:

   a. rib fractures.
   b. penetration of the diaphragm and injury to the spleen.
   c. a pneumothorax or hemothorax.
   d. an injury to the apex of the heart.

5.19. Patient #5 is a 28-y.o. female who is very upset and is complaining of numbness and tingling in her hands and feet. No obvious injuries are present. Her skin is warm and dry. Breath sounds are present and equal bilaterally. Vital signs are BP—132/92; P—114, strong, regular; R—30, deep, regular; and SaO_2—99% on room air. What is this patient's *most* likely problem?

   a. She is having difficulty maintaining her airway.
   b. She is hyperventilating because of anxiety.
   c. She has internal bleeding and is in the early stages of shock.
   d. She has a spinal injury with pressure on the spinal cord.

Scenario Four

A 7-y.o. male fell approximately 8 feet from a tree. He is A & O × 4 c/o right ankle and foot pain. His skin is pink, warm, and dry. Vital signs are BP—110/70; P—96, strong, regular; and R—22, regular, unlabored.

Your Plan of Action

Fill in the blank lines with your treatment plan for this patient. Then compare your plan with the questions, answers, and rationale.

1. _____
2. _____
3. _____
4. _____
5. _____
6. _____
7. _____
8. _____
9. _____

Multiple Choice

5.20. Which of the following statements about the anatomy of the ankle and foot is correct?
   a. The ankle is a ball and socket joint.
   b. The foot comprises the tarsals, metacarpals, and phalanges.
   c. The ankle is formed by the lateral malleolus and the medial malleolus.
   d. The ankle is formed by the distal tarsal bones.

5.21. The bone that forms the heel is the:
   a. calcaneus.
   b. talus.
   c. cuboid.
   d. cuneiform.

Scenario Five

Your patient is a 13-y.o. female with a history of asthma who obviously is in respiratory distress. She is sitting up and leaning forward, using her accessory muscles to help her breathe. Her skin is pale, warm, and moist. Expiratory wheezing can be heard throughout the lung fields. Vital signs are BP—110/66; P—128, strong, regular; R—32, regular, labored; and SaO_2—92%.

Your Plan of Action

Fill in the blank lines with your treatment plan for this patient. Then compare your plan with the questions, answers, and rationale.

1. _____
2. _____
3. _____
4. _____
5. _____
6. _____
7. _____
8. _____
9. _____

Multiple Choice

5.22. The muscles that move the ribs up and out during normal inhalation are the:
    a. sternocleidomastoids.
    b. trapezius.
    c. pectoralis.
    d. intercostals.

5.23. In the respiratory system, gas exchange with the blood occurs in the:
    a. trachea.
    b. mainstem bronchi.
    c. bronchioles.
    d. alveoli.

5.24. The cilia in the respiratory tract:
    a. filter, warm, and humidify inspired air.
    b. move the mucus layer that traps foreign particles.
    c. cover the trachea to prevent food and liquids from entering.
    d. help move oxygen into the alveoli.

5.25. Oxygen moves from the alveoli into the pulmonary capillaries because the capillaries contain:
    a. more oxygen than the alveoli.
    b. less oxygen than the alveoli.
    c. more carbon dioxide than the alveoli.
    d. less carbon dioxide than the alveoli.

5.26. The normal respiratory rate for a 13-y.o. child is:
    a. 12 to 20.
    b. 15 to 30.
    c. 20 to 30.
    d. 24 to 30.

5.27. The normal respiratory rate for an adult is:
  a. 12 to 20.
  b. 15 to 30.
  c. 20 to 30.
  d. 24 to 30.

5.28. The normal respiratory rate for an infant from birth to 5 months is:
  a. 12 to 20.
  b. 15 to 30.
  c. 25 to 40.
  d. 40 to 60.

5.29. Tidal volume is the amount of air:
  a. reaching the alveoli for gas exchange.
  b. inhaled and exhaled in a single respiratory cycle.
  c. remaining in the larger airways that is unavailable for gas exchange.
  d. remaining in the lungs at the end of a complete exhalation.

5.30. Room air contains:
  a. 79% carbon dioxide and 21% oxygen.
  b. 79% oxygen and 21% nitrogen.
  c. 79% nitrogen and 21% oxygen.
  d. 79% carbon dioxide and 21% oxygen.

Scenario Six

You are dispatched to a report of an "injured child." The patient is a 4-y.o. female who fell on a sidewalk, abrading the anterior surface of her right forearm. She is alert and oriented appropriately for her age. Bleeding from the abrasions has stopped. Distal circulation, sensation, and movement are intact with full range of motion in the extremity. Vital signs are BP—100/66; P—102, strong, regular; and R—24, regular, unlabored.

Your Plan of Action

Fill in the blank lines with your treatment plan for this patient. Then compare your plan with the questions, answers, and rationale.

1. _____
2. _____
3. _____
4. _____
5. _____
6. _____
7. _____
8. _____
9. _____

Multiple Choice

5.31. The *principal* concern with this patient's injury is:
   a. infection.
   b. blood loss.
   c. nerve damage.
   d. a possible underlying fracture.

5.32. The functions of the skin include:
   a. protection and support against gravity.
   b. temperature control and fluid absorption.
   c. protection and temperature regulation.
   d. temperature regulation and support against gravity.

5.33. From outermost to innermost, the layers of the skin are:
   a. dermis, epidermis, and subcutaneous.
   b. epidermis, subcutaneous, and dermis.
   c. subcutaneous, dermis, and epidermis.
   d. epidermis, dermis, and subcutaneous.

5.34. The ability of the human body to maintain a stable internal environment is:
   a. equifinality.
   b. homeostasis.
   c. physiologic equilibrium.
   d. hemostasis.

5.35. The basic unit of life is the:
   a. cell.
   b. tissue.
   c. organ.
   d. organ system.

5.36. The superior portion of the sternum is the:
   a. ischium.
   b. xiphoid.
   c. gladiolus.
   d. manubrium.

5.37. The part of the femur that is injured when a patient "breaks a hip" is the:
   a. head.
   b. neck.
   c. greater trochanter.
   d. shaft.

5.38. The bones of the pelvis include the:
   a. ischium.
   b. acetabulum.
   c. ileum.
   d. sacrum.

Labelling

Label the diagram with correct sections of the spine.

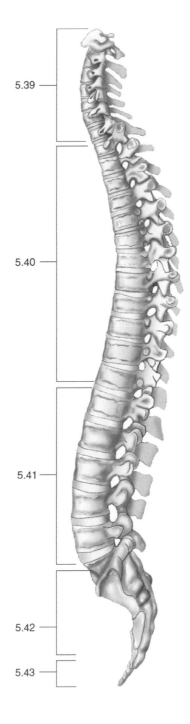

5.39. _____

5.40. _____

5.41. _____

5.42. _____

5.43. _____

Matching

Epithelial tissue   Connective tissue
Muscle tissue   Nerve tissue

5.44. _____ Has the ability to contract when stimulated; there are three types: skeletal, smooth, and cardiac

5.45. _____ Conducts electrical impulses throughout the body

5.46. _____ Lines body surfaces, provides protection, and performs specialized functions such as absorption, secretion, diffusion, and filtration

5.47. _____ Provides support and insulation for the body

Answer Key—Chapter 5

SCENARIO ONE

Plan of Action

1. <u>Body Substance Isolation (BSI)</u>

2. <u>Is the scene safe? Yes. Assess mechanism of injury, number of patients, and need for additional resources.</u>

3. <u>Manually stabilize head and neck. Assess mental status. Ensure open airway, assess breathing, apply oxygen 10 to 15 lpm, and assess circulation.</u>

4. <u>Determine priority and consider ALS.</u>

5. <u>Rapid trauma examination</u>

6. <u>Baseline vital signs</u>

7. <u>SAMPLE</u>

8. <u>Apply cervical collar, extricate to long spine board, and apply cervical immobilization device.</u>

9. <u>En route, perform detailed physical examination if time permits. Perform ongoing assessment.</u>

Rationale

The mechanism of injury involves significant injury and force. Although the initial assessment reveals no immediate life threats, the rapid trauma examination and the baseline vital signs suggest the possibility of bleeding into the abdomen, probably from an injury to the spleen. The patient should be rapidly extricated and transported to a facility with capabilities for immediate surgery. Bleeding from an injured spleen frequently irritates the diaphragm on the left side, producing pain referred to the left shoulder.

5.1. **A,** The left upper quadrant contains the left kidney, spleen, pancreas, and stomach. The gallbladder and liver are located in the right upper quadrant. The appendix is located in the right lower quadrant.

5.2. **A,** The organs most likely to be injured are the pancreas or spleen because they are located in the left upper quadrant. The gallbladder and liver are located in the right upper quadrant.

5.3. **B,** If the patient was having pain in the left flank, you would suspect injury to the kidney. The kidneys are located in the upper quadrant behind the peritoneum (abdominal cavity lining). Pain from kidney injury or disease tends to radiate (travel) from the lower back around the flank to the groin.

5.4. D, The right kidney, part of the pancreas, liver, and gallbladder are in the right upper quadrant. The spleen and stomach are in the left upper quadrant. The appendix is located in the right lower quadrant. The urinary bladder is in the lower abdomen in the midline. The descending colon is located in the left upper and left lower quadrants.

5.5. C, The liver and spleen are solid organs. The gallbladder, stomach, urinary bladder, and descending colon are hollow organs.

5.6. A, The gallbladder and stomach are hollow organs. The liver and spleen are solid organs.

5.7. C, From 1000 mL to 1500 mL of blood can be lost into the abdomen without noticeable distension.

5.8. C, One of the functions of the pancreas is to produce insulin, which is responsible for helping glucose move from the bloodstream into the cells. The pancreas also produces enzymes that assist with digesting food. The bone marrow produces red blood cells. The liver produces bile. The stomach produces gastric juices.

Scenario Two

Plan of Action
1. BSI
2. Is the scene safe? Yes. Assess mechanism of injury, number of patients, and need for additional resources.
3. Manually stabilize head and neck. Assess mental status. Ensure open airway, assess breathing, apply oxygen 10 to 15 lpm, and assess circulation.
4. Determine priority and consider ALS.
5. Rapid trauma examination
6. Baseline vital signs
7. SAMPLE
8. Apply cervical collar, long spine board, and cervical immobilization device.
9. En route, do a detailed physical examination if time permits and perform ongoing assessment.

Rationale
Motorcycle riders are especially prone to injury because they do not have any protection. The laceration of the right chest wall could be associated with a pneumothorax or hemothorax. The laceration should be covered with an occlusive dressing. The patient should be given oxygen by non-rebreather mask. If his breathing becomes labored or inadequate, it should be assisted with a bag-valve mask. The patient should be secured to a long spine board with a cervical collar and cervical immobilization device in place.

5.9. C, The formation of a blood clot resulting in a pulmonary embolus is not an immediate concern in thoracic trauma. Bruising of the myocardium (myocardial contusion) can result in effects similar to a heart attack. Injury to the pulmonary artery, pulmonary veins, venae cavae, or aorta can cause massive blood loss. Bruising of the lungs (pulmonary contusion) can interfere with gas exchange between the lungs and blood.

5.10. **C,** The axillary artery is located outside the chest cavity in the armpit (axilla).

5.11. **D,** A flail chest occurs when three or more ribs in a row are fractured in two or more places, creating a free-floating section of chest wall. The flail segment will move opposite from the rest of the chest wall as the patient breathes.

5.12. **C,** The sternum is the breastbone. The double-walled membrane that surrounds the lung is the pleura. The pericardium is the sac that surrounds the heart. The scapula, or shoulder blade, is the flat bone located in the shoulder.

5.13. **B,** The force that produces a flail chest also causes a bruise (pulmonary contusion) on the underlying lung. In the bruised areas, blood leaks from damaged vessels and surrounds or fills the alveoli, interfering with normal gas exchange.

SCENARIO THREE

Plan of Action

1. BSI

2. Is the scene safe to enter? Based on the initial assessment by the police, yes. However, appropriate protective equipment (helmet, gloves, boots, and turnout coat) should be worn. Extreme caution should be exercised because a secondary explosive device may be present.

3. Establish a command post in cooperation with ranking on-scene law enforcement and fire officers.

4. Begin triage of patients using the START method. Assess number of patients and need for additional resources.

5. Establish a staging area for additional ambulances.

6. Begin establishing treatment area for casualties.

Rationale

In a mass casualty incident, the responsibility of the first-arriving EMS unit is to establish a command structure that will allow effective, efficient management of the incident. One member of the crew should serve as initial EMS commander. The EMS commander should request a response by additional ambulances, establish a command post in cooperation with law enforcement and fire officials, designate a staging area for additional ambulances, and establish a treatment area for casualties. Another crewmember from the first-arriving EMS unit should initiate triage, the sorting of casualties for treatment based on the severity of their injuries. The START (Simple Triage and Rapid Treatment) system is a simple method for quickly evaluating large numbers of casualties.

5.14. **C,** The femur is located in the thigh. The upper arm has a bone called the humerus; the lower leg is composed of the tibia and fibula; and the bones of the ankles are tarsals.

5.15. **B,** The head of the femur sits in an indentation in the pelvis called the acetabulum.

5.16. A, The facial bones include the mandible (lower jaw), maxilla (upper jaw), and zygomatic bone (cheekbone). The scapula is part of the shoulder; the occipital bone is part of the skull; and the manubrium is part of the sternum.

5.17. B, The occipital bone is located on the posterior side of the skull just above the cervical spine. The frontal bone forms the forehead. The temporal bones form the sides of the skull. The top of the skull is composed of the parietal bones.

5.18. C, Your principal concern is that the patient has a pneumothorax or hemothorax that could interfere with his ability to breathe or produce shock. The spleen and the apex of the heart are located on the left side of the chest, so injury to these structures is less likely. Although a rib fracture may be present, the injury to the rib is less significant than associated trauma to the pleura, lung, or blood vessels and nerves of the chest wall.

5.19. B, The patient appears to have hyperventilation syndrome. She is moving air well, so there is no problem maintaining the airway. Her warm, dry skin and strong pulse suggest that blood loss and shock are not present. An injury to the spinal cord that is high enough to affect sensation in the upper and lower extremities would paralyze the chest wall, interfering with breathing.

SCENARIO FOUR

Plan of Action

1. BSI

2. Is the scene safe? Yes. Assess mechanism of injury, number of patients, and need for additional resources.

3. Manually stabilize head and neck. Assess mental status. Ensure open airway, assess breathing, apply oxygen 10 to 15 lpm, and assess circulation.

4. Determine the priority and consider ALS.

5. Rapid trauma assessment

6. Baseline vital signs

7. SAMPLE

8. Splint ankle with pillow splint. Secure patient to long spine board with cervical immobilization device in place. Assess pulses, movement, and sensation before and after splinting.

9. En route, perform detailed assessment if time allows. Perform ongoing assessment.

Rationale

In this situation, evaluation of mechanism of injury is important. Although the patient is complaining only of foot and ankle pain, a significant mechanism of injury is present if he fell from more than three times his height. A rapid trauma examination should be performed to identify any other injuries that might be present. The patient should be secured to a long board with a cervical collar and cervical immobilization device in place.

5.20. C, The ankle is formed by the lateral malleolus and the medial malleolus. An example of a ball-and-socket joint is the hip joint. The carpals and metacarpals are located in the upper extremity.

5.21. C, The calcaneus is the heel bone.

SCENARIO FIVE

Plan of Action

1. BSI
2. Is the scene safe? Yes. Assess nature of illness, number of patients, and need for additional resources.
3. Assess mental status. Ensure open airway, assess breathing, apply oxygen, assist ventilations with bag-valve mask if needed, and assess circulation.
4. Determine priority and consider ALS.
5. History of present illness; SAMPLE
6. Focused physical examination
7. Baseline vital signs
8. Request ALS or provide bronchodilator therapy as permitted by local protocol.
9. Transport and perform ongoing assessment.

Rationale

This patient is in severe respiratory distress. She needs high concentration oxygen. If she becomes tired or has difficulty ventilating adequately, her breathing should be assisted with a bag-valve mask. An ALS unit should be requested to provide therapy with bronchodilators. If your protocols allow, you may assist her with using her own inhaler or provide bronchodilator therapy using a small volume nebulizer.

5.22. D, The intercostal muscles pull the ribs up and out during normal respiration. The sternocleidomastoid muscles of the neck and the pectoralis muscles of the upper chest are used to assist the intercostal muscles during respiratory distress. The trapezius muscle is located in the upper back.

5.23. D, Gas exchange with the blood takes place in the alveoli.

5.24. B, Cilia are microscopic, hairlike structures on the surface of the cells that line the respiratory tract. They beat in a wavelike fashion, moving a layer of mucus that traps foreign material toward the pharynx, where the mucus and entrapped foreign material are swallowed.

5.25. B, Oxygen moves from the alveoli into the pulmonary capillaries because the concentration of oxygen is lower in the capillaries than in the alveoli.

5.26. A, A 13-y.o. child would be expected to have a respiratory rate of 12 to 20 breaths per minute. Adolescents normally have respiratory rates that fall into the adult range.

5.27. A, An adult's normal respiratory rate is 12 to 20 breaths per minute.

5.28. C, The respiratory rate of an infant from birth to 5 months is 25 to 40 breaths per minute.

5.29. B, Tidal volume is the amount of air inhaled and exhaled with each breath. The air remaining in the large airways that is unavailable for gas exchange is the dead space air. The air remaining in the lungs after a complete exhalation is the residual volume.

5.30. C, Room air contains approximately 21% oxygen and 79% nitrogen.

SCENARIO SIX

Plan of Action
1. BSI
2. Is the scene safe? Yes. Assess mechanism of injury, number of patients, and need for additional resources.
3. Assess mental status. Ensure open airway, assess breathing, and assess circulation.
4. Determine priority.
5. Focused trauma assessment
6. Baseline vital signs
7. SAMPLE
8. Transport

Rationale
The mechanism of injury is not significant. The initial assessment reveals no immediate life threats. The physical examination can focus on the abrasions on the patient's right forearm. This patient probably does not require transport. However, if the abrasions contain significant amounts of foreign materials, the parents should be encouraged to take the patient to their physician or to the emergency department by private vehicle. Foreign material in an abrasion can lead to a significant infection. Additionally, dirt can become incorporated into the skin as the abrasion heals, leaving a permanent discoloration called a "traumatic tattoo."

5.31. A, Your principal concern with this patient's injury is the potential for infection. When skin is abraded, the protective barrier that keeps out bacteria is lost, and infection of the underlying tissues can occur. Blood loss is not normally a concern with abrasions because larger blood vessels are usually not damaged. Abrasions typically are not deep enough to cause nerve damage. This patient has no signs or symptoms that suggest the presence of a fracture; however, because children's bones are still flexible, the possible presence of a "greenstick" fracture should be considered.

5.32. C, Protection and temperature regulation are skin's major functions. The skeletal system supports the body against gravity. Fluid is absorbed through the digestive system. One of skin's functions is to prevent excess fluid loss from evaporation by providing the body with a watertight seal.

5.33. D, Skin, from the outermost layer to the innermost layer, comprises the epidermis, the dermis, and the subcutaneous layers.

5.34. B, Homeostasis is the human body's ability to maintain a stable internal environment.

5.35. A, The *cell* is the basic unit of life. Cells group together to make tissue; tissues group together to make up organs; organs group together to make organ systems; and the organ systems group together to form the organism.

5.36. D, The superior portion of the sternum is the manubrium. The ischium is part of the pelvis. The xiphoid forms the inferior tip of the sternum. The gladiolus or body is the middle part of the sternum.

5.37. B, When a person "breaks a hip" he or she actually has fractured the neck of the femur. The neck is the portion of the femur that connects the rounded head, which joins the pelvis, to the vertical shaft. The greater trochanter is an area on the superior portion of the femur's shaft that provides an attachment point for the muscles of the hip.

5.38. A, The ischium is part of the pelvis. The acetabulum is the socket in the pelvis into which the head of the femur inserts. It is a structure formed by the bones of the pelvis but is not itself a bone. The ileum is part of the small bowel. It should not be confused with the ilium, one of the bones of the pelvis, which forms the iliac crest. The sacrum is the portion of the spinal column that joins with the pelvis.

5.39. Cervical spine

5.40. Thoracic spine

5.41. Lumbar spine

5.42. Sacrum

5.43. Coccyx

5.44. Muscle tissue has the ability to contract when stimulated. There are three types of muscle tissue: skeletal, smooth, and cardiac.

5.45. Nervous tissue conducts electrical impulses throughout the body.

5.46. Epithelial tissue lines body surfaces, provides protection for the body, and has specialized functions such as absorption, secretion, diffusion, and filtration.

5.47. Connective tissue provides support, connection, and insulation for the body.

6

Moving and Lifting Patients

BODY MECHANICS

- Position your feet approximately a shoulder width apart
- Lift with your legs, *not* with your back
- Keep your back straight
- When lifting, never twist
- Keep the weight as close to your body as possible
- When possible, push; do *not* pull
- Do *not* push or pull objects above your head
- Do *not* lean or extend from the waist to retrieve heavy objects

EMERGENCY MOVES

One-Rescuer Drags

- Clothes drag—Grab patient's clothing at shoulders. Pull patient in the direction of the long axis of body. Do not try to pull sideways (Figure 6-1).

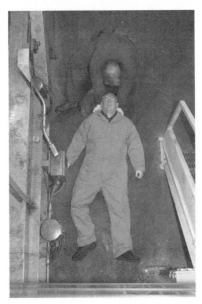

Figure 6-1   Clothing drag. (From Chapleau W: *Emergency first responder,* St Louis, 2004, Mosby.)

- Shoulder drag—Place your hands under the patient's armpits. Pull the patient along the long axis of body. Use caution not to injure head. Do not pull sideways (Figure 6-2).
- Firefighter's drag—Place the patient on his or her back. Tie the patient's wrists together. Straddle the patient. Place the patient's bound wrists over your head. Raise your body and crawl on your hands and knee, dragging the patient with you (Figure 6-3).
- Incline (bent-arm) drag—Squat behind the patient. Lift the patient to a semi-sitting position. Reach under the patient's armpits, and grab the patient's opposite wrist. Squeeze the patient's head and torso against your torso, and then stand up. Move the patient by walking backward (Figure 6-4).
- Foot drag—Position yourself at the patient's feet. Grip the patient's ankles and pull along the long axis of the body. Be careful not to bump the patient's head (Figure 6-5).

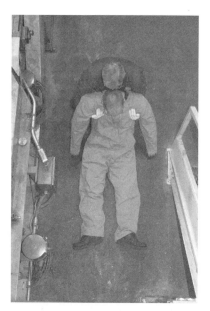

Figure 6-2   Shoulder (upper extremity) drag. (From Chapleau W: *Emergency first responder,* St Louis, 2004, Mosby.)

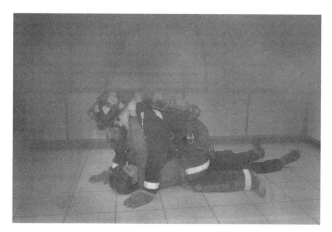

Figure 6-3   Firefighter's drag. (From Chapleau W: *Emergency first responder,* St Louis, 2004, Mosby.)

- Blanket drag—Place a rolled blanket alongside the patient. Gather half of the blanket up against the patient's side. Roll the patient toward your knees; place the blanket under the patient; and then gently roll the patient onto the blanket. Drag the patient by pulling the head end of blanket (Figure 6-6).

One-Rescuer Assists and Carries

- One-rescuer assist—Place the patient's arm around your neck, grasping the patient's hand in yours. Place your other arm around the patient's waist. Help the patient walk to safety (Figure 6-7).

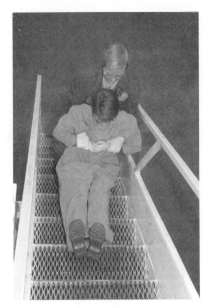

Figure 6-4 Incline drag. (From Chapleau W: *Emergency first responder,* St Louis, 2004, Mosby.)

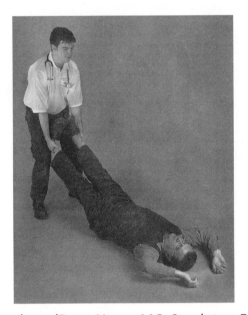

Figure 6-5 Foot drag. (From Henry MC, Stapleton ER: *EMT-prehospital care,* ed 3, St Louis, 2004, Mosby.)

- Cradle carry—Place one arm under the patient's back. Place your other arm under the patient's knees. Lift the patient, cradling him or her in your arms. This is appropriate only for very light patients (Figure 6-8).
- Pack-strap carry—Have the patient stand. Turn your back to the patient, bringing the patient's arms over your shoulders to cross your chest. Keep the patient's arms straight with his or her

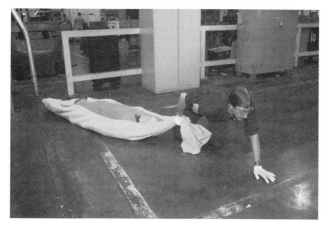

Figure 6-6   Blanket drag. (From Chapleau W: *Emergency first responder,* St Louis, 2004, Mosby.)

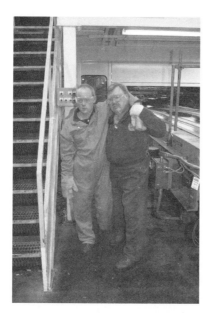

Figure 6-7   One-rescuer assist. (From Chapleau W: *Emergency first responder,* St Louis, 2004, Mosby.)

armpits over your shoulders. Hold the patient's wrists, bend, and pull the patient onto your back (Figure 6-9).

- Piggyback carry—Assist the patient to stand. Place the patient's arms over your shoulders so they cross your chest. Bend over and lift the patient. While the patient holds on, crouch and grab each leg. Use the lifting motion to move the patient onto your back. Pass your forearms under the patient's knees, and grasp the patient's wrists (Figure 6-10).
- Firefighter's carry—Place your feet against the patient's feet. Pull the patient toward you. Bend at the waist, and flex your knees. Pull the patient across your shoulders, keeping hold of one of the patient's wrists. Use your free arm to reach between the patient's legs, and grasp the thigh. Stand

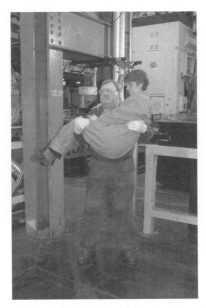

Figure 6-8   One-person cradle carry. (From Chapleau W: *Emergency first responder,* St Louis, 2004, Mosby.)

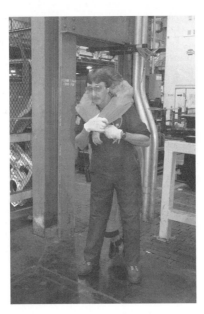

Figure 6-9   Pack-strap carry. (From Chapleau W: *Emergency first responder,* St Louis, 2004, Mosby.)

up supporting the patient's weight on your shoulders. Transfer your grip on the thigh to the patient's wrist (Figure 6-11).

Two-Rescuer Assists and Carries

- Two-rescuer assist—The patient's arms are placed around the shoulders of both rescuers. Each rescuer grips one of the patient's hands and places his or her free arm around the patient's waist (Figure 6-12).

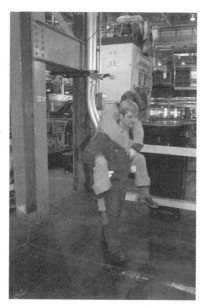

Figure 6-10   Piggyback carry. (From Chapleau W: *Emergency first responder,* St Louis, 2004, Mosby.)

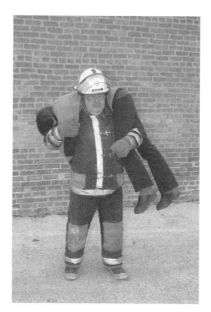

Figure 6-11   Firefighter's carry. (From Chapleau W: *Emergency first responder,* St Louis, 2004, Mosby.)

- Firefighter's carry with an assist—The second rescuer assists the first rescuer with positioning the patient (Figure 6-13).

NONURGENT MOVES (WITHOUT SUSPECTED SPINAL TRAUMA)

- Extremity carry—Place the patient on his or her back with knees flexed. EMT 1 kneels at the patient's head with his or her hands under the patient's shoulders. EMT 2 kneels at the patient's feet, grasps the patient's wrists, and pulls the patient to a sitting position. EMT 1 reaches under

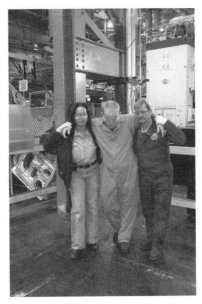

Figure 6-12 Two-rescuer assist. (From Chapleau W: *Emergency first responder,* St Louis, 2004, Mosby.)

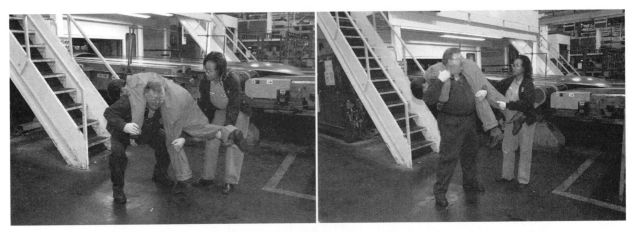

Figure 6-13 Firefighter carry with assist. The second provider assists the first provider to put the patient into position. (From Chapleau W: *Emergency first responder,* St Louis, 2004, Mosby.)

the patient's armpits and across the chest to grasp the patient's opposite wrist. EMT 2 then stands between the patient's legs and places his or her arms under the patient's knees. Rescuers stand to lift the patient (Figure 6-14).

- Draw sheet method—Loosen the bottom sheet of a bed and roll it from the sides toward the patient. Place the stretcher, rails lowered, parallel to and touching the side of the bed. Using their bodies to lock the stretcher against the side of the bed, EMTs pull on the sheet to move the patient onto the stretcher (Figure 6-15).

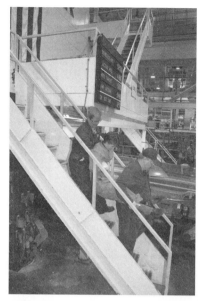

Figure 6-14 Extremity lift. (From *Mosby's 1st responder textbook*, St Louis, Mosby.)

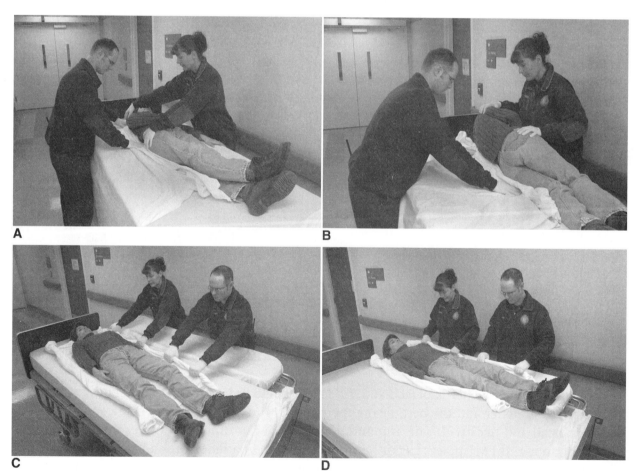

Figure 6-15 Draw sheet method. (From *Mosby's 1st responder textbook,* St Louis, Mosby.)

- Direct ground lift—The stretcher is set in the lowest position on the opposite side of the patient. The EMTs face the patient and drop to one knee. The head-end EMT cradles the patient's head and neck with one arm and places his or her other arm under the patient's back. The foot-end EMT slides one arm under the patient's knees and the other just above the buttocks. On signal, the EMTs lift the patient to his or her knees. On signal, the EMTs stand and carry the patient to the stretcher, drop to one knee, and roll forward to place the patient on the mattress (Figure 6-16).

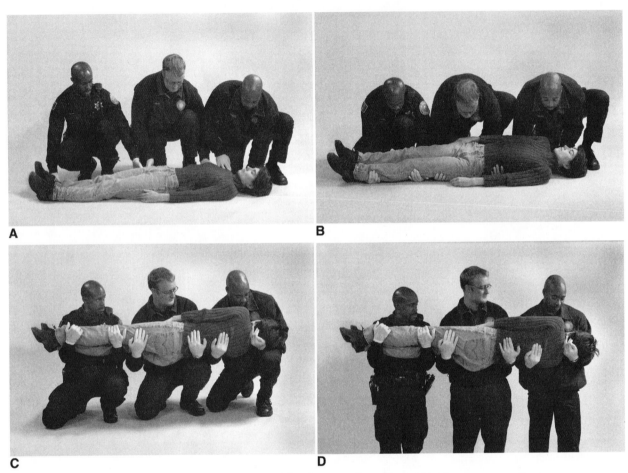

Figure 6-16   Direct ground lift. (From Chapleau W: *Emergency first responder*, St Louis, 2004, Mosby.)

- Direct carry—The stretcher is placed at a 90-degree angle to bed. Both EMTs stand between the stretcher and the bed, facing the patient. The head-end EMT cradles the patient's head and neck with one arm and places his or her other arm under the patient's back. The foot-end EMT places his or her arms under the patient's hips and calves. The EMTs lift and curl the patient to their chests and return to the standing position. They rotate and then slide the patient onto the stretcher (Figure 6-17).

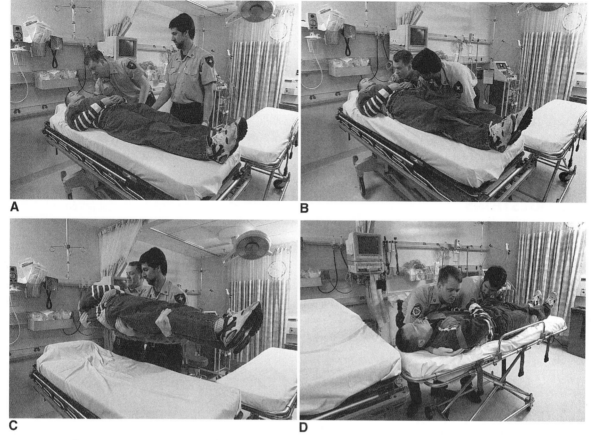

Figure 6-17   Direct carry. (From *Mosby's 1st responder textbook*, St Louis, Mosby.)

PATIENT-CARRYING DEVICES

- Wheeled ambulance stretcher—"Stretcher," "cot," or "gurney." It extends to the ground and folds for loading into the ambulance. It has small side rails, lightweight mattress, and wheels. There are lift-in (two-man) and roll-in (one-man) types.
- Portable ambulance stretcher—Does not have leg extensions or wheels. This stretcher must be carried by hand and is usually made of canvas, aluminum, coated fabric, or plastic. Some have a continuous metal frame, whereas others fold.
- Stair chair—Lightweight chair with an aluminum frame. It has wheels for rolling the chair on the ground. Some models have straps to secure the patient. Useful to move patients down stairs or through narrow or winding corridors. The patient must be able to sit upright.
- Scoop stretcher—Constructed of aluminum or lightweight steel. It splits apart at the head and feet for placement under the patient from the sides. The device is then locked together, so the patient is literally "scooped" up.
- Long spine board—Designed to immobilize the full length of a patient's body and is made of wood, plastic, or aluminum.
- Short spine board—Designed to ensure head, neck, and torso move as a unit. It is useful to extricate patients from a sitting position in vehicles and is made of wood, plastic, or aluminum.

- Vest-type extrication device—Designed to ensure head, neck, and torso move as a unit. It is useful to extricate patients from a sitting position in vehicles. The lower portion of the device wraps around the torso like a vest for greater limitation of movement than short spine boards.
- Basket stretcher or Stokes basket—Made of wire mesh with a metal frame or of plastic. It is designed to carry a patient long distances over rough terrain. The patient may be immobilized on a long spine board first and then secured in a basket stretcher.
- Flexible stretcher (Reeves stretcher)—Made of canvas or other flexible material, often with wooden slats sewn into pockets and three carrying handles on each side. It is useful in confined spaces and narrow hallways.

REVIEW QUESTIONS

Scenario One

Your patient is a 31-y.o. female who lives on the third floor of an apartment building that has no elevators. She has been experiencing nausea, vomiting, and diarrhea for 3 days. She is awake and alert. Her skin is cool and dry. Capillary refill is 3 seconds. Vital signs with the patient in a sitting position are pulse (P)—106, weak, regular; respiration (R)—14, shallow, regular; and blood pressure (BP)—106/88.

Your Plan of Action

Fill in the blank lines with your treatment plan for this patient. Then compare your plan with the questions, answers, and rationale.

1. _____
2. _____
3. _____
4. _____
5. _____
6. _____
7. _____
8. _____
9. _____

Multiple Choice

6.1. The *best* way to move this patient from her apartment to the ambulance would be:
- **a.** carrying her on a spine board.
- **b.** having her walk down the stairs.
- **c.** using a stair chair.
- **d.** using a scoop stretcher.

6.2. When you lift patients, you should *avoid* using your:
- **a.** abdominal muscles.
- **b.** lower back muscles.
- **c.** gluteal muscles.
- **d.** trapezius muscles.

6.3. Before lifting, your feet should be placed:
- **a.** with the ankles together.
- **b.** a shoulder width apart.
- **c.** with the right foot ahead of the left foot.
- **d.** flat on the floor 6 inches apart.

6.4. All of the following are correct procedures for moving a patient down stairs *except:*
- **a.** the patient should be moved feet first, facing down the stairs.
- **b.** keep your back straight and bend at your knees.
- **c.** use some personnel as "spotters" to direct the move and assist with navigation.
- **d.** use a minimum number of personnel to reduce the risk of tripping or falling.

Scenario Two

You have been called to a house fire. A patient has been found by firefighters unconscious in a bedroom near the back of the house. The structure is still on fire. A narrow hallway leads from the bedroom to the living room and outside.

Multiple Choice

6.5. The carry or device the firefighters would be *most likely* to use to move this patient is:
- **a.** a long spine board.
- **b.** a direct ground lift.
- **c.** the draw sheet method.
- **d.** the extremity carry.

6.6. All of the following are examples of emergency carries *except:*
- **a.** an extremity lift.
- **b.** a pack-strap carry.
- **c.** the power lift.
- **d.** a cradle carry.

Scenario Three

You have been dispatched to a report of a collapse at a construction site where one worker has been trapped. When you arrive, you discover the fire department and construction company personnel have been able to clear a 3- to 4-foot diameter tunnel to a void space where the patient is located. After you put on appropriate protective equipment, you crawl to the patient, who is a 38-y.o. male. The patient is awake and alert. He has abrasions and superficial lacerations on his face and upper extremities and complains of pain in his left thigh, which is swollen and deformed. He denies any head, neck, or back pain. His skin is pale, cool, and moist. Radial pulses are 124, weak, regular. Capillary refill is 4 seconds. The patient does not appear to be pinned in the debris, but he is unable to crawl because of pain in his left thigh.

Your Plan of Action

Fill in the blank lines with your treatment plan for this patient. Then compare your plan with the questions, answers, and rationale.

1. _____
2. _____
3. _____
4. _____
5. _____
6. _____
7. _____
8. _____
9. _____

Multiple Choice

6.7. After you describe the situation to the fire chief, a decision is made to extricate the patient through the access tunnel as quickly as possible. The simplest way to accomplish this would be with:

   a. an incline drag.
   b. a blanket drag or fireman's drag.
   c. a scoop stretcher.
   d. a foot drag.

6.8. Which of the following statements about the fireman's drag is *correct*?

   a. Grip the patient's ankles, pull by the long axis of the body, being careful not to bump his head.
   b. Move the patient feet-first to protect his head.
   c. Grip the patient under his armpits, and be careful to also cradle his head.
   d. Straddle the patient, and pass your head through his bound wrists; then raise your body, and crawl on your hands and knees.

6.9. If you used the foot drag, which of the following statements would be *correct*?

   a. Grip the patient's ankles, and be careful not to bump his head.
   b. Always move the patient head-first.
   c. Grip the patient under the armpits, and be careful to cradle and support the head.
   d. Straddle the patient, and pass your head through his bound wrists; then raise your body, and crawl on your hands and knees.

6.10. Which of the following statements about the incline drag is *correct*?

   a. Drag the patient by pulling on his ankles, being careful not to bump his head.
   b. Always move the patient head-first.
   c. Grip the patient around the waist, and move slowly.
   d. Straddle the patient, and pass your head through his bound wrists; then raise your body, and crawl up the incline on your hands and knees.

Scenario Four

A 16-y.o. male had been hiking in a national forest on a very hot summer day when he began to experience weakness, dizziness, and nausea. Because of the dizziness, he tripped, spraining his right ankle. Unable to walk, he sat on a rock by the side of the trail. Approximately 10 minutes later another hiker found him and went for help at a ranger station located approximately 3 miles away. You respond in your ambulance to a location on a roadway approximately 2 miles from the patient's location, meet a ranger and the rescue team, and hike approximately 2 miles to the patient. The patient is awake but does not know what day it is or what has happened to him. His skin is pale, cool, and dry. Radial pulses are weak and rapid. He does not appear to have been carrying a canteen with him. His right ankle is painful, swollen, and discolored. You call for an advanced life support (ALS) unit to meet you where your vehicle is parked and begin the task of extricating the patient from the woods.

Your Plan of Action

Fill in the blank lines with your treatment plan for this patient. Then compare your plan with the questions, answers, and rationale.

1. _____
2. _____
3. _____
4. _____
5. _____
6. _____
7. _____
8. _____
9. _____

Multiple Choice

6.11. The *best* way to move this patient through the woods over rough terrain would be the:
   a. scoop stretcher.
   b. cradle carry.
   c. Stokes basket.
   d. stair chair.

6.12. Which of these statements about the device you would use in Question 6.11 is *correct?*
   a. This device is usually made of wire mesh with a metal frame or a plastic material. The patient may be immobilized on a spine board first before being secured in the device.
   b. This device is also called an orthopedic stretcher and is commonly used at sporting events. It may also be used for patients with hip injuries.
   c. This device is extremely useful to move patients up and down stairs or through narrow areas that a stretcher may not move through easily.
   d. This device is commonly used, has different models, and can be adjusted to varying heights.

Scenario Five

You respond to a report of a small explosion in the chemistry lab at the high school. The fire department also is en route. On arrival you learn that four students are in the lab. Two appear to be unconscious but are breathing without difficulty. The other two are awake but are confused and unable to remove themselves from the lab.

> **Your Plan of Action**
>
> *Fill in the blank lines with your treatment plan for these patients. Then compare your plan with the questions, answers, and rationale.*
>
> 1. _____
> 2. _____
> 3. _____
> 4. _____
> 5. _____
> 6. _____
> 7. _____
> 8. _____
> 9. _____

Multiple Choice

6.13. After donning the proper rescue equipment, the firefighters remove the students. Which of the following methods would be the best under these circumstances?

    a. Give high-concentration oxygen to the students; then remove them with regular stretchers.

    b. Use either the blanket drag or the fireman's carry to remove the students from the lab; then give high-concentration oxygen.

    c. Give high-concentration oxygen to all four patients; perform a rapid trauma examination; and then remove them using the incline drag.

    d. Secure the patients to long spine boards because they may have been injured during the explosion; remove them from the lab, and then give high-concentration oxygen.

6.14. The *highest* priority in this case is to:

    a. immediately assess the ABCs.

    b. remove the patients from the dangerous environment.

    c. avoid worsening any injuries that may have been caused by the explosion.

    d. immediately notify the proper authorities because there are chemicals involved.

Scenario Six

You are relaxing at home when you see what looks like smoke from the neighbor's house. You know she is 81 y.o. and may not be able to get out on her own. You call the fire department and then rush over. The patient is in an upstairs bedroom. She is confused and disoriented but does not appear to have any injuries.

Multiple Choice

6.15. The patient weighs more than 200 pounds and cannot walk without her cane. The *best* way to get her downstairs would be to use the:
    a. blanket drag.
    b. pack-strap carry.
    c. one-rescuer assist.
    d. cradle carry.

6.16. An emergency move is used when:
    a. there are no spinal injuries.
    b. there is no one else available to help.
    c. the patient's condition may suddenly deteriorate.
    d. there is an immediate threat to the patient's life.

Scenario Seven

You are dispatched to "an unknown illness." On arrival you find a 62-y.o. male sitting on the roof of his house. You notice a ladder set against the side of the house. Because there appear to be no immediate hazards, you climb up to evaluate your patient. The patient tells you he was repairing some roof damage when he developed squeezing pain in the center of his chest, accompanied by nausea and weakness. He is diaphoretic, pale, and short of breath. His vital signs are P—132, strong, regular; R—24, shallow, regular; and BP—148/96. By this time the fire department's rescue truck has arrived. Unfortunately the aerial ladder truck is busy at a fire scene and is unavailable.

Your Plan of Action

Fill in the blank lines with your treatment plan for this patient. Then compare your plan with the questions, answers, and rationale.

1. _____
2. _____
3. _____
4. _____
5. _____
6. _____
7. _____
8. _____
9. _____

Multiple Choice

6.17. The *best* way to get the patient down would be to:
   a. have him climb down the ladder by himself.
   b. use the cradle carry to assist him down the ladder.
   c. place him in the Stokes basket, and lower it to the ground.
   d. immobilize him on a long spine board, and lower it to the ground.

6.18. All of the following statements about the power lift are correct *except:*
   a. it is used when the patient is extremely heavy.
   b. the back is kept straight and locked in position.
   c. the person lifting squats before lifting.
   d. the person lifting bends from the waist, not from the knees.

6.19. If you must choose between pushing and pulling, you should:
   a. push rather than pull the patient.
   b. keep the knees and elbows locked.
   c. try to keep the majority of the patient's weight below waist level.
   d. always pull the patient feet-first.

6.20. You have two patients from a motor vehicle collision (MVC). Both are immobilized on long spine boards. Only one ambulance is available. You should:
   a. put the more critically injured patient on the stretcher, and load him first.
   b. place the less critically injured patient on the stretcher, and load her second.
   c. load the less critically injured patient first, and place her on the bench seat.
   d. load the more critically injured patient first, and place him on the bench seat.

SCENARIO ONE

Plan of Action

1. Body Substance Isolation (BSI)

2. Is the scene safe? Yes. Assess nature of illness, number of patients, and need for additional resources.

3. Assess mental status, assess airway, assess breathing, apply oxygen 10-15 lpm by non-rebreather mask, and assess circulation.

4. Determine priority, consider ALS.

5. HPI, SAMPLE

6. Focused physical examination

7. Baseline vital signs

8. En route, do detailed physical examination if time permits, and perform ongoing assessment.

Rationale

The patient has flu symptoms and does not appear to be in distress. Vital signs suggest that she is mildly hypovolemic. She needs to be taken to the emergency department for fluid replacement and to stop any nausea, vomiting, or diarrhea. Because she is dehydrated, she probably should not walk because there is a possibility of a syncopal episode. The best way to move her to the ambulance would be to use a stair chair and carry her downstairs.

6.1. C, The best way to move the patient downstairs is to use the stair chair because it maneuvers well through narrow areas and around tight corners. The patient must be able to sit upright for the stair chair to be used.

6.2. B, Avoid using your lower back muscles. Keep your back straight, and lift with your legs. Back injuries are the most common work-related injury in EMS today.

6.3. B, When lifting from a squatting position, place your feet a shoulder width apart. This will help provide firm footing and a good base from which to lift.

6.4. D, Use as many people as you need to lift the patient. Trying to lift a large patient with too little help is more likely to cause someone to be injured than having too many people attempt to move the patient.

6.5. **D,** Because the patient needs to be moved away from danger down a long, narrow hallway, the extremity carry is the best option. One person takes hold of the patient under the shoulders, and the other places his or her hands and arms under the patient's legs.

6.6. **C,** The power lift is not an example of an emergency carry. The extremity lift, pack-strap carry, and cradle carry are emergency carries. When using the power lift, stand as close to the object as possible. Stand with your feet a shoulder width apart with the feet planted firmly on the floor. Keep the back straight and locked in. Lift with your arms locked—raising the upper body by extension of the back. Never bend at the waist!

SCENARIO THREE

Plan of Action
1. BSI
2. Is the scene safe? No. Remove the patient from the dangerous environment. Assess mechanism of injury, number of patients, and need for additional resources.
3. Assess mental status, assess airway, assess breathing, apply oxygen at 10-15 lpm, and assess circulation.
4. Determine priority, consider ALS.
5. Reconsider mechanism of injury, and consider spinal immobilization.
6. Rapid trauma examination
7. Baseline vital signs
8. En route, do a detailed physical examination if time permits, and perform ongoing assessment.

Rationale
The patient is in a potentially dangerous environment because of the risk of further structural collapse. He appears to have a fractured femur and is showing signs and symptoms of hypovolemic shock. The most important immediate consideration is to remove the patient from the place where he is trapped. Consider connecting with ALS for fluid replacement and pain medications.

6.7. **B,** Because the patient needs to be evacuated quickly through a narrow opening and does not appear to have any spinal injuries, you would use the blanket drag or fireman's drag. With the blanket drag, place the patient on the blanket with a log roll, positioning the blanket under the patient as you go. Drag the patient by grasping the top of the blanket. To perform the fireman's drag, tie the patient's wrists together with a cravat. Straddle the patient, and pass your head through the patient's bound wrists. Then raise your body to a crawl position, and crawl on your hands and knees, dragging the patient along as you go.

6.8. D, To perform a fireman's drag, tie the patient's wrists together with a cravat or whatever is accessible. Position yourself in a crawling position, straddling the patient. Pass the patient's bound wrists over your head. Raise your body, and crawl, bringing the patient with you as you crawl along.

6.9. A, To perform a foot drag, position yourself at the patient's feet. Grip the patient's ankles, and pull by the long axis of the body. Be careful not to bump the patient's head.

6.10. B, To perform an incline drag, your body should be in a standing position. Then grip the patient around the waist. The patient's head will be against your abdomen. Pull the patient head-first.

SCENARIO FOUR

Plan of Action

1. BSI

2. Is the scene safe? Yes. Assess mechanism of injury, nature of illness, number of patients, and need for additional resources.

3. Assess the mental status, assess airway, assess breathing, apply oxygen at 10-15 lpm, and assess circulation.

4. Determine priority, consider ALS.

5. Rapid trauma examination

6. Baseline vital signs

7. Extricate the patient from wooded area.

8. En route, do ongoing assessment.

Rationale

The patient appears to be dehydrated from hiking all day without water. The injured ankle should be splinted, but he probably does not need full spinal precautions because there is no neck or back pain and the mechanism of injury is unlikely to cause a spinal injury. The Stokes basket is the best way to carry him out of the woods over the rough terrain because it will allow multiple rescuers to move the patient and also will secure the patient more completely than other types of carrying devices.

6.11. C, The best way to carry the patient over rough terrain is with the Stokes basket. If necessary, the patient may be immobilized in the basket before transport with a cervical collar and spine board. Then at least six rescuers can grasp the handholds along the sides of the stretcher to carry the patient.

6.12. A, The basket stretcher or Stokes basket is made of wire mesh with a metal frame or of plastic polymer. It is designed to carry a patient long distances over rough terrain. The patient first may be immobilized on a long spine board. Then the patient is secured in the basket with straps.

SCENARIO FIVE

Plan of Action

1. BSI

2. Is the scene safe? No. Entry should be attempted only with proper personal protective equipment. Attempt to evaluate mechanism of injury, nature of illness, number of patients, and need for additional resources without entering danger area.

3. Extricate victims as soon as possible.

4. Assess mental status. Ensure open airway, assess breathing, apply oxygen at 10-15 lpm, and assess circulation.

5. Determine priority, consider ALS.

6. HPI, SAMPLE

7. Focused physical examination

8. Baseline vital signs

9. En route, do detailed physical examination if time permits, and perform ongoing assessment.

Rationale

The most important thing is to remove the victims from the dangerous environment. Put on protective equipment, and quickly open some windows; then staying as close to the floor as possible, remove the students. Care for the ABCs, and transport as quickly as possible because you do not know what chemicals were involved.

6.13. **B,** Because the air is full of vapors and the students are showing altered mental status, they need to be removed to a safe location as quickly as possible. Two are unconscious but do not appear to have injuries, and the other two are groggy. Use either the blanket drag, staying as close to the floor as possible, or the fireman's carry. The important thing is to get the patients to a safe area before beginning treatment.

6.14. **B,** These patients are in a hazardous environment. The highest priority must be given to moving them to a safe area before beginning treatment.

6.15. **C,** The patient is disoriented but appears to be uninjured and is able to walk. Using a one-rescuer assist will be the best way to help her outside while ensuring she does not fall on the way.

6.16. **D,** An emergency move is made when there is an immediate danger to the patient's life (e.g., fire, impending building collapse, potential for explosion).

SCENARIO SEVEN

Plan of Action

1. BSI

2. Is the scene safe? Yes, just do not fall off the roof! Assess nature of illness, number of patients, and need for additional resources.

3. Assess mental status. Ensure open airway, assess breathing, apply oxygen at 10-15 lpm, and assess circulation.

4. Determine priority, consider ALS.

5. HPI, SAMPLE

6. Focused physical examination

7. Baseline vital signs

8. Keep warm, reassure, and assist with or give nitroglycerin.

9. Remove from roof as soon as possible. En route to hospital, do ongoing assessment.

Rationale

This patient is most likely having an acute myocardial infarction. Allowing him to climb down the ladder would increase the workload on his heart. The safest way to move him is to ask the firefighters to secure the patient in a Stokes basket and lower him to the ground. ALS is definitely needed to monitor the patient's cardiac rhythm and for IV and drug therapy.

6.17. C, Because the patient is experiencing chest pain and dyspnea, he cannot climb down a ladder. It would place further stress on the heart. Place him in a Stokes basket, strap him in, and lower him to the ground as rapidly and safely as possible.

6.18. D, To use the power lift, the EMT squats before lifting. This way he or she lifts with the legs, not the back.

6.19. A, In a situation in which you may have a choice of whether to push or pull, it is easier to push than to pull a heavy object.

6.20. C, When you are transporting two patients in the same ambulance, the one on the bench seat is loaded first. Then the most critically injured patient (usually) is placed on the stretcher. It is easier to tend to the patient on the stretcher because you have access from both sides. In addition, the patient on the stretcher will be unloaded first at the hospital and the first patient the hospital receives for treatment.

7

Scene Size-Up, Initial Assessment, and SAMPLE

SCENE SIZE-UP

Assessment of the scene to determine presence of threats to responders, bystanders, or patients, the nature of the call, the number of patients, and the need for additional resources

- Safety
  - Dispatch information
  - Observations of scene
    - Unstable vehicles or structures
    - Downed electrical lines
    - Leaking gasoline
    - Traffic flow
    - Pedestrians, bystanders in or near roadway
    - Smoke, fire
    - Clues for presence of hazardous materials
    - Hostile persons
    - Signs of violence
  - Body substance isolation (BSI) procedures
- Danger zones
  - Motor vehicle crashes
    - No apparent hazards—Park unit 50 feet away from wreckage
    - Fuel spilled—Park unit at least 100 feet away from wreckage, upwind, uphill, or as far from flowing fuel as possible
    - Fire involved—Park unit at least 100 feet away from wreckage
    - Downed power lines—Park unit at least one full span of wires from pole with broken wires
  - Hazardous materials
    - Consult *North American Emergency Response Guidebook* or CHEMTREC for appropriate distances
    - If possibility of explosion, park at least 2000 feet away
    - Notify dispatch and other responding agencies
    - Do NOT approach scene unless properly trained
- Nature of call
  - Mechanism of injury (MOI)
    - Motor vehicle crashes—Head-on, rear-end, side-impact, rollover, and rotational impact
    - Penetrating vs. blunt trauma
  - Nature of illness
    - Patient
    - Family members or bystanders
    - Scene
- Number and location(s) of patients
- Need for additional or specialized resources
  - Additional ambulances
  - A supervisor
  - Fire suppression units
  - Extrication/rescue units
  - Law enforcement
  - Utility company units

THE INITIAL ASSESSMENT

Assessment to identify any immediately life-threatening problems. *Always* is *first* element in total assessment of patient. If life-threatening problems are found, correct them before proceeding with assessment.

- General impression—What seems to have happened? Medical, trauma, or both? How sick does the patient look?
  - Observations of scene
  - Patient's appearance—People who look sick, ARE sick!
  - Chief complaint—What the patient says the problem is
- Mental status—Use AVPU scale
  - Alert—Patient knows who he or she is, location or where he or she is, the date, and events that led up to the injury or illness. Alert and oriented × 4 = PPTE
  - Verbal stimulus—Patient's eyes do not open spontaneously but do open to verbal stimuli. May not be oriented to PPTE
  - Painful stimuli—Patient's eyes open spontaneously and patient responds by moving or crying out in response to painful stimuli such as the sternal rub or firmly pinching the patient's skin.
  - Unresponsive—Patient does not respond to painful stimuli such as the sternal rub or the pinch test.
- Airway
  - Is patient alert and talking clearly or crying, or is airway partially or completely obstructed?
  - Noisy breathing is obstructed breathing, but all obstructed breathing is not noisy! (For example, if the airway is completely obstructed or the patient is not breathing at all.)
  - Open airway using
    - Head-tilt chin-lift if no spinal injury suspected
    - Jaw thrust for patients with suspected spinal injuries
  - Clear airway with manual finger sweeps or suctioning
  - Maintain airway by inserting oropharyngeal or nasopharyngeal airway
- Breathing
  - Is patient breathing? Is patient moving air adequately? Is oxygen reaching the blood and the tissues?
  - Assess air movement at mouth and nose, chest rise, and skin color
  - If patient is in respiratory arrest, perform rescue breathing
  - Assist ventilations if the respiratory rate is:
    - less than 8 or greater than 24 breaths/min in adults
    - less than 15 or greater than 30 breaths/min in children
    - less than 25 or greater than 40 in infants
- Circulation
  - Is the patient's heart beating? Is blood circulating adequately? Is there any life-threatening external bleeding?
  - If patient unresponsive, check for a carotid pulse. If carotid pulse is absent, begin cardiopulmonary resuscitation (CPR)
  - Check peripheral pulses, skin color and temperature, and capillary refill
    - Radial pulse = systolic blood pressure (BP) > 80 mm Hg; femoral pulse = systolic BP > 70 mm Hg; carotid pulse = systolic BP > 60 mm Hg
    - Pale, cool, moist skin indicates poor circulation, possible shock.
    - Slow capillary refill (>2 seconds) indicates poor circulation, possible shock.
  - Check for and control severe external bleeding

- Determine priority, consider requesting advanced life support (ALS)
  - Immediate transport vs. further on-scene assessment and care
  - High-priority conditions
    - Poor general impression
    - Unresponsive
    - Responsive but unable to follow commands
    - Difficulty in breathing
    - Poor perfusion (shock)
    - Complicated childbirth
    - Uncontrolled bleeding
    - Severe pain in any area

VITAL SIGNS

Outward indicators of the adequacy of a patient's cardiopulmonary function and metabolism. Taken after initial assessment is performed and any life-threatening problems are corrected

- Pulse—Indicates adequacy of heart's pumping action
  - Count number of beats for 30 seconds and multiply by 2
  - Note and report rhythm, strength, and rate
  - Normal ranges
    - Adults and adolescents—60 to 100 beats/min
    - School-aged children—70 to 110 beats/min
    - Preschoolers—80 to 120 beats/min
    - Toddlers—80 to 130 beats/min
    - Infants aged 6 to 12 months—80 to 140 beats/min
    - Infants aged 0 to 6 months—90 to 140 beats/min
    - Newborns—120 to 160 beats/min
- Respirations—Indicates adequacy of breathing
  - Count number of breaths for 30 seconds and multiply by 2
  - Note and report rhythm, quality, and rate
  - Note presence of abnormal sounds (stridor, wheezes, rhonchi, and crackles)
  - Normal ranges
    - Adults and adolescents—12 to 24 breaths/min
    - School-aged children—15 to 30 breaths/min
    - Preschoolers and toddlers—20 to 30 breaths/min
    - Infants aged 6 to 12 months—20 to 30 breaths/min
    - Infants aged 0 to 6 months—25 to 40 breaths/min
    - Newborns—30 to 50 breaths/min
- Skin color, temperature, and moisture—Indicate adequacy of circulation
  - Check color at lips, nail beds, and inside lower eyelids and cheek
  - Check temperature using back of hand. Compare temperature of trunk to extremities
  - Skin color, temperature may be affected by environmental temperatures.
  - Skin color significance
    - Pink—Normal in light-skinned patients, or lips, nail beds, and mucosa of dark-skinned patients
    - Pale—Constricted blood vessels from blood loss, emotional distress, hypotension, or shock
    - Cyanotic (blue-gray)—Inadequate oxygenation of blood

- Flushed (red)—Exposure to heat, fever, or allergic reaction
- Jaundiced (yellow)—Liver disease
- Mottling (blotchiness)—Poor perfusion
  - ○ Skin temperature, moisture significance
    - Cool, moist (clammy)—Shock, anxiety
    - Cold, dry—Exposure to cold
    - Hot, dry—High fever, heat exposure
    - Hot, moist—High fever, heat exposure
- Capillary refill—Indicates adequacy of circulation. Most reliable in infants and children aged less than 6 years
  - ○ Press on nail bed, top of hand, or top of foot. Observe time for normal color to return
  - ○ Normal is less than 2 seconds.
  - ○ Prolonged capillary refill indicates poor circulation or exposure to cold temperatures.
- Pupils—Indicate adequacy of brain oxygenation and function
  - ○ Check size, equality, and reactivity to light
  - ○ Pupil signs significance
    - Dilated—Fright, blood loss, or drug effects
    - Constricted—Narcotics, glaucoma medications; or some strokes
    - Unequal—Stroke, head injury, eye injury, artificial eye, or use of medications in one eye
    - Lack of reactivity—Drugs, lack of oxygen to brain, head injury, or stroke
- BP—Indicates adequacy of circulation by measuring pressure of blood against walls of arteries
  - ○ Components
    - Systolic—Pressure generated when ventricles contract
    - Diastolic—Pressure generated when ventricles relax
  - ○ Methods for obtaining
    - Auscultation—Requires use of stethoscope and sphygmomanometer. Provides systolic and diastolic pressures
    - Palpation—Requires use of sphygmomanometer only. Provides only systolic pressure
  - ○ Normal ranges
    - Adults—Systolic—90 to 150; diastolic—60 to 90
    - Infants and children—Systolic—80 + (2 × age in years); diastolic—2/3 × systolic

SAMPLE HISTORY

Basic information about the patient's present problem and past history needed to begin care in the field and continue it at the hospital

- Signs and symptoms—What is wrong?
  - ○ Signs—Objective information. Something you can see, hear, feel, or smell
  - ○ Symptom—Subjective information. Something the patient tells you
- Allergies—Do you have any allergies?
- Medications—What medications are you currently taking (prescription, over-the-counter, recreational)?
- Pertinent past history—Have you been having any medical problems? Have you recently had any surgery or injury? Have you been seeing a doctor? What is your doctor's name?
- Last oral intake—When did you last eat or drink? What did you last eat or drink?
- Events leading to the injury or illness—What sequence of events led up to today's problem?

REVIEW QUESTIONS
Scenario One

You have been dispatched to a stabbing at a medium security prison. The patient is a 28-y.o. male with a small wound to the upper left chest. He is conscious but is not oriented to place or time. Bleeding has been partially controlled, but blood still is seeping through the dressings. The patient has no significant past medical history, is not taking any medications, and has no known allergies. Vital signs are BP—106/66; pulse (P)—116, weak, regular; respiration (R)—24, regular, nonlabored; SaO_2—95%.

Your Plan of Action

Fill in the blank lines with your treatment plan for this patient. Then compare your plan with the questions, answers, and rationale.

1. _____
2. _____
3. _____
4. _____
5. _____
6. _____
7. _____
8. _____
9. _____

Multiple Choice

7.1. What should your *first* action be when you arrive at the scene of this call?
   a. Ensure that the patient's airway is open.
   b. Make sure the scene is safe.
   c. Obtain a report from the nurse at the facility.
   d. Call for an ALS ambulance.

7.2. The *most important* action after arriving on a scene is to:
   a. do a focused history and physical examination.
   b. assess the patient's airway, breathing, and circulation.
   c. ensure the safety of your crew, the patient, and any bystanders.
   d. determine if the patient is responsive or unresponsive.

7.3. Removing the patient's clothing while you do the rapid trauma assessment may:
   a. make assessment of the ABCs easier to perform.
   b. worsen shock by increasing loss of body heat.
   c. allow hidden life-threatening injuries to be identified.
   d. delay life-saving treatment.

7.4. If a life-threatening problem is discovered during the *initial* assessment, you would:

    a. immediately apply a cervical collar and spine board.

    b. correct the problem as you advance through the detailed physical examination.

    c. treat the problem immediately.

    d. reassess airway, breathing, and circulation.

7.5. Which of this patient's organ systems are you *most* concerned about?

    a. Neurologic system

    b. Cardiovascular system

    c. Muscular system

    d. Respiratory system

7.6. The *most important* sign to monitor with this patient is the:

    a. pulse rate.

    b. mental status.

    c. respiratory rate.

    d. amount of bleeding from the wound.

7.7. The *initial* assessment would include evaluation of:

    a. mental status, airway, breathing, and circulation.

    b. mental status, respiratory rate, heart rate, and BP.

    c. mental status, airway, breathing, and initiation of spinal precautions.

    d. mental status, airway, circulation, and initiation of spinal precautions.

7.8. Which of the following pieces of information would be *most* helpful to evaluate this patient's MOI?

    a. Patient's past medical history

    b. Whether the patient is taking any medications

    c. Whether the patient fell

    d. The length of the knife or object involved

7.9. A scene size-up is done to:

    a. determine where to safely park your vehicle.

    b. identify BSI and other protective equipment needed for the call.

    c. obtain information useful to ensure safety or manage the call.

    d. determine quickly what is wrong with the patient.

Scenario Two

You have just cleared from the previous call when you are dispatched to a "train derailment with possible injuries." The fire department and additional ambulances are en route. When you arrive, you find approximately eight railcars overturned and piled like logs. When you step out of the ambulance, you smell a peculiar odor.

Your Plan of Action

Fill in the blank lines with your treatment plan for this patient. Then compare your plan with the questions, answers, and rationale.

1. _____

2. _____

3. _____

4. _____

5. _____

6. _____

7. _____

8. _____

9. _____

Multiple Choice

7.10. Your *first* action should be to:
   a. assess the scene to determine the number of patients.
   b. move to a safe location, and inform the dispatcher of a hazardous materials release.
   c. put on a helmet, turnout coat, and SCBA, and assess the scene.
   d. begin triage of any patients in the immediate area.

7.11. Which of the following statements about where to park is *most* correct?
   a. Upwind and uphill from the spill
   b. Downwind and uphill from the spill
   c. Upwind and downhill from the spill
   d. Downwind and downhill from the spill

7.12. Steps to identify the spilled material should include all of the following *except:*
   a. using binoculars to look for placards on the railcars.
   b. contacting the railroad dispatcher.
   c. interviewing any train crew who have left the danger area.
   d. attempting to locate the shipping papers.

7.13. The fire chief has established an on-scene incident management system (IMS). Under IMS, EMS personnel are *most* likely to be responsible to the:
   a. finance-administration chief.
   b. logistics chief.
   c. operations chief.
   d. plans chief.

7.14. You have requested additional ambulances. Unless directed otherwise, these ambulances should respond to the:
   a. command post.
   b. staging area.
   c. treatment area.
   d. transport area.

Scenario Three

You have received a call for a "possible shooting." As you pull up to the scene you see a young male lying on the ground with another person bending over him. The area is poorly lit, so it is difficult to see exactly what is happening.

Multiple Choice

7.15. Your *most appropriate* action at this time would be to:
   a. immediately go to the patient, and perform an initial assessment.
   b. call for backup because you may have two patients.
   c. pull back and wait for the police because you do not know where the assailant is.
   d. advise dispatch you are on the scene and may need an ALS unit.

Scenario Three—cont'd

The police have arrived and secured the scene. The patient is a 28-y.o. male with a gunshot wound to the LLQ. He responds to verbal stimuli and is oriented to person and place. His skin is pale, cool, and moist. He complains of thirst. Vital signs are BP—96/58; P—128, weak, regular; and R—28, labored, regular.

Your Plan of Action

Fill in the blank lines with your treatment plan for this patient. Then compare your plan with the questions, answers, and rationale.

1. _____
2. _____
3. _____
4. _____
5. _____
6. _____
7. _____
8. _____
9. _____

Multiple Choice

7.16. Which of the following pieces of information would be *most* useful to evaluate the MOI?
   a. How long ago the shooting took place
   b. How many assailants were involved
   c. When the patient last ate
   d. What type of gun was used

7.17. A rapid trauma assessment should be performed on what type of patient?
   a. All trauma patients
   b. Any trauma patient with significant MOI
   c. Any patient who requires spinal precautions
   d. All unresponsive patients

7.18. Which of the following patients has *early* signs of shock?
   a. A 28-y.o. male with a gunshot wound. BP—104/86; P—128, weak, regular; and R—28, regular, labored. Skin—cool, pale, and moist.
   b. A 59-y.o. male c/o chest pain. BP—100/68; P—90, weak, regular; and R—20, regular, labored. Skin—warm, moist.
   c. A 6-y.o. male who crashed his bicycle into a parked car. BP—92/56; P—116, strong, regular; and R—24, deep, regular, and unlabored. Skin—cool, dry.
   d. A 70-y.o. female c/o dysuria. BP—96/50; P—78, weak, regular; and R—10, regular, unlabored. Skin—hot, dry.

7.19. Which of the following pieces of information about the patient in Scenario Three is a symptom?
   a. He is complaining of thirst.
   b. His blood pressure is 96/58.
   c. His skin is cool and moist.
   d. His respirations are 28 and labored.

7.20. How often should you assess this patient's vital signs en route to the hospital?
   a. Every 5 minutes
   b. Every 10 minutes
   c. Every 15 minutes
   d. Whenever you note a change in the patient's mental status

7.21. The "P" on the AVPU scale stands for:
   a. amount of pain the patient feels when assessing the injury.
   b. provoking factors that led up to the injury.
   c. painful sensation felt when assessing the neurologic status.
   d. painful stimuli arouse the patient.

Scenario Four

You have been called for a "fall" at a construction site. You find three patients who fell about 25 feet when the scaffold they were working on collapsed.

- Patient #1 is a 20-y.o. male who landed on his feet and then fell forward to the ground. He is c/o right lower leg pain. Vital signs are BP—118/78; P—98, strong, regular; and R—20, nonlabored, regular. He is alert and oriented to PPTE.
- Patient #2 is a 28-y.o. male c/o left wrist pain. He says he reached out to stop the fall. Vital signs are BP—136/94; P—82, strong, regular; and R—22, nonlabored, regular. He is alert and oriented to PPTE.
- Patient #3 is a 34-y.o. male who is c/o lower back pain. He says he thinks he landed on his feet but is not sure. Vital signs are BP—150/88; P—92, strong, regular; and R—20, regular, nonlabored. He is alert and oriented to PPT.

Your Plan of Action

Fill in the blank lines with your treatment plan for this patient. Then compare your plan with the questions, answers, and rationale.

1. _____
2. _____
3. _____
4. _____
5. _____
6. _____
7. _____
8. _____
9. _____

Multiple Choice

7.22. The fall described in this scenario would be a:
   a. insignificant MOI.
   b. traumatic but non–life-threatening MOI.
   c. significant MOI.
   d. moderate MOI.

7.23. Patient #3 has back pain after landing on his feet. The mechanism of his back injury is:
   a. direct force.
   b. indirect force.
   c. indeterminate force.
   d. twisting force.

7.24. Spinal precautions for these patients should be initiated:
   a. before starting the detailed physical examination.
   b. while assessing the mental status and ABCs.
   c. after the scene size-up is completed.
   d. after the initial assessment is done.

7.25. The "D" in DCAP-BTLS means:
   a. disability.
   b. distance of the fall.
   c. deformities.
   d. dilatation of the pupils.

7.26. The "C" in DCAP-BTLS stands for:
   a. contusions.
   b. circulation.
   c. correct life-threatening problems.
   d. chest injuries.

7.27. Patient #2 is c/o wrist pain. He remembers hitting his wrist against something when he reached out to stop his fall. This is an example of what MOI?
  a. Direct force
  b. Indirect force
  c. Indeterminate force
  d. Twisting force

7.28. You are performing a rapid trauma survey on Patient #1. The *next* step after examining the neck would be to:
  a. assess the chest, listen to breath sounds, and apply oxygen.
  b. assess the clavicles, scapula, and arms.
  c. apply a cervical collar.
  d. apply oxygen and continue on with the trauma survey.

7.29. For these patients, the *next* step after the initial assessment would be to:
  a. obtain and assess the baseline vital signs.
  b. perform a rapid trauma assessment.
  c. perform a detailed trauma assessment.
  d. perform a focused trauma history and physical examination.

Scenario Five

You have been called to restaurant for a customer who is complaining of chest pain. The patient is a 68-y.o. male who developed midsternal chest pain approximately 5 minutes ago. He says he has never had pain like this before. The patient has a history of a transient ischemic attack (TIA) 5 years ago and colon cancer 8 years ago. He takes no medications at this time and has no known drug allergies.

Your Plan of Action

Fill in the blank lines with your treatment plan for this patient. Then compare your plan with the questions, answers, and rationale.

1. _____
2. _____
3. _____
4. _____
5. _____
6. _____
7. _____
8. _____
9. _____

Multiple Choice

7.30. Your *first* step to assess this patient would be to:
   - **a.** ask him what the pain feels like.
   - **b.** form an initial impression.
   - **c.** perform an initial assessment.
   - **d.** apply oxygen to the patient at 10 lpm.

7.31. While you ask the patient about his chest pain, you review the OPQRST mnemonic. The "R" reminds you to ask:
   - **a.** how he would rate the pain on a scale of 1 to 10.
   - **b.** in what region is the pain located.
   - **c.** if the pain radiates to any other part of his body.
   - **d.** if rest makes it better.

Scenario Five—cont'd

The vital signs are BP—188/110; P—110, strong, irregular; and R—24, regular, slightly labored. The patient's skin is warm, dry, and pink.

7.32. Which of the following would be the *best* location to check this patient's pulse?
   - **a.** Brachial
   - **b.** Radial
   - **c.** Carotid
   - **d.** Femoral

7.33. A normal pulse rate for an adult is:
   - **a.** 40 to 60 beats/min.
   - **b.** 50 to 60 beats/min.
   - **c.** 60 to 100 beats/min.
   - **d.** 100 to 180 beats/min.

7.34. Why is this patient's irregular pulse significant?
   - **a.** He is hypertensive.
   - **b.** He is anxious.
   - **c.** He is in the early stages of shock.
   - **d.** His heart is not maintaining a steady rhythm.

7.35. When you evaluate the quality of a patient's pulse, you ask yourself:
   - **a.** Is it regular or irregular?
   - **b.** Is the rate within the normal range?
   - **c.** Is it weak or strong?
   - **d.** Is it present or absent?

7.36. This patient's skin color and temperature would help provide information about his:
   - **a.** perfusion.
   - **b.** capillary refill status.
   - **c.** heart rate.
   - **d.** BP.

7.37. The systolic pressure is the pressure against the walls of the arteries when the:
   - **a.** atria relax.
   - **b.** atria contract.
   - **c.** ventricles relax.
   - **d.** ventricles contract.

7.38. The diastolic pressure is the pressure against the walls of the arteries when the:
    a. atria contract.
    b. atria relax.
    c. ventricles contract.
    d. ventricles relax.

7.39. The patient's heart rate of 110 would be described as:
    a. tachycardia.
    b. bradycardia.
    c. normocardia.
    d. dyscardia.

Scenario Six

A 46-y.o. female was at a shopping mall when she experienced an episode of weakness and dizziness leading to a fall. When you arrive the patient is conscious, alert, and oriented to person, place, time, and events. She says she still feels weak, but the dizziness is gone. She is not experiencing any pain associated with the fall. She has a past history of diabetes mellitus controlled by diet and of leukemia that has been in remission for 3 years. She takes no medications but is allergic to sulfa drugs. Vital signs are BP—102/56; P—96, weak, regular; R—20, regular, nonlabored; and SaO_2—98%.

Your Plan of Action

Fill in the blank lines with your treatment plan for this patient. Then compare your plan with the questions, answers, and rationale.

1. _____
2. _____
3. _____
4. _____
5. _____
6. _____
7. _____
8. _____
9. _____

Multiple Choice

7.40. After completing your *initial* assessment of this patient, you would perform a:
    a. detailed physical examination.
    b. focused history and physical examination.
    c. SAMPLE history.
    d. rapid physical examination.

7.41. The SAMPLE history for this patient would include all of the following information *except* the fact that she:
  a. has diabetes that is diet controlled.
  b. is alert and oriented.
  c. had leukemia several years ago.
  d. is not on any medications and has no allergies.

7.42. On which of the following body systems would you focus your assessment?
  a. The respiratory system because she is dizzy and weak
  b. The gastrointestinal system because she probably has not eaten recently
  c. The cardiovascular system because she is dizzy and weak
  d. The neurologic system because she is dizzy and weak

7.43. The "S" in SAMPLE refers to:
  a. specific chief complaint.
  b. significant past medical history.
  c. signs and symptoms of the current problem.
  d. scene size-up.

7.44. The "A" in SAMPLE refers to:
  a. abdominal quadrants.
  b. alertness.
  c. airway.
  d. allergies.

7.45. The "M" in SAMPLE refers to:
  a. musculoskeletal system.
  b. MOI.
  c. medications.
  d. mental status.

7.46. The "P" in SAMPLE refers to:
  a. pertinent past medical history.
  b. pain status.
  c. provoking factors.
  d. pulse rate and quality.

7.47. The "L" in SAMPLE refers to:
  a. lacerations.
  b. list of medications the patient takes.
  c. last oral intake.
  d. lung sounds.

7.48. The "E" in SAMPLE refers to:
  a. EMS available—your time of arrival on the scene.
  b. events leading up to the injury or illness.
  c. expose as needed.
  d. examination—perform the head-to-toe detailed examination.

Answer Key—Chapter 7

SCENARIO ONE

Plan of Action

1. Body Substance Isolation (BSI)

2. Is the scene safe? Yes. Assess MOI, number of patients, and need for additional resources.

3. Assess mental status. Ensure open airway, assess breathing, cover chest wound with occlusive dressing, give oxygen at 10-15 lpm by non-rebreather mask, and assess circulatory status.

4. Determine priority, consider requesting ALS.

5. Perform rapid trauma assessment (significant MOI—penetrating chest trauma).

6. Baseline vital signs

7. SAMPLE history

8. Transport

9. Perform detailed physical examination en route if time permits, and provide ongoing assessment.

Rationale

The patient has been stabbed in the chest. Without an x-ray, there is no way to know just how deep the wound is. He is not having respiratory distress at this time, but he needs to be carefully observed for a pneumothorax or hemothorax. Cover the wound with an occlusive dressing. Control any external bleeding. Monitor the vital signs for signs of internal bleeding. A rapid head-to-toe assessment is indicated because of the significant MOI (penetrating trauma to the thorax). The wound track possibly could extend through the diaphragm into the abdominal cavity. Also, the patient may have other stab wounds.

7.1. **B,** Before entering any scene, you should check for hazards to you and your partner. Scene safety comes before airway, obtaining a report from the nurse, or calling for an ALS assist.

7.2. **B,** Because the patient is awake and oriented to person, place, and time, you should perform an initial assessment by checking airway, breathing, and circulation. You already made sure the scene was safe, and the focused examination comes later.

7.3. **C,** Removing the patient's clothing during the rapid trauma assessment increases your chances of identifying hidden life-threatening injuries. The ABCs should already have been checked during the initial assessment before you begin the rapid trauma survey. Although removing the patient's clothing can increase loss of body heat and worsen shock, he should be covered with a blanket when you finish the rapid trauma assessment. He will not be undressed long enough to become hypothermic. Because treatment can be performed at the same time the patient is being undressed, life-saving care will not be delayed.

7.4. **C,** If a life-threatening problem is discovered during the initial assessment, it should be corrected immediately. During the initial assessment, movement of the head and neck can be limited by manual stabilization. A cervical collar and spine board are not needed yet, and attempting to apply them would delay treatment of the life-threatening problem. The detailed physical examination is performed en route to the hospital after life-threatening problems have been corrected. Reassessment of the ABCs would be performed after you have corrected the life-threatening problem.

7.5. **D,** Because of the location of the wound you should be most concerned about the respiratory system. The patient may have a pneumothorax or hemothorax. The vital signs and physical examination findings do not indicate any problems with perfusion or cardiovascular function. The location of the wound makes significant neurologic injuries unlikely. Although the stab wound may have damaged muscle tissue, this problem is less potentially life threatening than a respiratory system injury.

7.6. **C,** Because you suspect an injury that involves the respiratory system, the patient's respiratory rate and effort would be the best indicator of a worsening problem. Pulse rate and quality would be more closely related to cardiovascular function and quality of perfusion. Mental status could suggest a change either in respiratory function or cardiovascular function. The amount of external bleeding at this patient's wound site is the least significant of the possible internal injuries.

7.7. **A,** The *initial assessment* includes developing a general impression; assessing mental status, airway, breathing, and circulation; and determining the patient's priority for immediate transport. Answer "A" is the correct choice because it contains the greatest number of these steps.

7.8. **D,** Of the options provided, the length of the knife would be most helpful to evaluate the MOI in a stab wound. Blade length can be useful to estimate the depth of the wound. However, it is important to remember that soft tissues can compress along the object with which the patient was stabbed. Therefore, the wound may be significantly longer than the blade.

7.9. **C,** A scene size-up is done to obtain information useful to ensure safety and manage the call. Information to assist with safely parking the vehicle and selecting protective equipment may be obtained during the scene size-up. However, the size-up should also provide additional information useful to call management, such as number and location of patients or MOI. Attempting to determine what is wrong with the patient is not part of the scene size-up.

SCENARIO TWO

Plan of Action

1. BSI

2. This scene is not safe.

3. Move to a position upwind and uphill of the chemical release. Take all steps necessary to avoid exposure to or contamination by the chemical.

4. Establish EMS command, request additional units, and coordinate your activities with those of initial fire department and law enforcement commanders.

5. Work with the fire department to identify the spilled material(s); designate hot, warm, and cold zones; and establish facilities for patient and rescuer decontamination, triage, treatment, and transport.

6. Patients self-extricating from the incident who make their way to the cold zone may be treated, but steps should be taken first to ensure they do not contaminate personnel or equipment.

Rationale

The type of incident and presence of unusual odors suggest that a hazardous material release has occurred. Highest priority must be given to avoid exposure or contamination of responding personnel and their equipment. EMS, fire, and law enforcement personnel must establish an IMS to coordinate their activities. Personnel entering the scene to control the chemical release or rescue patients must wear protective equipment appropriate for the chemical involved. Patients brought out of the hot zone must be appropriately decontaminated to avoid spread of the spilled chemical off the scene.

7.10. **B,** The type of incident and the presence of a peculiar odor suggest the release of a hazardous material. Attempting to determine the number of patients or beginning triage could be hazardous until the spilled material can be identified. Standard protective equipment used for firefighting or rescue operations is not adequate for many hazardous materials. Return to your vehicle, advise the dispatcher of the nature of the incident, establish command, and begin attempts to safely identify the spilled material(s) using the *Emergency Response Guidebook*.

7.11. **A,** You should park the vehicle uphill and upwind from the spill. Take as many precautions as possible to keep the ambulance or rescue vehicle from becoming contaminated.

7.12. **D,** Although the shipping papers would provide exact information on the product or products involved in the spill, attempting to enter the danger area at this time is not advisable. Placards on the railcars may provide enough information to make initial decisions about managing the incident. The railroad dispatcher can provide information about the materials the train was carrying. Members of the train crew also can provide information about the products they are transporting and may have taken the shipping papers with them when they left the train.

7.13. C, In the IMS, the operations chief is responsible for determining and executing the tactics needed to meet the incident commander's strategic objectives for managing an emergency. Because care of the injured and medical support of the hazardous material team are operational issues, the officer in charge of EMS will report to and receive direction from the operations chief.

7.14. B, Unless directed otherwise, all additional resources should report to the staging area and remain there until given specific assignments.

7.15. C, Pull back and wait for the police to arrive. If the person bending over the victim is the assailant, you could be the next victim.

SCENARIO THREE

Plan of Action

1. BSI
2. The scene is not safe. Do not approach until the police have secured the scene.
3. Assess mental status. Ensure open airway, assess breathing, give oxygen at 10-15 lpm by non-rebreather mask, consider assisted breathing, assess circulatory status, control any external bleeding, and position patient on back with lower extremities elevated 12 inches.
4. Determine priority, consider requesting ALS.
5. Transport
6. Perform rapid trauma assessment en route (significant MOI—penetrating abdominal trauma).
7. Baseline vital signs
8. SAMPLE history
9. Perform detailed physical examination en route if time allows; provide ongoing assessment.

Rationale

Until the police secure the scene, approaching the patient would be unsafe. This patient has penetrating trauma to the abdomen from a gunshot wound. His signs and symptoms suggest he has hypovolemic shock. The only definitive treatment for his problem is surgery to stop the internal bleeding. After you apply oxygen, control external bleeding, and begin treatment for shock, the patient should be transported. An ALS unit could be met en route, but there should be as few delays as possible moving this patient toward the operating room. The head-to-toe rapid trauma assessment, baseline vital signs, and SAMPLE history can be obtained en route.

7.16. D, Because the MOI is a shooting, the most useful information would be what type of gun was involved.

7.17. B, A rapid trauma assessment is performed on any patient with a significant MOI.

7.18. A, This patient has rapid, weak pulses; rapid breathing; and cool, most skin—most characteristic of shock.

7.19. A, A symptom is something the patient tells you. Signs are things you can see, feel, or hear.

7.20. A, A critically injured patient's vital signs should be assessed at least every 5 minutes en route to the hospital.

7.21. D, A "P" on the AVPU scale indicates the patient will respond to painful stimuli.

SCENARIO FOUR

Plan of Action

1. BSI

2. Is the scene safe? Yes. Consider MOI, number of patients, and need for additional resources. Request additional units.

3. Initial spinal precautions with manual stabilization. Assess mental status. Ensure open airway, evaluate breathing, apply oxygen 10-15 lpm by non-rebreather mask, and assess circulatory status for each patient.

4. Determine priority, consider ALS.

5. Rapid trauma examination on each patient (significant mechanism—fall greater than 20 feet)

6. Baseline vital signs

7. SAMPLE

8. Cervical collar, spine board, and cervical immobilizer (head blocks) are needed for each patient. Splint other injuries appropriately.

9. Transport

10. Perform detailed physical examination if time permits; provide ongoing assessment.

Rationale

Because of the number of patients and MOI, additional ambulances should be requested. Each patient appears to have only an isolated injury and no obvious problems involving mental status, airway, breathing, or circulation. However, the MOI, a fall of greater than 15 feet or three times a patient's height, is significant. Therefore, each patient should receive a head-to-toe rapid trauma assessment. Because the MOI suggests spinal injuries, each patient should be placed on long spine board with a cervical collar and cervical immobilizer in place. Because the patients are stable all fractures should be splinted before transport.

7.22. C, A fall of greater than 15 feet or three times a patient's height is a significant MOI for an adult.

7.23. B, Indirect force caused this patient's back injury. Indirect force is present when the force from an impact to one area of the body is transmitted to another area, causing injury there.

7.24. B, Spinal precautions should be initiated at the same time the initial assessment is performed.

7.25. C, The "D" in DCAP-BTLS stands for deformities.

7.26. A, The "C" in DCAP-BTLS stands for contusions.

7.27. A, Direct force is the mechanism that caused this patient's wrist injury. Direct force is present when an injury occurs at a point of impact on the body.

7.28. C, After examining the neck you should apply a cervical collar.

7.29. B, Perform a rapid trauma assessment. The rapid trauma assessment should be performed on patients with a significant MOI.

SCENARIO FIVE

Plan of Action

1. BSI

2. Is the scene safe? Yes. Assess nature of illness, number of patients, and need for additional resources.

3. Assess mental status. Ensure an open airway, assess breathing, apply oxygen at 10-15 lpm by non-rebreather mask, and assess circulatory status.

4. Determine priority, consider ALS.

5. Assess chief complaint plus signs and symptoms (OPQRST).

6. SAMPLE history

7. Perform a focused medical assessment based on the chief complaint and history.

8. Baseline vital signs

9. Transport; provide ongoing assessment, meet ALS unit.

Rationale

The patient's ABCs appear to be stable, and he is able to communicate with you. Therefore, you can focus your history and physical examination on the body system(s) and area(s) associated with the chief complaint and history. The location and quality of the patient's chest pain suggest he is having an acute myocardial infarction (a heart attack). He should receive oxygen, be placed in a semi-sitting position, and be made as comfortable as possible. ALS backup for monitoring of the cardiac rhythm and drug therapy should be requested unless transport time to the hospital is shorter than the estimated time of arrival for ALS. Use of lights and sirens during transport should be avoided to prevent the patient from becoming anxious and increasing his heart rate.

7.30. C, An initial assessment of mental status, airway, breathing, and circulation should always be your first step with every patient.

7.31. C, The "R" in OPQRST is a reminder to ask whether a pain radiates (travels) to any other part of the body.

7.32. B, Because the patient is responsive, the radial pulse should be checked first. If the patient is unresponsive or if you cannot feel a radial pulse, then check for a carotid pulse.

7.33. C, The normal pulse rate for an adult is 60 to 100 beats/min.

7.34. D, An irregular pulse indicates that the heart is not maintaining a regular rhythm. This could result from the heart being irritable and producing extra abnormal beats. Because the patient appears to have cardiac chest pain, this is significant. Most patients who die of heart attacks die because their heart becomes very irritable and develops ventricular fibrillation.

7.35. C, The quality of the patient's pulse refers to its strength. Is it weak, strong, bounding, or thready?

7.36. A, Skin color and temperature are indicators of the patient's perfusion. One cannot assess heart rate and BP by checking skin color and temperature. Capillary refill time also cannot be inferred from skin color and temperature. However, it also is a good indicator of perfusion for children and infants.

7.37. D, Systolic pressure is the pressure generated against the walls of the arteries when the ventricles contract.

7.38. D, Diastolic pressure is the pressure remaining in the arteries when the ventricles relax.

7.39. A, A pulse rate of 110 is tachycardic. Tachycardia is a pulse rate greater than 100 beats/min.

SCENARIO SIX

Plan of Action

1. BSI
2. Is the scene safe? Yes. Assess nature of illness, number of patients, and need for additional resources.
3. Assess mental status. Ensure an open airway, assess breathing, apply oxygen at 10-15 lpm by non-rebreather mask, and assess circulatory status.
4. Determine priority, consider ALS.
5. Assess chief complaint plus signs and symptoms (OPQRST).
6. SAMPLE history
7. Perform a focused medical assessment based on the chief complaint and history.
8. Baseline vital signs
9. Transport; perform ongoing assessment, meet ALS unit.

Rationale

The patient's ABCs appear to be stable, and she is able to communicate with you. Therefore, you can focus your history and physical examination on the body system(s) and area(s) associated with the chief complaint and history. Because this patient has a past history of diabetes and leukemia, it will be difficult to identify the exact cause for her weakness and dizziness in the field. However, her presentation suggests a temporary problem with perfusion. She should receive oxygen and be made as comfortable as possible. Because she may have problems with perfusion, she should be moved in a supine position. ALS backup for monitoring of the cardiac rhythm and drug therapy should be requested unless transport time to the hospital is shorter than the estimated time of arrival for ALS.

7.40. B, Because the patient has no immediate life-threatening problems and is able to provide a history, you should perform a focused history and physical examination based on her chief complaint. If the patient had been unable to provide specific information about her complaints, a rapid head-to-toe physical examination would have been indicated.

7.41. B, The patient's alertness and orientation would have been identified during the initial assessment. Diabetes and leukemia are part of the "P" in SAMPLE. Medications are the "M" in SAMPLE, and allergies are the "A."

7.42. C, You would focus initially on the cardiovascular system. The weakness and dizziness suggest a temporary episode of poor perfusion.

7.43. C, Signs and symptoms of the current problem

7.44. D, Allergies

7.45. C, Medications

7.46. A, Pertinent past medical history

7.47. C, Last oral intake

7.48. B, Events leading up to the injury or illness

8

Airway Management

RESPIRATORY ANATOMY

- Upper airway
  - Mouth—Oral cavity
  - Nose—Anterior openings are called nares.
  - Pharynx (throat)
    - Nasopharynx—Posterior to nasal cavity
    - Oropharynx—Posterior to oral cavity
    - Laryngopharynx—Inferior to oropharynx, adjacent to epiglottis and glottic opening
  - Epiglottis—Flaplike structure. Closes during swallowing, covering and protecting glottic opening
- Lower airway
  - Larynx—Voice box or Adam's apple. Contains vocal cords. Includes thyroid and cricoid cartilages
  - Trachea—Windpipe. Extends from inferior border of larynx into chest cavity behind upper portion of sternum (manubrium)
  - Mainstem bronchi—Branch from trachea to carry gases to right and left lungs. Divide into lobar, segmental, and subsegmental bronchi, and bronchioles
  - Bronchioles—Smallest airways. Contain no cartilage in wall. Carry air to alveoli
  - Alveoli—Air sacs surrounded by capillaries where gas exchange with blood occurs
    - Inhaled air has high oxygen, low carbon dioxide concentration
    - Blood pumped to pulmonary capillaries from right side of heart has low oxygen, high carbon dioxide concentration
    - Oxygen diffuses from alveoli into blood for transport to body
    - Carbon dioxide diffuses from blood to alveoli to be exhaled

MECHANICS OF VENTILATION

- Inhalation
  - Active phase of breathing, requires muscular effort
  - Diaphragm contracts and moves downward, increasing vertical size of chest cavity
  - Intercostal muscles contract and pull ribs up and out, increasing horizontal size of chest cavity
  - Increase in chest cavity size causes intrathoracic pressure to become less than atmospheric pressure
  - Air flows in through airways until pressures equalize
- Exhalation
  - Passive phase of breathing, does not require muscular effort
  - Diaphragm and intercostal muscles relax
  - Elasticity of lungs pulls chest wall back to resting position
  - Size of thoracic cavity decreases
  - Decrease in chest cavity size causes intrathoracic pressure to increase above atmospheric pressure
  - Air flows out through airway until pressures equalize
- Tidal volume—Amount of air moved with each breath. Approximately 8 mL/kg body weight or approximately 500 mL in the average adult male
- Minute volume—Amount of air inhaled and exhaled per minute
  - Respiratory rate × Tidal volume

CONTROL OF BREATHING

- Breathing is controlled by respiratory center in brain stem.
- Normal stimulus to breathe is carbon dioxide level in arterial blood (respiratory drive).
  - Increase in arterial carbon dioxide stimulates respiratory drive.
  - Respiratory center produces nerve impulses that cause diaphragm and intercostal muscles to contract.
  - Carbon dioxide is exhaled from body.
- Oxygen levels in arterial blood provide backup to respiratory drive (hypoxic drive).
  - Decrease in arterial oxygen stimulates hypoxic (low oxygen) drive.
  - Respiratory center produces nerve impulses that cause diaphragm and intercostal muscles to contract.
  - Oxygen is inhaled.
  - Hypoxic drive may be active in patients with chronic obstructive pulmonary disease who have chronically high arterial carbon dioxide levels.

ASSESSMENT OF BREATHING

- Adequate breathing
  - Rate
    - Adults and adolescents—12 to 24 breaths/min
    - School-aged children—15 to 30 breaths/min
    - Preschoolers and toddlers—20 to 30 breaths/min
    - Infants aged 6 to 12 months—20 to 30 breaths/min
    - Infants aged 0 to 6 months—25 to 45 breaths/min
    - Newborns—30 to 50 breaths/min
  - Rhythm
    - Regular
  - Depth
    - Normal tidal volume
    - Not unusually shallow or deep
  - Quality
    - Breath sounds present in both lung fields and equal
    - Chest expansion adequate and equal
    - Minimum effort
- Inadequate breathing
  - Rate
    - Tachypnea—Rapid respirations
    - Bradypnea—Slow respirations
    - Agonal breathing—Occasional gasps for air, seen just before death
  - Rhythm
    - Irregular respiratory pattern
  - Depth
    - Very shallow or very deep
    - Air movement felt at mouth or nose is absent or below normal.
  - Quality
    - Breath sounds diminished, not present, or unequal
    - Inadequate or uneven chest expansion
    - Muscles of neck and upper chest used to assist air movement

- Retractions of soft tissue between ribs, over clavicles, or over upper abdomen
- Nasal flaring
- Wheezing, crowing, stridor, snoring, gurgling, or gasping
  - Cyanosis
  - Patient unable to speak in complete sentences

OPENING THE AIRWAY

- Head-tilt/chin-lift—Used to lift tongue from back of throat in patients who do not have possible cervical spine injuries
- Jaw-thrust—Used to lift tongue from back of throat in patients who may have possible cervical spine injuries, including unconscious patients when no history of the mechanism of injury is available

AIRWAY ADJUNCTS

- Oropharyngeal airway
  - Keeps tongue from blocking pharynx
  - Used only for unconscious persons with no gag reflex
  - Measure from the tip of earlobe to the corner of the mouth
  - Depress tongue, slide airway into mouth with concave side facing upward, and rotate 180 degrees until flange rests on lips
- Nasopharyngeal airway
  - Also called nasal trumpet
  - Used for unconscious persons who have gag reflex but who have difficulty maintaining airway
  - Measure from tip of nose to earlobe
  - Use water-soluble lubricant before inserting
  - Insert into nostril with bevel away from septum, advance until flange rests against nostril

SUCTIONING

- Used to clear blood, vomitus, or secretions from upper airway
- Indicated whenever gurgling sounds are heard during ventilation
- Devices
  - Mounted (fixed) suction—At head of stretcher in patient compartment
  - Portable suction—Electrically or manually operated. Can be taken to patient
  - Either mounted or portable devices must be able to generate at least a 300-mm Hg vacuum.
- Tips and catheters
  - Rigid
    - Yankauer or tonsil-tip suctions
    - Allow for good control of catheter
    - Large enough to move thick secretions
    - May trigger gag reflex
  - Soft
    - Can be inserted through oral airways or endotracheal tubes
    - Less likely to trigger gag reflex
    - Kinks easily
    - Will not move thick secretions
- Suctioning technique
  - Use appropriate infection-control practices

○ Suction with patient or patient's head turned to side so gravity helps drain secretions
○ Never suction for >15 seconds at a time
○ Place catheter tip where you want to begin to suction and suction on the way out
○ Large particles may have to be removed with manual finger sweeps.

SUPPLEMENTAL OXYGEN

- Oxygen cylinders
  ○ Seamless steel or aluminum cylinders filled with oxygen under pressure
  ○ Common sizes
    ■ D cylinder—350 liters (most often used to carry oxygen to patient)
    ■ E cylinder—625 liters
    ■ M cylinder—3000 liters (most often used as fixed supply on ambulance)
    ■ G cylinder—5300 liters
    ■ H cylinder—6900 liters
- Pressure regulators
  ○ Pressure in full tank is 2000 pounds per square inch (psi)
  ○ Pressure regulators reduce pressure to useful range, 40 to 70 psi
- Flowmeters
  ○ Bourdon gauge—Rugged, operates at any angle. Inaccurate at low flows. Cannot compensate for backpressure from kinked lines
  ○ Pressure-compensated (Thorpe) flowmeter—Must be upright to operate. Indicates actual flow at all times
  ○ Constant flow selector valve—Allows adjustment of flow in set increments
  ○ Open or "crack" the cylinder before attaching the regulator to blow dust and other debris out of the cylinder's head
- Oxygen delivery devices
  ○ Non-rebreather mask
    ■ Flow should be set at 10 to 15 lpm.
    ■ Will deliver 90% oxygen with good face seal
  ○ Nasal cannula
    ■ Flow should be set at 1 to 6 lpm.
    ■ Do not exceed more than 6 lpm
    ■ Will deliver 24% to 44% oxygen. Each liter per minute increases inspired oxygen by approximately 4% above room air (1 lpm = 24%, 2 lpm = 28%, 3 lpm = 32%, 4 lpm = 36%, 5 lpm = 40%, and 6 lpm = 44%).

ARTIFICIAL VENTILATION DEVICES

- Pocket mask
  ○ Protects rescuer from exposure to communicable disease while ventilations are delivered
  ○ Connect to oxygen if available
  ○ Open airway using head-tilt/chin-lift or jaw-thrust method
  ○ Place pocket mask over the patient's mouth and nose
  ○ Take normal breath and ventilate through mask for 1 second
  ○ Watch for chest rise
- Bag-valve mask (BVM)
  ○ A self-refilling bag connected to transparent face mask by one-way valve
  ○ Adult-size bags contain 1600 mL of gas

○ When connected to oxygen can deliver 95% to 100% oxygen

○ Devices with pop-off valves may cause inadequate ventilation of patients with high airway resistance

○ Use with an oral or nasal airway to ensure open airway when bagging

○ Difficult for single rescuers to squeeze bag while maintaining mask seal

○ Two-rescuer technique with one rescuer sealing the mask while the other squeezes the bag may improve ventilations

- Flow-restricted oxygen-powered ventilation device

○ Uses oxygen under pressure to deliver artificial ventilations through mask placed on patient's face

○ Peak flow rate of 100% oxygen at up to 40 lpm

○ Easier to operate for single rescuer than BVM

○ Higher ventilation pressures may cause gastric distension

○ Should *not* be used on pediatric patients

REVIEW QUESTIONS
Scenario One

You have just finished restocking the ambulance and checking the on-board oxygen supply when a call comes in for a "5-y.o. with a history of asthma having difficulty breathing."

Multiple Choice

8.1. The large oxygen tank on your ambulance that holds 3000 liters of oxygen is:
   a. an "H" cylinder.
   b. a "D" cylinder.
   c. an "M" cylinder.
   d. an "E" cylinder.

8.2. A full oxygen tank normally has a pressure of approximately:
   a. 625 liters of oxygen.
   b. 2000 psi.
   c. 2000 liters of oxygen.
   d. 2800 psi.

Matching

8.3. _____ D cylinder   **a.** 3000 liters of oxygen
8.4. _____ E cylinder   **b.** 6900 liters of oxygen
8.5. _____ M cylinder   **c.** 350 liters of oxygen
8.6. _____ G cylinder   **d.** 625 liters of oxygen
8.7. _____ H cylinder   **e.** 5300 liters of oxygen

Multiple Choice

8.8. An oxygen tank must be hydrostatically tested every:
   a. 6 months.
   b. 3 years.
   c. 5 years.
   d. 10 years.

8.9. The date that an oxygen tank must be hydrostatically tested is indicated by the:
  a. yellow plastic tape around the top of the tank.
  b. date on the tank (e.g., Aug. 2001).
  c. date on the tank (e.g., 4M99M*).
  d. date on the tank (e.g., 8M2002M) and the yellow tape.

8.10. When you "crack" the valve of an oxygen tank, you are:
  a. emptying the tank of all oxygen and refilling it.
  b. quickly opening and closing the tank to blow out any dust.
  c. turning the flowmeter to 15 lpm to remove any debris.
  d. sealing the tank with a band of yellow tape to prevent dust from entering.

8.11. All of the following statements are correct *except:*
  a. fire risks increase when oxygen is used because oxygen supports combustion, causing a fire to burn and spread more rapidly.
  b. the optimal flow of oxygen through a non-rebreather mask is 10 to 15 lpm.
  c. when the BVM is used, the patient should receive at least 800 mL of air, and the volume of the BVM is approximately 1600 mL of air.
  d. the oxygen tank and adjunctive equipment should be oiled periodically to prevent rust from forming.

8.12. You have arrived on the scene of a 5-y.o. asthmatic male with difficulty breathing. Which of the following indicate he is in moderate respiratory distress?
  a. Nasal flaring; retractions between the ribs and below the rib cage; shallow or inadequate breathing; and a seesaw-breathing pattern, with the chest and abdomen moving in opposite directions
  b. A respiratory rate of 26 breaths/min; nasal flaring; retractions between the ribs and also below the rib cage; shallow or inadequate breathing; and quiet but easy respirations
  c. A respiratory rate of 26 breaths/min; nasal flaring; shallow or inadequate breathing; a seesaw-breathing pattern, with the chest and abdomen moving in opposite directions; and quiet but easy respirations
  d. A respiratory rate of 26 breaths/min; nasal flaring; retractions between the ribs and also below the rib cage; shallow or inadequate breathing; a seesaw-breathing pattern, with the chest and abdomen moving in opposite directions; and quiet but easy respirations

8.13. Cyanosis is:
  a. an early sign of difficulty breathing.
  b. a late sign of hypoxia.
  c. an indication that agonal respirations will be present shortly.
  d. an indication of an irregular respiratory pattern.

8.14. The normal respiratory rate for a 5-y.o. child would be:
  a. 10 to 15 breaths/min.
  b. 15 to 20 breaths/min.
  c. 20 to 30 breaths/min.
  d. 30 to 40 breaths/min.

8.15. Rescue breaths for a child should be given at a rate of:
  a. 8-10 breaths/min.
  b. 12-20 breaths/min.
  c. 22-28 breaths/min.
  d. 30-40 breaths/min.

Scenario Two

You have been dispatched to a "52-y.o. female not breathing." When you arrive, the patient is unresponsive. Firefighters have inserted an oral airway and are ventilating her with a BVM. The patient's pulse (P) is 102, weak and regular. Her blood pressure (BP) is 92/60. No family members are present to give a medical history.

Your Plan of Action

Fill in the blank lines with your treatment plan for this patient. Then compare your plan with the questions, answers, and rationale.

1. _____
2. _____
3. _____
4. _____
5. _____
6. _____
7. _____
8. _____
9. _____

Multiple Choice

8.16. When an oral airway is inserted into an adult, it is inserted by:
   a. pushing the tip along the tongue until it reaches the back of the throat.
   b. holding the airway upside down and rotating it 180 degrees.
   c. placing it in the position of function with the tip facing the posterior oropharynx and advancing it slowly into place.
   d. advancing the airway until the gag reflex is stimulated, then pulling back slightly.

8.17. To select the proper size of a nasal airway, you would measure from the:
   a. corner of the patient's mouth to the bottom of the earlobe.
   b. tip of the patient's nose to the bottom of the earlobe.
   c. patient's upper lip to the Adam's apple.
   d. tip of the nose to the Adam's apple.

8.18. When selecting the proper size of an oral airway, you would measure from the:
   a. corner of the patient's mouth to the patient's earlobe.
   b. middle of the lips to the angle of the jaw.
   c. tip of the patient's nose to the bottom of the earlobe.
   d. corner of the patient's mouth to the back of the throat.

8.19. When a pocket mask is used to ventilate an adult, each ventilation should be delivered for:
   a. ½ second.
   b. 1 second.
   c. 2 seconds.
   d. 3 seconds.

8.20. A patient's ventilations should be assisted if the rate falls below:
  a. 6 breaths/min.
  b. 8 breaths/min.
  c. 10 breaths/min.
  d. 12 breaths/min.

8.21. The medical term for "difficulty breathing" is:
  a. dysphagia.
  b. dyspnea.
  c. apnea.
  d. dyspulmonia.

8.22. The suction unit provides a vacuum of:
  a. no more than 30 mm Hg of positive pressure.
  b. at least 300 mm Hg of negative pressure.
  c. at least 100 mm Hg of negative pressure.
  d. no more than 200 mm Hg of negative pressure.

8.23. All of the following statements about suctioning are true *except:*
  a. suction is not applied until after the catheter has been fully inserted.
  b. suctioning helps prevent foreign materials from entering the trachea.
  c. finger sweeps may have to be used to remove large pieces of material that cannot pass through the suction catheter.
  d. suctioning reduces the patient's need for supplemental oxygen.

8.24. Signs of respiratory distress include all of the following *except:*
  a. use of the shoulder or neck muscles when the patient inhales.
  b. retraction of the tissue between the ribs when the patient inhales.
  c. flaring of the nostrils when the patient inhales.
  d. movement of the chest and abdominal walls in the same direction when the patient inhales.

8.25. The maximum period for which an adult should be suctioned is:
  a. 5 seconds.
  b. 15 seconds.
  c. 20 seconds.
  d. 30 seconds.

8.26. All of the following statements about suctioning are true *except:*
  a. it may be performed safely on infants and children using proper equipment and technique.
  b. it may cause hypoxia if performed incorrectly.
  c. it may help remove excess fluid from the alveoli.
  d. it may cause vomiting if the patient has a gag reflex.

8.27. To obtain an accurate respiratory rate, you should count the number of breaths the patient takes in:
  a. 6 seconds and multiply by 10.
  b. 10 seconds and multiply by 6.
  c. 15 seconds and multiply by 4.
  d. 30 seconds and multiply by 2.

8.28. The two types of suction catheters are:
   a. rigid and semi-rigid.
   b. rigid and soft.
   c. curved and straight.
   d. French and soft Yankauer.

8.29. Which of the following statements *best* describes proper suctioning technique?
   a. Insert the catheter without applying suction.
   b. Suction only while advancing the catheter.
   c. Remove the airway and insert the suction catheter, applying suction as you withdraw the suction catheter.
   d. Insert a rigid catheter to the back of the mouth, applying suction while inserting.

Scenario Three

You respond to a report of a patient in respiratory distress at a nursing home. When you arrive, you discover you actually have two patients.

- Patient #1 is an 80-y.o. male who is unresponsive. Vital signs are BP—168/90; P—102, weak, regular; and respirations (R)—8, shallow, regular.

Your Plan of Action

Fill in the blank lines with your treatment plan for this patient. Then compare your plan with the questions, answers, and rationale.

1. _____
2. _____
3. _____
4. _____
5. _____
6. _____
7. _____
8. _____
9. _____

- Patient #2 is a 71-y.o. female who has a history of congestive heart failure and is having difficulty breathing. Vital signs are BP—188/94; P—148, weak, regular; and R—34, regular, labored. You immediately call for additional assistance and advanced life support (ALS). You then continue to assess and care for the patients.

Your Plan of Action

Fill in the blank lines with your treatment plan for this patient. Then compare your plan with the questions, answers, and rationale.

1. _____

2. _____

3. _____

4. _____

5. _____

6. _____

7. _____

8. _____

9. _____

Multiple Choice

8.30. To ventilate Patient #1 with a BVM, you should:
   a. give 30 ventilations/min to compensate for difficulty sealing the mask.
   b. insert a nasopharyngeal airway.
   c. use an oral airway if the patient tolerates it.
   d. not use an oral or nasal airway because these devices are designed for pediatric patients.

8.31. The advantage of using a flow-restricted oxygen-powered ventilation device instead of a BVM is that:
   a. it may be used without a face mask.
   b. no additional airway adjunctive equipment is required.
   c. it makes ventilating the patient easier for the single rescuer.
   d. it reduces the risk of gastric distension.

8.32. Which of the following statements about the BVM is *correct*?
   a. It may only be used in apneic patients.
   b. It provides an oxygen concentration of approximately 50% with oxygen flow rates of 10 to 15 lpm.
   c. It should have a pop-off valve to overcome increased air resistance in pediatric patients.
   d. It may provide an inadequate ventilation volume if a good mask seal is not maintained.

8.33. Which statement *best* describes the design and function of an oropharyngeal airway?
   a. It is a curved plastic device designed to hold the tongue away from the posterior wall of the throat.
   b. It is designed so the distal tip sits in the pharynx and the proximal tip rests on the external nares.
   c. It is a plastic tube with several small holes on each side and a port for delivery of supplemental oxygen.
   d. It is a piece of plastic tubing containing two ports designed to deliver supplemental oxygen through the nares.

8.34. During inspiration the:
  a. diaphragm contracts and the intercostal muscles contract.
  b. diaphragm contracts and the intercostal muscles relax.
  c. diaphragm relaxes and the intercostal muscles contract.
  d. diaphragm relaxes and the intercostal muscles relax.

8.35. Tidal volume is the amount of air:
  a. moved in and out of the respiratory tract per minute.
  b. that remains in the respiratory system after forced expiration.
  c. in the lungs at the end of a maximal inspiration.
  d. inhaled and exhaled with each breath.

8.36. Gurgling respirations generally indicate:
  a. an upper airway obstruction that usually can be relieved with an oral airway.
  b. fluid in the upper airway that requires use of suction.
  c. swelling in the upper airway that will require placement of an endotracheal tube by a paramedic.
  d. fluid in the lower airway that will require endotracheal intubation and drug therapy by a paramedic.

Matching

8.37. _____ Cyanosis
8.38. _____ Gag reflex
8.39. _____ Head-tilt/chin-lift
8.40. _____ Hypoxia
8.41. _____ Jaw-thrust
8.42. _____ Pressure regulator

a. A device connected to an oxygen cylinder and used to reduce cylinder pressure so oxygen can be delivered to a patient safely
b. The response by the body that causes vomiting or retching when something is inserted into the throat
c. A maneuver used to correct airway blockage caused by the tongue when trauma is not suspected
d. Blue-gray skin color that results from a lack of oxygen in the body
e. A maneuver used to correct airway blockage caused by the tongue when trauma is suspected
f. An insufficient supply of oxygen in the body's tissues

True/False

8.43. There are three types of oxygen flowmeters: the Bourdon gauge flowmeter, the pressure-compensated flowmeter, and the constant flowmeter.
  a. True
  b. False

Multiple Choice

8.44. The average volume of air in an adult BVM device is:
  a. 500 mL.
  b. 800 mL.
  c. 1200 mL.
  d. 1600 mL.

8.45. The portion of the inhaled air that never reaches the alveoli is the:
    a. minute ventilation.
    b. dead space air.
    c. tidal volume.
    d. accessory space air.

8.46. When you assess a patient's respirations, which of the following should be noted?
    a. Quality, quantity, and rate
    b. Rate, rhythm, and whether any noises are present
    c. Rate, rhythm, quality, and depth
    d. Rate, chest expansion

8.47. Which of the following statements about respiration is *correct?*
    a. Oxygen binds to hemoglobin in the tissue capillary beds.
    b. Blood releases oxygen and takes up carbon dioxide in the pulmonary capillary beds.
    c. Blood takes up carbon dioxide and releases oxygen in the tissue capillary beds.
    d. Carbon dioxide binds to hemoglobin in the pulmonary capillary beds.

8.48. A nasal cannula connected to oxygen at 4 lpm delivers what percentage of inspired oxygen?
    a. 24%
    b. 35%
    c. 90%
    d. 100%

8.49. The non-rebreather mask connected to oxygen at 10 to 15 lpm delivers what percentage of inspired oxygen?
    a. 24%
    b. 50%
    c. 60%
    d. 90%

8.50. A BVM with an oxygen reservoir connected to oxygen at 15 lpm delivers what percentage of inspired oxygen?
    a. 45%
    b. 55%
    c. 65%
    d. 95%

8.1. C, The large oxygen tanks on ambulances are M cylinders, which hold approximately 3000 liters of oxygen. D cylinders hold approximately 350 liters of oxygen. E cylinders hold approximately 625 liters. D and E cylinders are carried on ambulances to provide a portable oxygen source. An H cylinder holds 6900 liters of oxygen.

8.2. B, A full oxygen tank normally has a pressure of approximately 2000 psi.

8.3. C, D cylinders contain 350 liters of oxygen when full.

8.4. D, E cylinders contain 625 liters of oxygen when full.

8.5. A, M cylinders contain 3000 liters of oxygen when full.

8.6. E, G cylinders contain 5300 liters of oxygen when full.

8.7. B, H cylinders contain 6900 liters of oxygen when full.

8.8. C, Oxygen cylinders must be tested every 5 years.

8.9. C, The test date is stamped on the cylinder and will have a "star" after it (e.g., 5M88MM˙).

8.10. B, Cracking the valve on an oxygen cylinder means quickly opening and closing the tank to clear any dirt and dust from the delivery port before attaching a regulator.

8.11. D, Oil-based products should never be applied to oxygen tanks and equipment. Because oxygen vigorously supports combustion, applying oil to oxygen cylinders or equipment increases the risk of an explosion or fire.

8.12. A, Nasal flaring, intercostal or subcostal retractions, shallow or inadequate breathing, and seesaw movement of the chest and abdomen indicate respiratory distress. A respiratory rate of 26 breaths/min and quiet, easy respirations would be normal findings in a 5-y.o. child.

8.13. B, Cyanosis is a late sign of hypoxia. Presence of cyanosis is not necessarily associated with an irregular respiratory pattern. It also does not necessarily indicate that agonal breathing will be present shortly.

8.14. C, A 5-y.o. child's respiratory rate normally would be 20 to 30 breaths/min.

8.15. B, Rescue breaths for a child should be given at a rate of 12 to 20 breaths/min (one every 3 to 5 seconds).

SCENARIO TWO

Plan of Action

1. Body Substance Isolation (BSI)

2. Is the scene safe? Yes

3. Ensure open airway, assess ventilations, continue ventilating the patient with BVM and oxygen, and assess circulation.

4. Determine priority, call for ALS.

5. Rapid physical examination

6. Baseline vital signs

7. HPI, SAMPLE (if any family are present)

8. Transport, perform ongoing assessment, and meet ALS unit.

Rationale

The patient is not breathing but has a pulse. You should continue to ventilate her with high-concentration oxygen. A rapid physical examination and history should be obtained to identify possible causes of the respiratory arrest. Ongoing assessment should be performed to identify changes in the patient's condition, particularly inadequate perfusion and cardiac arrest.

8.16. B, Oral airways are inserted in adults by beginning with the airway upside down and rotating it 180 degrees. This maneuver reduces the risk of pushing the tongue into the airway and causing an obstruction.

8.17. B, Nasal airways are measured from the tip of the patient's nose to the bottom of the earlobe.

8.18. A, Oral airways are measured from the corner of the mouth to the bottom of the earlobe.

8.19. B, Pocket mask ventilations for adults should be delivered for 1 second. The volume of air delivered should be sufficient to cause visible chest rise.

8.20. B, A patient's ventilations may need to be assisted if the rate is <8 breaths/min.

8.21. B, Dyspnea means "difficulty breathing."

8.22. B, A suction unit should provide a vacuum of at least 300 mm Hg of negative pressure.

8.23. D, Suctioning does not decrease a patient's need for supplemental oxygen. Suctioning time must be limited because supplemental oxygen cannot be given while a suction catheter is in the patient's airway.

8.24. D, The chest wall and abdomen normally move in the same direction when the patient breathes. A seesaw pattern in which the chest and abdomen move in opposite directions is an indication of respiratory distress.

8.25. B, The maximum time for suctioning an adult is 10 to 15 seconds.

8.26. C, Suctioning will not remove excess fluid from the alveoli. It is performed to remove fluid from the mouth and throat.

8.27. D, To obtain the respiratory rate, count the number of breaths taken in 30 seconds and multiply by 2.

8.28. B, The two principal types of suction catheters are rigid and soft.

8.29. A, The catheter should be inserted without applying suction. Once the catheter is in place, suction is applied as it is withdrawn from the airway.

SCENARIO THREE

Plan of Action

Patient #1

1. BSI

2. Is the scene safe? Yes. Assess nature of illness, number of patients, and need for additional resources. Request additional help because of number of patients.

3. Assess mental status. Ensure an open airway, assess breathing, insert oral airway, assist ventilation with BVM connected to oxygen at 15 lpm, and assess circulatory status.

4. Determine priority, call for ALS unit.

5. Rapid physical examination

6. Baseline vital signs

7. HPI, SAMPLE

8. Transport as soon as possible to meet ALS unit. Continue ongoing assessment for any changes in respirations or pulse.

Patient #2

1. BSI

2. Is the scene safe? Yes. Assess nature of illness, number of patients, and need for additional resources. Request additional help because of number of patients.

3. Assess mental status. Ensure open airway, assess breathing, apply oxygen at 10-15 lpm with non-rebreather mask, and assess circulation.

4. Determine priority, call for a second ALS unit.

5. HPI, SAMPLE

6. Focused physical examination

7. Baseline vital signs

8. Transport, meet the ALS unit, and continue the ongoing assessment.

Rationale

Because you have two patients who are both experiencing life-threatening respiratory emergencies, additional help should be requested immediately.

Patient #1 is unresponsive and has a respiratory rate of only 8 breaths/min. This is too slow; therefore, his ventilations must be assisted with a BVM and oxygen. His perfusion appears to be adequate. If possible a rapid physical examination should be performed and a history taken to identify possible causes of his respiratory arrest. Assisted ventilations should be continued, and ongoing assessment should be performed until ALS unit personnel take over care.

Patient #2 is having difficulty breathing. She should be given high-concentration oxygen by non-rebreather mask. A history should be taken and used as the basis for a focused physical examination to help identify the cause of the difficulty breathing. High-concentration oxygen should be continued, and ongoing assessment should be performed until ALS personnel take over care.

8.30. **C,** Because Patient #1 is unresponsive, an oral airway should be inserted to help keep the tongue out of the pharynx. A ventilation of 30 breaths/min is too rapid. The nasal airway is most useful for patients who have a gag reflex but need help to keep the tongue out of the airway. Nasal and oral airways are produced in sizes for use in adult and pediatric patients.

8.31. **C,** A flow-restricted, oxygen-powered ventilator is easier for a single rescuer to operate than a BVM. A mask is required to seal a flow-restricted, oxygen-powered ventilator to a patient's face. An oral airway should be inserted to help hold the patient's tongue out of the pharynx. Because this device generates higher pressure than a BVM, there is an increased risk of gastric distension.

8.32. **D,** If you do not maintain a good mask-to-face seal, a BVM may provide inadequate ventilation volume. The BVM can be used for apneic patients and for patients who are breathing but who need assistance. At flow rates of 10 to 15 lpm, the BVM provides in excess of 90% oxygen. BVMs used with pediatric patients should not have pop-off valves because the high airway resistance present in these patients can cause the valve to open, producing inadequate ventilation volumes.

8.33. **A,** The oropharyngeal airway is a curved piece of plastic inserted into the airway to hold the tongue away from the back of the throat.

8.34. **A,** During inspiration the diaphragm and intercostal muscles contract. As the diaphragm moves down and the intercostal muscles pull the ribs up and out, the volume of the chest cavity increases. The increase in chest volume causes intrathoracic pressure to decrease below atmospheric pressure, and air flows into the lungs until the pressures equalize.

8.35. **D,** Tidal volume is the amount of air inhaled and exhaled with each breath. The amount of air moved in and out of the respiratory tract per minute is the minute volume. The amount of air remaining in the respiratory system after a forced exhalation is the residual volume. The amount of air in the lungs at the end of a maximum inhalation is the total lung capacity.

8.36. **B,** Gurgling indicates there is fluid in the upper airway that should be removed by suctioning.

8.37. **D,** Cyanosis is a blue-gray skin color that results from a lack of oxygen in the body.

8.38. **B,** The gag reflex is the body's response that causes vomiting or retching when something is inserted into the throat.

8.39. **C,** The head-tilt/chin-lift is a maneuver used to correct airway blockage caused by the tongue when trauma is NOT suspected.

8.40. **F,** Hypoxia is an insufficient supply of oxygen in the body's tissues.

8.41. **E,** The jaw-thrust maneuver is a maneuver used to correct airway blockage caused by the tongue when trauma is suspected.

8.42. **A,** A pressure regulator is a device connected to an oxygen cylinder used to reduce cylinder pressure so oxygen can be delivered to a patient safely.

8.43. **A,** The three types of oxygen flowmeter are the Bourdon gauge flowmeter, the pressure-compensated flowmeter, and the constant flowmeter.

8.44. **D,** The average volume of air contained in an adult BVM is 1600 mL.

8.45. **B,** The dead space air is the part of the inhaled air that fills the larger airways and never reaches the alveoli to take part in gas exchange.

8.46. **C,** When you assess a patient's respirations, you should note and record the rate, rhythm, quality, and depth.

8.47. **C,** The blood takes up carbon dioxide and releases oxygen in the tissue capillary beds. Oxygen binds to hemoglobin in the pulmonary capillary beds. Carbon dioxide enters the blood in tissue capillary beds and is transported primarily in the blood plasma, not on the hemoglobin.

8.48. **B,** A nasal cannula connected to oxygen at 4 lpm delivers approximately 35% inspired oxygen.

8.49. **D,** A non-rebreather mask connected to oxygen at 10 to 15 lpm delivers approximately 90% inspired oxygen.

8.50. **D,** A BVM connected to supplemental oxygen at 15 lpm delivers approximately 95% inspired oxygen.

9

Trauma Assessment

SCENE SIZE-UP

- Scene safety—Dangers to responders, bystanders, and patients
- Nature of call—Mechanism of injury (MOI)
- Number and location of patients
- Adequacy of resources

BODY SUBSTANCE ISOLATION (BSI)

- Necessary on every call
- Use gloves, mask, gown, and eyewear as needed

INITIAL ASSESSMENT

Identify and correct immediate life-threatening problems (Figure 9-1)
- Form general impression (scene, chief complaint, and patient appearance)
- Assess mental status—AVPU
- Assess airway with manual stabilization of cervical spine
- Assess breathing
- Assess circulation (pulses, perfusion, and hemorrhage)
- Identify priority of patient and make transport decision

RECONSIDER MECHANISM OF INJURY

- Is MOI significant or not significant?
- Significant MOIs
  - Ejection from a motor vehicle
  - Motor vehicle collision (MVC) with death in same passenger compartment as patient
  - Fall of greater than 15 feet or three times patient's height
  - Rollover of vehicle
  - High-speed collision
  - Pedestrian struck by motor vehicle
  - MVC involving a motorcycle
  - Unresponsive or altered mental status
  - Penetrating trauma to head, chest, or abdomen
- Significant MOI—Children
  - Fall of greater than 10 feet
  - MVC involving bicycle
  - MVC at medium speed or high speed

If No Significant Mechanism of Injury

  - Determine chief complaint
  - Perform focused physical examination based on chief complaint and MOI. Assess areas of patient's body with possible injuries for DCAP-BTLS:
    - Deformities
    - Contusions
    - Abrasions
    - Punctures/penetrations
    - Burns
    - Tenderness
    - Lacerations

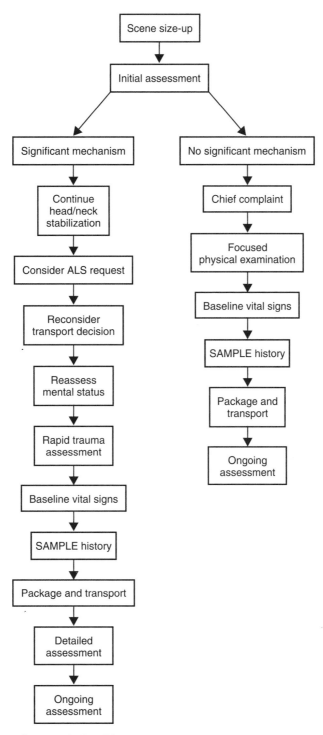

Figure 9-1   The trauma assessment process.

■ Swelling
○ Assess baseline vital signs
○ Obtain SAMPLE history
○ Package and transport
○ Ongoing assessment

- Repeat initial assessment (general impression, mental status, and ABCs)
- Reassess vital signs
- Repeat focused assessment
- Check interventions

If Significant Mechanism of Injury

- ○ Continue manual stabilization of head and neck
- ○ Consider requesting advanced life support (ALS)
- ○ Reconsider transport decision
- ○ Reassess mental status
- ○ Perform rapid trauma assessment
  - Begin with head. Work down body, checking extremities last
  - Systemically check all regions of the body. Inspect, palpate for DCAP-BTLS
- ○ Head
  - Inspect, palpate the skull and scalp for DCAP-BTLS, crepitation
  - Inspect face, ears, nose for DCAP-BTLS
  - Check eyes and pupils
  - Recheck airway
- ○ Neck
  - Inspect, palpate for DCAP-BTLS, crepitation, and jugular distension
  - Check back of neck, then apply cervical collar
- ○ Chest
  - Inspect, palpate for DCAP-BTLS, crepitation
  - Look for equal chest expansion with each breath
  - Look for paradoxical motion
  - Auscultate for presence, equality of breath sounds
- ○ Abdomen
  - Inspect for DCAP-BTLS, distension
  - Palpate for rigidity, tenderness
- ○ Pelvis
  - Inspect for DCAP-BTLS
  - Gently compress for tenderness, instability
- ○ Extremities
  - Inspect for DCAP-BTLS
  - Check distal pulses, motor function, and sensation
- ○ Back
  - Inspect for DCAP-BTLS
- Obtain baseline vital signs
- Obtain SAMPLE history
- Package and transport
- Perform detailed physical examination
  - ○ Only after all critical interventions have been performed
  - ○ Only en route to hospital or while waiting on air transport
  - ○ Repeat rapid trauma assessment adding examination of the ears, nose, and mouth
- Ongoing assessment

REVIEW QUESTIONS
Scenario One
You have been dispatched to a report of a person "over the falls" at Fillmore Glen State Park. The location you are responding to has a large waterfall that is approximately 50 feet from top to bottom. A 16-y.o. male is apparently unconscious at the bottom of the falls. A bystander tells you the patient fell approximately 30 feet, landing in the water. A hiker pulled him out of the water, and he now is lying on a flat rock.

Your Plan of Action

Fill in the blank lines with your treatment plan for this patient. Then compare your plan with the questions, answers, and rationale.

1. _____
2. _____
3. _____
4. _____
5. _____
6. _____
7. _____
8. _____
9. _____

Multiple Choice
9.1. The *first* step in the assessment process would be to perform:
   a. an initial assessment.
   b. a scene size-up.
   c. a check of the airway.
   d. an assessment of the patient's mental status.
9.2. If the patient did not respond to any stimuli, he would be at what point on the AVPU scale?
   a. A
   b. V
   c. P
   d. U
9.3. A patient who is at "V" on the AVPU scale:
   a. is able to respond verbally by answering questions appropriately.
   b. responds to stimulation verbally by at least moaning.
   c. responds to verbal stimuli such as saying his or her name.
   d. is able to answer questions, although the answers may not be appropriate.
9.4. As you assess the patient's mental status, you should also:
   a. check the airway.
   b. feel for a carotid pulse.
   c. initiate spinal precautions.
   d. form a general impression of the environment.

Scenario One—cont'd

The patient's airway is open. His breathing is labored and shallow. Radial pulses are absent. Carotid pulses are rapid and weak. The skin is pale, cool, and moist.

9.5. The next step to assess this patient would be to:

    a. do a focused history and physical examination.

    b. perform a rapid trauma examination.

    c. reconsider the MOI and transport decision.

    d. perform the DCAP-BTLS.

9.6. As you assess and treat this patient you would do all of the following *except:*

    a. perform a rapid trauma survey.

    b. do thorough detailed examination on scene.

    c. initiate spinal motion restriction.

    d. consider air transport.

9.7. Stabilization of this patient's cervical spine should begin:

    a. while you are performing the rapid trauma examination.

    b. during the detailed examination to ensure all body areas are adequately examined first.

    c. while you perform the initial assessment.

    d. just before air transport.

Scenario Two

You have been called to an MVC. When you arrive, fire/rescue tells you the patients are two teenagers who were driving home from a party when they missed a curve and struck a tree at high speed. The front end of the vehicle has been displaced backward at least 3 feet. The 18-y.o. male driver is unconscious and is pinned in the vehicle. The 16-y.o. female passenger is lying on the ground moaning. Her right thigh is swollen and deformed.

Your Plan of Action

Fill in the blank lines with your treatment plan for this patient. Then compare your plan with the questions, answers, and rationale.

1. _____

2. _____

3. _____

4. _____

5. _____

6. _____

7. _____

8. _____

9. _____

Multiple Choice

9.8. During what part of the assessment process do you decide whether to call for additional ambulances?

   a. The initial assessment

   b. The rapid trauma assessment

   c. The scene size-up

   d. After reconsidering the MOI

9.9. The driver has a Glasgow Coma Score of 8. What is the Glasgow Coma Score?

   a. A part of the AVPU examination used to determine neurologic status

   b. A system that will dictate the transport priority of the patient

   c. A description of whether the patient is conscious, semiconscious, or unconscious

   d. A numerical system to assess and describe patient neurologic status

9.10. What technique will you use to open the passenger's airway?

   a. Modified jaw-thrust

   b. Head-tilt/chin-lift

   c. Head-tilt without chin-lift

   d. Modified head-tilt

9.11. As you examine the driver, it would be important to do which of the following?

   a. Only remove clothing around obvious injuries

   b. Remove all clothing, then cover the patient with a blanket to avoid hypothermia

   c. Remove a piece of clothing, examine, and replace the clothing to avoid hypothermia

   d. Remove clothing only after securing the patient to a long spine board

9.12. All of the following are part of the initial assessment *except:*

   a. forming a general impression.

   b. assessing breathing and applying oxygen or assisting ventilation.

   c. obtaining a blood pressure, pulse, and respiratory rate.

   d. determining the patient's priority.

Scenario Three

You have been dispatched to an MVC in a residential area. A 40-y.o. female swerved to miss a dog and went off the road into a hedge. She was traveling approximately 20 mph and was wearing a seat belt. She is alert and oriented × 4. Her airway is open. Her breathing is unlabored. Radial pulses are present. She is c/o back and neck pain. She has no significant past medical history and is allergic to Ceclor. Vital signs are BP—120/76; P—82, strong, regular; and R—16, regular, unlabored.

Your Plan of Action

Fill in the blank lines with your treatment plan for this patient. Then compare your plan with the questions, answers, and rationale.

1. _____

2. _____

3. _____

4. _____

5. _____

6. _____

7. _____

8. _____

9. _____

Multiple Choice

9.13. Based on the MOI and initial assessment findings, what kind of assessment would you perform?

   a. A rapid trauma examination

   b. A focused physical examination

   c. A detailed physical examination

   d. An ongoing assessment

9.14. Which of the following patients has a significant MOI?

   a. A 10-y.o. male who fell off his bicycle

   b. An 18-y.o. female whose vehicle was struck from behind by another vehicle traveling at 25 mph

   c. A 16-y.o. male pedestrian who was struck by a vehicle traveling 35 mph

   d. A 40-y.o. female whose vehicle was traveling at 20 mph when she lost control and struck a hedge

Order

9.15. Arrange the steps to assess the patient in Scenario Three in order from the time you arrive on the scene until the time you reach the hospital.

   a. _____ Assess baseline vital signs

   b. _____ Perform a focused physical examination

   c. _____ Obtain the SAMPLE history

   d. _____ Perform the ongoing assessment

   e. _____ Perform the initial assessment

   f. _____ Call in the radio report

Multiple Choice

9.16. When you perform the rapid trauma assessment, what mnemonic do you use to remind you of the problems you are checking for?
   a. BTLS
   b. PSDE
   c. DCAP-BTLS
   d. OPQRST

9.17. The "S" in the correct answer to the previous question refers to:
   a. severity.
   b. swelling.
   c. signs/symptoms.
   d. significant MOI.

Scenario Four

You have been called to a car vs. deer collision. On arrival you find a 31-y.o. female still in the car. The vehicle's front end is dented, and the airbag has deployed. The patient has several minor abrasions and lacerations and is c/o pain in her right ankle. The right ankle is swollen and deformed. She tells you she was traveling approximately 35 mph when a deer darted onto the roadway in front of her. She has no significant past medical history, no known allergies, and takes ibuprofen occasionally for headaches as needed. Vital signs are BP—110/72; P—86, strong, regular; and R—20, shallow, nonlabored.

Your Plan of Action

Fill in the blank lines with your treatment plan for this patient. Then compare your plan with the questions, answers, and rationale.

1. _____
2. _____
3. _____
4. _____
5. _____
6. _____
7. _____
8. _____
9. _____

Multiple Choice

9.18. The *first* step as you begin to assess the patient would be to:
   a. remove her from the vehicle using a Kendrick extrication device (KED).
   b. assess the airway.
   c. assess the level of consciousness.
   d. form a general impression.

9.19. Because the airbag was deployed, you should:
  a. lift the airbag and check the steering wheel.
  b. check the patient's abdomen for seat belt bruising.
  c. wait for the fire department to extricate the patient.
  d. be less concerned about a significant MOI.

9.20. When you examine the patient's abdomen, you should:
  a. palpate first, then inspect, and auscultate.
  b. check for rebound tenderness.
  c. inform the patient which part of the examination you are doing.
  d. palpate using only the palm of your hand.

9.21. To evaluate the patient's mental status, you should ask her:
  a. who she is, where she is, and what day it is.
  b. who she is, where she is, and where she is employed.
  c. what day it is, who she is, and what happened.
  d. who she is, where she is, what day it is, and what happened.

Scenario Five

You have been dispatched to a car vs. motorcycle accident. A 28-y.o. male struck the car broadside and was ejected from his motorcycle. Bystanders tell you the car and motorcycle were both traveling at approximately 40 mph. The patient opens his eyes spontaneously and answers your questions appropriately. He is able to follow your instructions. Sensation and movement are present in all four extremities. His right thigh is painful, swollen, and deformed. Vital signs are BP—108/54; P—106, weak, regular; and R—22, shallow, regular.

> **Your Plan of Action**
> *Fill in the blank lines with your treatment plan for this patient. Then compare your plan with the questions, answers, and rationale.*
> 1. _____
> 2. _____
> 3. _____
> 4. _____
> 5. _____
> 6. _____
> 7. _____
> 8. _____
> 9. _____

Multiple Choice

9.22. The MOI of the motorcyclist would be a:
  a. lateral collision.
  b. rotational collision.
  c. head-on collision.
  d. rollover.

9.23. The motorcyclist's MOI is:
  a. not significant because he is conscious and alert.
  b. significant because of the speed.
  c. not significant because of the speed.
  d. significant because he is conscious and alert.

9.24. Which of these statements about the patient's extremity injury is *correct?*
  a. Femur fracture is frequently associated with a blood loss up to 1 liter.
  b. There is no reason for concern because distal movement and sensation are intact.
  c. Shock is unlikely because this is a closed injury.
  d. A traction splint should not be applied because this will delay transport.

9.25. The patient's Glasgow Coma Score is:
  a. 8.
  b. 11.
  c. 13.
  d. 15.

9.26. While you are transporting the patient to the hospital, you would:
  a. do a focused trauma examination and ongoing assessment every 15 minutes.
  b. perform an ongoing assessment every 5 minutes.
  c. do a detailed trauma examination, then perform an ongoing assessment every 5 minutes.
  d. perform an ongoing assessment every 10 minutes and contact the emergency department if there are any changes.

9.27. The "Golden Hour" is the time from:
  a. your arrival on scene until the patient is in surgery.
  b. receiving the call until the patient is at the hospital.
  c. when the injury occurs until the patient is in surgery.
  d. your arrival on scene until the patient is at the hospital.

9.28. All of these patients are candidates for air transport *except:*
  a. a 16-y.o. female involved in a high-speed MVC. She was ejected and is unconscious. Radial pulses are absent. Carotid pulses are rapid and weak.
  b. a 31-y.o. farmer who was riding a tractor when he rolled down an embankment. He has bruising across the chest and abdomen. He is unresponsive, pulseless, and apneic.
  c. a 5-y.o. male who was burned in a house fire. He is conscious but has 35% second-degree burns on his chest, abdomen, and extremities. His respirations are labored with wheezing and rhonchi in both lung fields.
  d. a 40-y.o. male who was just diagnosed with an abdominal aortic aneurysm. He is conscious and in extreme pain.

Answer Key—Chapter 9

SCENARIO ONE

Plan of Action

1. Body Substance Isolation (BSI)

2. Is the scene safe? Yes. (However, extreme caution should be exercised to reach this patient, and personnel involved in the rescue should wear appropriate protective equipment.) Assess MOI, number of patients, and need for additional resources.

3. Manually stabilize head and neck. Assess mental status. Ensure open airway, assess breathing, apply oxygen at 10-15 lpm, assist ventilations as needed, assess circulation, and begin treatment for shock as needed (external bleeding control, positioning, pneumatic antishock garment [PASG], and body heat conservation).

4. Determine priority, call for ALS, and consider air transport.

5. Apply cervical collar, long spine board, and cervical immobilization device.

6. Rapid trauma examination either en route to hospital or while waiting for air transport

7. Baseline vital signs en route to hospital or while waiting for air transport

8. SAMPLE en route to hospital or while waiting for air transport

9. Do detailed physical examination en route to hospital if time allows, continue ongoing assessment.

Rationale

The MOI and the patient's altered mental status indicate critical trauma. This patient should be transported as soon as possible so he can reach the operating room within the Golden Hour. After steps are taken on scene to ensure adequate airway, breathing, and circulation, the patient should be secured to a long spine board and transported. The rapid trauma assessment and care of specific injuries, such as splinting extremity fractures, can be performed en route as time allows.

9.1. B, The first step in the assessment process would be to do a scene size-up. Are there any dangers to you and your crew? Are there obstacles to reaching the patient? Is any additional equipment going to be needed? The initial assessment, including assessment of mental status and a check of the airway, would not be performed until you reach the patient.

9.2. D, An unresponsive patient would be at "U" on the AVPU scale.

9.3. C, A patient who is at "V" on the AVPU scale responds to verbal stimuli such as saying his or her name.

9.4. **C,** Spinal precautions should be initiated by manually stabilizing the head and neck at the same time the patient's mental status is assessed.

9.5. **C,** At this point the MOI and the transport decision should be reevaluated. Before the rapid trauma examination is performed, a decision must be made whether to assess the patient on the scene or to transport immediately and perform the examination en route. A focused history and physical examination would not be appropriate for this patient because of the MOI.

9.6. **B,** This patient fell a significant distance and therefore should be transported as soon as possible. A rapid trauma examination for any potentially life-threatening injuries is indicated, and spinal motion restriction should be performed before the patient is moved. However, this patient does not need to remain on scene for the time required to perform a detailed examination. If time allows, the detailed examination can be performed en route to the hospital.

9.7. **C,** Manual stabilization of the head and neck is initiated as soon as you begin to perform the initial assessment.

SCENARIO TWO

Plan of Action

1. BSI

2. Is the scene safe? Yes. Assess MOI, number of patients, and need for additional resources. Request additional ambulance or air transport because of number of patients.

3. Manually stabilize head and neck. Assess mental status. Ensure open airway, assess breathing, apply oxygen at 10-15 lpm, assist ventilations as needed, assess circulation, and begin treatment for shock as needed (external bleeding control, positioning, PASG, and body heat conservation).

4. Determine priority, call for ALS, and consider air transport.

5. Apply cervical collar, long spine board, and cervical immobilization device.

6. Rapid trauma examination either en route to hospital or while waiting for air transport

7. Baseline vital signs en route to hospital or while waiting for air transport

8. SAMPLE en route to hospital or while waiting for air transport

9. Do detailed physical examination en route to hospital if time allows, continue ongoing assessment.

Rationale

The MOI and initial presentation of both patients suggest critical trauma. Because the driver is unconscious, a head injury should be suspected. The passenger appears to have a femur fracture and probably has other significant trauma caused by her being ejected. Because both patients are critically injured, an additional ambulance or a helicopter should be requested. After initial care to stabilize the ABCs is performed, both patients should be rapidly transported to the hospital. The rapid trauma examination and management of specific injuries can be performed en route. Management of this call should be directed toward getting both patients to the operating room as quickly as possible.

9.8. C, The number of additional ambulances required is determined during the scene size-up.

9.9. D, The Glasgow Coma Scale is a numerical system to describe the patient's neurologic status.

Eye opening response	Spontaneous	4
	To voice	3
	To pain	2
	None	1
Best verbal response	Oriented × 4	5
	Confused	4
	Inappropriate words	3
	Incomprehensible words	2
	None	1
Best motor response	Obeys commands	6
	Localizes pain	5
	Withdraws from pain	4
	Flexion to pain	3
	Extension to pain	2
	None	1

9.10. A, You would open the airway using the modified jaw-thrust to limit movement of the cervical spine.

9.11. B, Critical trauma patients should have all of their clothing removed during the physical examination. If the patient is not undressed, injuries may be missed. When the examination is completed, the patient should be covered with a blanket to avoid hypothermia from loss of body heat.

9.12. C, Obtaining a pulse, blood pressure, and respiratory rate is *not* part of the initial assessment. The initial assessment includes forming a general impression, ensuring an open airway, assessing breathing, assessing circulation, and making a transport decision. Vital signs are not taken until after the initial assessment is completed and any life-threatening problems have been corrected.

SCENARIO THREE

Plan of Action

1. BSI
2. Is the scene safe? Yes. Evaluate MOI, number of patients, and need for additional resources.
3. Manually stabilize head and neck. Assess mental status. Ensure open airway, assess breathing, apply oxygen at 10-15 lpm, and assess circulation.
4. Determine priority, consider ALS.

Continued

SCENARIO THREE—cont'd

Plan of Action

5. Perform focused trauma assessment of back, neck, abdomen, and extremity motor/sensory function.

6. Baseline vital signs

7. SAMPLE

8. Apply cervical collar, extricate to long spine board using KED, cervical immobilization device.

9. Transport, perform ongoing assessment.

Rationale

The MOI is minor. The patient was traveling at only 20 mph and was wearing a seat belt. The vehicle did not impact a substantial object. The examination should focus on the patient's neck, back, and extremity motor/sensory function. Because she was wearing a seat belt, she also should be examined for restraint-related injuries. This patient should be extricated using the KED because she is stable but is complaining of neck and back pain.

9.13. **B,** A focused examination of the patient's neck, back, and abdomen would be appropriate. The patient was not traveling a high speed and did not strike a substantial fixed object. The examination should focus on her neck and back because she is experiencing pain there. Her abdomen should be examined for possible injuries caused by the seat belt. Because there is no significant MOI, the rapid trauma examination and detailed physical examination do not need to be performed. The ongoing examination would not be performed until the patient was en route to the hospital.

9.14. **C,** A vehicle-pedestrian accident would be a significant MOI. The other mechanisms described do not involve sufficient energy to be considered significant.

9.15. 3. **a.** Assess baseline vital signs
    2. **b.** Perform a focused physical examination
    4. **c.** Obtain the SAMPLE history
    6. **d.** Perform the ongoing assessment
    1. **e.** Perform the initial assessment
    5. **f.** Call in the radio report

9.16. **C,** Use DCAP-BTLS to remind you of problems to look for during the physical examination. Answer "A" is simply basic trauma life support. Answer "B" is painful, swollen, and deformed extremity. Answer "D" is a memory aid for questions to ask when you evaluate a chief complaint of pain.

9.17. **B,** The "S" in DCAP-BTLS refers to swelling.

SCENARIO FOUR

Plan of Action

1. BSI

2. Is the scene safe? Yes. Evaluate MOI, number of patients, and need for additional resources.

3. Manually stabilize head and neck. Assess mental status. Ensure open airway, assess breathing, apply oxygen at 10-15 lpm, and assess circulation.

4. Determine priority, consider ALS.

5. Focused trauma assessment focusing on injured ankle and superficial soft tissue injuries

6. Baseline vital signs

7. SAMPLE

8. Apply cervical collar, extricate to long spine board using KED, cervical immobilization device.

9. Transport, perform detailed physical examination, ongoing assessment en route.

Rationale

Because this patient was traveling at low speed and was wearing a seat belt, the trauma is not significant. The physical examination should focus on the injured ankle and the superficial abrasions and lacerations. Because the patient is stable, she can be extricated to a long spine board using a KED. In some EMS systems, this patient may be cleared of spinal injuries on the scene.

9.18. **D,** The first step in the initial assessment is to form a general impression. What happened to the patient? Is this a medical call or a trauma? What is the MOI? How badly sick or hurt does the patient appear to be? The general impression is a quick evaluation of the patient's overall appearance before you begin to look at the specifics of the initial assessment.

9.19. **A,** You should lift the airbag and check the steering wheel for damage.

9.20. **C,** You should tell the patient what you are doing and why you are doing it as you perform the examination. Confidence is gained when there are no surprises, and the patient feels more in control by being informed and being allowed to give consent for each step. During the abdominal examination auscultation should precede palpation because palpating the abdomen may cause the bowel to become falsely hyperactive. Rebound tenderness should *not* be checked in the field because the patient may become apprehensive when the examination must be repeated at the hospital. The fingers should be used for palpation instead of the palm because they are more sensitive.

9.21. **D,** To evaluate mental status you should check the patient's orientation to person, place, time, and events. Does she know who she is, where she is, what day it is, and what happened?

SCENARIO FIVE

Plan of Action

1. BSI
2. Is the scene safe? Yes. Assess MOI, number of patients, and need for additional resources.
3. Manually stabilize head and neck. Assess mental status. Ensure open airway, evaluate breathing, apply oxygen at 10-15 lpm, and assess circulation.
4. Determine priority, consider ALS.
5. Rapid trauma examination
6. Apply traction splint to right leg
7. Baseline vital signs
8. SAMPLE
9. Apply cervical collar, long spine board, and cervical immobilization device.
10. Transport, perform detailed physical examination, ongoing assessment en route.

Rationale

The MOI is significant because motorcyclists have almost no protection from impact and because both vehicles were traveling at 40 mph. The initial assessment of the patient suggests no immediate life-threatening injuries. However, his rapid, weak pulse and rapid, shallow respirations may indicate early shock caused by the femur fracture or undetected internal injuries. A rapid head-to-toe trauma examination should be performed to identify other injuries. A traction splint should be applied to the patient's leg to limit movement of the bone ends and help control bleeding at the fracture site. Application of the traction splint on scene is appropriate because the patient's ABCs are stable and the benefits of immobilizing the femur fracture outweigh the risks of a prolonged scene time.

9.22. **C,** The MOI for the motorcyclist is a head-on collision because the front of his motorcycle was the point of impact. The driver of the vehicle that the motorcycle hit suffered a lateral collision.

9.23. **B,** The MOI is significant because of the speed at which he and the car were traveling. In addition, motorcycle riders have much less protection than occupants of automobiles; therefore, the chance of injuries is much greater.

9.24. **A,** A femur fracture may cause up to 1 liter of blood loss into the soft tissues of the thigh. Although distal movement and sensation are intact, this injury is cause for concern because of the potential for blood loss. Shock can result from a closed femur fracture because of internal hemorrhaging at the fracture site. Because this patient appears to be stable, a traction splint should be applied before he is transported. Stabilizing the fractured femur with traction will reduce bleeding at the fracture site and decrease the risk of nerve and blood vessel damage.

9.25. D, The Glasgow Coma Score is 15. He opens his eyes spontaneously, scoring a 4. He answers questions appropriately and is oriented to person, place, time, and events, which rates a 5. He is able to follow your commands, scoring a 6. His total score is 4 + 5 + 6 = 15.

9.26. C, Because of the significant MOI and the nature of the patient's injuries, you would perform a detailed physical examination (if time permits) en route to the hospital, and do an ongoing assessment every 5 minutes.

9.27. C, The Golden Hour is the time from when the incident occurred until the patient is in surgery. Critical trauma patients have the greatest chance to survive if they reach the operating room within the Golden Hour.

9.28. B, This patient is in cardiac arrest from blunt trauma. Patients in cardiac arrest usually are not candidates for air transport.

10

Musculoskeletal Injuries

ANATOMY

The musculoskeletal system consists of bones, joints, muscles, tendons, ligaments, and cartilage.

- Bones—Connective tissue; living cells surrounded by a calcium phosphate matrix
  - Provide framework and support for the body
  - Provide protection of vital organs
  - Produce blood cells
  - Store calcium and phosphorus
  - Diaphysis—Hollow shaft of long bones. Contains yellow bone marrow
  - Metaphysis—The region between the diaphysis and the epiphysis
  - Epiphysis—Weight-bearing end of the bone
  - Periosteum—A white fibrous connective tissue covering the bone
- Muscles—Specialized tissue capable of contraction; produces movement
  - Skeletal muscle—Voluntary movements
  - Smooth muscle—Involuntary movements of body organs
  - Cardiac muscle—Heart beat; stimulates own contractions without outside stimulation (automaticity)
- Tendons—Connective tissue that joins muscle to bone (muscle—tendon—bone)
- Ligaments—Connective tissue that joins bone-to-bone at joints (bone—ligament—bone)
- Cartilage—Connective tissue; covers bone ends, aids in movement at joints
- Joints—Places where bones meet and articulate
- Axial skeleton—Forms central axis of body
  - Skull
    - Cranium—Brain case
    - Face
  - Spinal column
    - Cervical spine—Seven vertebrae
    - Thoracic spine—12 vertebrae
    - Lumbar spine—Five vertebrae
    - Sacral spine—Five fused vertebrae
    - Coccygeal spine—Three to five fused vertebrae; the "tail bone"
  - Thoracic cage
    - Ribs—12 pairs
    - Sternum—Breastbone
- Appendicular skeleton—Forms extremities; connects them to body
  - Shoulder girdle
    - Clavicle—Collarbone
    - Scapula—Shoulder blade
  - Upper extremity
    - Humerus—Upper arm
    - Radius—Thumb side of forearm
    - Ulna—Little finger side of forearm
    - Carpals—Wrist
    - Metacarpals—Palm of hand
    - Phalanges—Fingers
  - Pelvic girdle
    - Ilium
    - Ischium

- Pubis
○ Lower extremity
  - Femur—Thigh
  - Tibia—Shin; medial side of lower leg
  - Fibula—Lateral side of lower leg
  - Patella—Kneecap
  - Talus—Largest of the ankle bones
  - Calcaneus—Heel bone
  - Tarsals—Ankle
  - Metatarsals—Foot
  - Phalanges—Toes

TYPES OF MUSCULOSKELETAL INJURIES

- Closed extremity injury—An injury to a bone, ligament, or muscle with no break in the overlying skin
- Open extremity injury—An injury to a bone, ligament, or muscle with a break in the overlying skin. May be caused by a broken bone or a penetrating object
- Fracture—A break in a bone; may be open or closed
- Dislocation—Movement of the bone ends out of their normal positions at a joint
- Strain—Overstretching of a muscle
- Sprain—Overstretching or tearing of ligaments at a joint

SIGNS AND SYMPTOMS OF MUSCULOSKELETAL INJURIES

- Edema (swelling)
- Pain
- Tenderness
- Crepitation (grating from movement of the bone ends)
- Ecchymosis (bruising of the overlying skin)
- Deformity
- Joints "locked" out of position—Dislocation
- Nerve and blood vessel compromise—Examine for sensation, movement, pulses, distal skin color and temperature, and capillary refill

TYPES OF SPLINTS

- Padded board splints
- Conforming splints
- Vacuum splints
- Sling and swathe
- Pillow splint
- Traction splint

REVIEW QUESTIONS
Scenario One

A 7-y.o. male was rollerblading when he hit a hole in the pavement and fell. When you arrive he is c/o left elbow pain. The elbow is swollen, and the patient cannot straighten it. A 3-inch laceration on the left forearm is bleeding profusely. Bone fragments are visible in the laceration. The patient's skin is pale, cool, and dry. Vital signs are blood pressure (BP)—98/66; pulse (P)—120, weak, regular; and respiration (R)—24, shallow, regular. The patient can feel but cannot move his left hand. A weak radial pulse is present at the left wrist, but capillary refill in the left hand is 3 seconds. His parents are not present.

Your Plan of Action

Fill in the blank lines with your treatment plan for this patient. Then compare your plan with the questions, answers, and rationale.

1. _____
2. _____
3. _____
4. _____
5. _____
6. _____
7. _____
8. _____
9. _____

Multiple Choice

10.1. The structures that make up the musculoskeletal system include:
   a. muscles, bones, joints, and blood vessels.
   b. muscle, bones, and joints.
   c. muscles, bones, joints, connective tissue, and nerves.
   d. muscles, joints, bones, ligaments, and tendons.

10.2. If you are unable to easily determine whether a patient has a fracture, dislocation, or sprain involving an extremity, you may describe the situation by saying the patient has a:
   a. partially swollen deformed extremity.
   b. partially swollen disabled extremity.
   c. painful swollen deformed extremity.
   d. painful swollen dislocated extremity.

10.3. Careful assessment and management of extremity injuries can help to:
   a. reduce blood loss and prevent nerve injury.
   b. prevent nerve injury and avoid loss of function.
   c. prevent loss of function and reduce blood loss.
   d. reduce blood loss, prevent nerve injury, and prevent loss of function.

10.4. Your *initial* action to care for this patient would be to:
   a. assess for blood loss.
   b. assess for responsiveness.
   c. assess for circulation, sensation, and motion in the injured extremity.
   d. splint the extremity as found because the elbow is involved.

10.5. Which of the following would be your *most immediate* concern with this patient?
  a. His inability to move his elbow
  b. The bleeding
  c. His pale skin
  d. Your inability to reach his parents

10.6. All of the following statements about the musculoskeletal system are correct *except:*
  a. bones provide support for the body, acting as a framework.
  b. tendons hold bones together at joints.
  c. bones protect vital organs such as the brain, heart, and lungs.
  d. some bones produce blood cells.

10.7. How should you stabilize this patient's injured elbow?
  a. Apply a sling and swathe, elevating the wrist above the elbow.
  b. Place a splint from the shoulder to wrist, securing the joint above and the joint below. Apply a sling and swathe to support the limb, keeping the extremity in the position found.
  c. Place a rigid splint from the armpit to the fingertips. Using a roller bandage, secure the arm to the splint in the position most comfortable for the patient.
  d. Splint with an arm board from the elbow to beyond the fingertips, and use a sling and swathe for support and elevation.

10.8. Which of the following bones are found in the upper extremity?
  a. Humerus, radius, and fibula
  b. Humerus, ulna, and tarsals
  c. Radius, ulna, and humerus
  d. Ulna, radius, and metatarsals

10.9. During transport you should monitor this patient's:
  a. vital signs.
  b. capillary refill, motion, and sensation in the left hand.
  c. skin color, capillary refill, sensation, and movement of the left hand.
  d. blood pressure, pulse, respirations, skin color, and sensation and movement in the left hand.

Scenario Two

An 8-y.o. female was hiking with her parents in the Smoky Mountains when she fell over an 8-foot embankment, landing on her feet. Although she had a 2-inch laceration on her lower right leg, she was able to walk. However, 4 hours later she began to limp and to c/o pain in her right hip. The patient's skin is pink, warm, and dry. Capillary refill is <2 seconds. Her right thigh now seems swollen and discolored. As you immobilize her, you notice the right leg appears to be slightly shorter than the left, but no lateral rotation is present. Vital signs are BP—100/58; P—98, strong, regular; and R—22, shallow, nonlabored.

Your Plan of Action

Fill in the blank lines with your treatment plan for this patient. Then compare your plan with the questions, answers, and rationale.

1. _____
2. _____
3. _____
4. _____
5. _____
6. _____
7. _____
8. _____
9. _____

Multiple Choice

10.10. All of the following statements about splinting are correct *except:*
   a. splinting minimizes movement of broken bones.
   b. splinting decreases blood loss.
   c. splinting prevents further soft tissue and nerve damage.
   d. splinting increases the patient's pain.

True/False

10.11. The proximal pulse should be evaluated before and after splinting.
   a. True
   b. False

Multiple Choice

10.12. Where would you find the popliteal pulse?
   a. On the lateral aspect of the wrist
   b. On the dorsal surface of the foot
   c. Just inferior to the ankle
   d. Posterior to the knee

10.13. How much blood can be lost from a closed femur fracture?
   a. 100 mL
   b. 250 mL
   c. 500 mL
   d. 1000 mL

10.14. The hip is an example of which type of joint?
   a. Ball and socket
   b. Hinge
   c. Pivot
   d. Gliding

10.15. Circulation distal to this patient's injury would *best* be assessed by:
  a. asking her to move her fingers or toes.
  b. assessing sensation in the lower leg and foot.
  c. evaluating the distal skin temperature and color.
  d. palpating the femoral pulse.
10.16. This patient's *most likely* injury is a:
  a. fractured femur.
  b. dislocated hip.
  c. fractured hip.
  d. fractured fibula.
10.17. The finding that supports this diagnosis is the:
  a. swelling in the thigh.
  b. shortening of the leg.
  c. minimal amount of pain.
  d. laceration on the lower leg.
10.18. The mechanism of injury (MOI) in this case would be:
  a. direct force.
  b. indirect force.
  c. blunt force.
  d. torsion.

Matching

10.19. **a.** Epithelial tissue
  b. Muscle tissue
  c. Nervous tissue
  d. Connective tissue
  _____ Ligaments, tendons, blood, bone, fat, and cartilage
  _____ Comprises linings that cover internal and external body surfaces
  _____ Can contract, generating movement
  _____ Conducts electrical impulses that control and coordinate body functions

10.20. **a.** Bone
  b. Cartilage
  c. Tendons
  d. Ligaments
  _____ Attaches muscles to bones
  _____ Firm but flexible tissue that cushions bone ends at joints
  _____ Hard connective tissue consisting of living cells in a mineralized matrix
  _____ Attaches bones to other bones

Listing

10.21. List four functions of the skeletal system:
  1. _____
  2. _____
  3. _____
  4. _____

Scenario Three

Six-y.o. twin girls, Taylor and Jordan, were learning to ride the new bikes they had received for their birthday when they lost control on a hill and crashed into a wooden fence. They were wearing helmets. Jordan is complaining of left wrist and elbow pain. She is unable to move the extremity, but you are unable to assess sensation because she is crying loudly from the pain. Jordan's vital signs are BP—94/48; P—124, strong, regular; R—24, shallow, regular, and nonlabored; SaO_2—99%; and capillary refill—2 to 3 seconds. Taylor has profuse bright red bleeding from a laceration of the posterior right lower leg, just below the knee. She is c/o of little pain and has good sensation in the right foot. Taylor's vital signs are BP—74/44; P—136, weak, regular; R—26, shallow, regular, and nonlabored; SaO_2—95%; and capillary refill—4 seconds.

Your Plan of Action

Fill in the blank lines with your treatment plan for Taylor. Then compare your plan with the questions, answers, and rationale.

1. _____
2. _____
3. _____
4. _____
5. _____
6. _____
7. _____
8. _____
9. _____

Your Plan of Action

Fill in the blank lines with your treatment plan for Jordan. Then compare your plan with the questions, answers, and rationale.

1. _____
2. _____
3. _____
4. _____
5. _____
6. _____
7. _____
8. _____
9. _____

Multiple Choice

10.22. After completing initial assessment on both girls your *first* action should be to:
  a. immobilize Jordan's left arm and wrist.
  b. call the police to find the parents and get permission to treat and transport.
  c. immobilize Taylor's right leg because you suspect a knee injury.
  d. place a pressure dressing on the laceration just below Taylor's right knee.

10.23. The *most important* reason to splint a closed painful, swollen, and deformed extremity is to:
  a. cover any open soft tissue injuries.
  b. prevent further nerve, blood vessel, or soft tissue damage.
  c. allow the patient to move the injured extremity without pain.
  d. make the patient more comfortable and to make transportation easier.

10.24. General rules of splinting include:
  a. realigning open fractures by ensuring the bone ends are under the skin.
  b. splinting of all injuries before transport.
  c. avoiding extra padding because this may decrease the splint's effectiveness.
  d. checking for motor function, sensory response, and circulation before and after splinting.

10.25. A properly applied splint will immobilize the:
  a. injury site only.
  b. injury site and adjacent joints.
  c. entire body.
  d. injury site and one joint below if circulation is impaired.

10.26. Your *first* priority when treating a patient with an extremity injury is:
  a. ensuring the patient's airway, breathing, and circulation are adequate.
  b. splinting the injury and the bones and joints proximal and distal to the injury.
  c. applying direct pressure to stop all bleeding.
  d. assessing distal circulation, sensation, and movement in all injured extremities.

10.27. A significant MOI in a pediatric patient includes all of the following *except:*
  a. an event causing the death of another person in the same vehicle.
  b. any fall greater than 8 to 10 feet.
  c. any penetrating wounds to the trunk of the body.
  d. any bicycle accident.

10.28. Taylor keeps telling you not to touch her. Neither of her parents is available to give consent. You should:
  a. leave Taylor with the police until they find her parents.
  b. give Taylor some time to calm down and hope she will change her mind.
  c. send the police to find Taylor's parents.
  d. assume implied consent from Taylor's parents and treat her.

10.29. What is the anatomic relationship of the elbow to the hand?
  a. Distal
  b. Posterior
  c. Proximal
  d. Anterior

10.30. The two bones located in the lower leg are the:
  a. tibia, radius.
  b. humerus, fibula.
  c. ulna, tibia.
  d. tibia, fibula.

10.31. An injury to Jordan's metacarpals may interfere with her ability to:

    a. jump.

    b. write.

    c. walk.

    d. squat.

10.32. If Jordan fractured her humerus, which artery may be involved?

    a. Subclavian

    b. Radial

    c. Ulnar

    d. Brachial

Scenario Four

A 48-y.o. female was walking to work when she slipped and fell on the ice. She put her right arm out to catch herself and now is c/o severe right wrist and forearm pain. An obvious deformity of the right wrist is present. The patient is alert and oriented × 4. Her skin is pink, cool, and dry. She has no significant past medical history and no known allergies. The vital signs reported to you by fire department first responders are BP—148/98; P—122, strong, regular; and R—18, shallow, regular, and nonlabored.

Your Plan of Action

Fill in the blank lines with your treatment plan for this patient. Then compare your plan with the questions, answers, and rationale.

1. _____

2. _____

3. _____

4. _____

5. _____

6. _____

7. _____

8. _____

9. _____

Multiple Choice

10.33. Your *first* action to care for this patient would be to:

    a. obtain a new set of vital signs.

    b. apply an ice pack to reduce the swelling.

    c. elevate the wrist and hand to reduce the swelling.

    d. manually stabilize the right arm and hand, then apply a splint.

10.34. When you examine the injured extremity, crepitation is present. Crepitation is:

    a. discoloration of the skin caused by bleeding.

    b. usually present when a distal pulse is absent.

    c. the sound or sensation caused by broken bone ends rubbing together.

    d. caused by edema associated with a closed fracture.

True/False

10.35. A dislocation is an injury to muscles, ligaments, and tendons.
- **a.** True
- **b.** False

Multiple Choice

10.36. When a closed fracture is present:
- **a.** there is a break in the bone, but the overlying skin is intact.
- **b.** the bone ends have separated at the fracture site.
- **c.** the bone ends have separated at a joint, causing obvious deformity.
- **d.** there is always a hematoma from bleeding under the skin.

10.37. Circulation, sensation, and movement distal to a fracture site should be checked:
- **a.** after manual stabilization is applied.
- **b.** before manual stabilization is applied.
- **c.** before the splint is applied.
- **d.** before any bandages are applied.

10.38. A traction splint would be used to immobilize a fracture of the:
- **a.** femur or humerus.
- **b.** femur or tibia and fibula.
- **c.** tibia and fibula.
- **d.** femur.

10.39. The *best* splint to use for the patient described in Scenario Four would be:
- **a.** a padded short board splint, sling, and swathe.
- **b.** a padded long board splint.
- **c.** an air splint.
- **d.** a pillow splint.

10.40. You would expect to find all of the following in a patient with a musculoskeletal injury *except:*
- **a.** pain, tenderness at the injury site.
- **b.** swelling.
- **c.** crepitation on movement.
- **d.** full range of motion in the injured extremity.

10.41. Which of the following *best* describes anatomic position?
- **a.** Lying in the supine position, with the palms facing downward
- **b.** Standing, facing forward, with the palms facing forward
- **c.** Lying in the prone position, with the palms facing upward
- **d.** Standing, facing backward, with the palms facing backward

10.42. The major artery in the thigh is the:
- **a.** posterior tibial.
- **b.** femoral.
- **c.** popliteal.
- **d.** dorsal pedal.

Scenario Five

A 24-y.o. male who was involved in a motorcycle crash is complaining of pain in his left thigh. During the crash, he separated from his motorcycle. Examination reveals ecchymosis and swelling of the left thigh with external rotation of the extremity. Vital signs are BP—110/58; P—116, weak regular; R—22, shallow, regular, and nonlabored; and SaO$_2$—97%. He has no known allergies and takes no medications.

Your Plan of Action

Fill in the blank lines with your treatment plan for this patient. Then compare your plan with the questions, answers, and rationale.

1. _____
2. _____
3. _____
4. _____
5. _____
6. _____
7. _____
8. _____
9. _____

Multiple Choice

10.43. The *best* technique to immobilize this patient's injury would be to:
   a. apply pillow splint.
   b. apply a traction splint.
   c. apply a long padded board splint.
   d. secure the injured leg to the uninjured leg.

10.44. Ecchymosis near the injury site suggests:
   a. bleeding underneath the skin surface.
   b. impaired circulation to the distal extremity.
   c. infection of the tissue around the injury site.
   d. abnormal neurologic response of the injured extremity.

10.45. Which end of the femur is closer to the knee?
   a. Distal
   b. Proximal
   c. Lateral
   d. Medial

10.46. When a traction splint is being applied, manual traction should be maintained until:
   a. the traction splint has been placed under the injured leg.
   b. the ankle hitch is secured to the splint.
   c. mechanical traction has been applied, and all straps are secured.
   d. distal pulses, color, sensation, and movement have been rechecked.

Scenario Six

An 86-y.o. female fell when getting out of bed. You find her on the floor, conscious, alert, and oriented × 4. Her right leg appears shortened and is laterally rotated. Vital signs are BP—136/82; R—86, strong, regular; and R—16, regular, nonlabored.

Your Plan of Action

Fill in the blank lines with your treatment plan for this patient. Then compare your plan with the questions, answers, and rationale.

1. _____
2. _____
3. _____
4. _____
5. _____
6. _____
7. _____
8. _____
9. _____

Multiple Choice

10.47. You should suspect a:
    a. fractured right femur.
    b. fractured right hip.
    c. dislocated right hip.
    d. dislocated right knee.

10.48. You would immobilize this patient by applying a:
    a. traction splint on the right leg.
    b. pillow splint on the right foot and ankle.
    c. long board splint for the right leg.
    d. long spine board for full body immobilization.

10.49. An open fracture is defined as a break in the continuity of a bone with:
    a. associated tissue and nerve damage.
    b. an associated break in the skin.
    c. associated loss of movement.
    d. associated ecchymosis and swelling.

10.50. After you checked this patient's level of consciousness, airway, breathing, and circulation, your *next* action should have been to:
    a. take a complete set of vital signs.
    b. begin spinal motion restriction using a cervical collar and long spine board.
    c. begin a head-to-toe trauma assessment.
    d. identify her priority for transport.

10.51. The bones of the lower extremity include the:
    a. tibia, acetabulum, calcaneus, and phalanges.
    b. femur, tibia, phalanges, and fibula.
    c. femur, ulna, tibia, and phalanges.
    d. femur, tibia, fibula, tarsals, and metatarsals.

Answer Key—Chapter 10

SCENARIO ONE

Plan of Action

1. Body Substance Isolation (BSI)

2. Is the scene safe? Yes. Assess MOI, number of patients, and need for additional resources.

3. Manually stabilize head and neck. Assess mental status. Ensure open airway, assess breathing, apply oxygen at 10-15 lpm, assess circulation, and control bleeding.

4. Determine priority. Consider advanced life support (ALS).

5. Focused assessment of left upper extremity

6. Baseline vital signs

7. SAMPLE

8. Splint left upper extremity.

9. Apply cervical collar, long spine board, and cervical immobilization device.

10. Transport, provide ongoing assessment.

Rationale

The most immediate objective in this case is to control the bleeding from the forearm laceration. Because children have smaller blood volumes than adults, smaller amounts of blood loss can cause hypovolemic shock. Because the MOI is not significant, the assessment can focus on the elbow and forearm injury, which should be splinted before the patient is transported.

10.1. **D,** Muscles, joints, bones, ligaments, and tendons are musculoskeletal system structures. Cartilage also is part of the musculoskeletal system. Blood vessels are part of the circulatory system. Nerves are part of the nervous system.

10.2. **C,** "Painful, swollen, deformed extremity" is a phrase that can be used to describe an injury when you cannot easily distinguish between a fracture, a dislocation, and a sprain.

10.3. **D,** Careful assessment and management of extremity injuries can reduce blood loss, prevent nerve injury, and prevent loss of extremity function.

10.4. **B,** The first step to care for any patient is to perform an initial assessment, beginning with mental status. This involves assessing responsiveness, ensuring an open airway, and checking for effective breathing and circulation. Although extremity injuries frequently are dramatic and tend to attract your attention, life-threatening problems must always be identified and corrected first.

10.5. **B,** Your most immediate concern with this patient is the bleeding at the injury site. Because children have smaller blood volumes, less blood loss is required to produce hypovolemic shock. The external bleeding should be controlled as quickly as possible by applying direct pressure. The patient's inability to move his elbow may be a result of the fracture or dislocation, but it is not as immediate a concern as the bleeding. The patient's pale skin may indicate he is in the early stages of shock, a problem you can help begin to correct by controlling the bleeding. Your inability to locate the patient's parents is not an immediate concern because their consent to treat him is implied.

10.6. **B,** The tough fibrous tissues that hold bones together at joints are ligaments, not tendons.

10.7. **B,** Because he has an injury to the elbow, you must splint the elbow and the bones above and below the elbow. This means the wrist and shoulder also must be immobilized. A splint secured from the shoulder to the wrist will limit movement of the elbow. A sling and swathe will hold the arm to the body, limiting movement of the shoulder and the wrist.

10.8. **C,** The upper extremity includes the radius, ulna, and humerus. The fibula, tarsals, and metatarsals are found in the lower extremity.

10.9. **D,** During transport, you want to keep track of the patient's vital signs and skin color and the motor and sensory function in his left hand.

SCENARIO TWO

Plan of Action

1. BSI

2. Is the scene safe? Yes. Assess MOI, number of patients, and need for additional resources.

3. Assess mental status. Ensure open airway, assess breathing, apply oxygen at 10-15 lpm, and assess circulatory status.

4. Determine priority. Consider ALS, air transport.

5. Focused trauma assessment of left lower extremity

6. Baseline vital signs

7. SAMPLE

8. Splint left lower extremity.

9. Secure patient to long spine board.

10. Transport, provide ongoing assessment.

Rationale

Because the patient has shortening of her right thigh associated with pain and swelling, she may have suffered a greenstick fracture of her femur. The right leg should be splinted, and the patient should be placed on a long spine board or in a basket stretcher to make moving her from the mountain easier. Depending on your location, air transport may be considered. Although the patient shows no signs of poor perfusion, she should receive ongoing monitoring during transport for shock caused by bleeding at the fracture site.

10.10. D, Splinting *decreases* the patient's pain by limiting movement at the injury site.

10.11. B, You should evaluate the *distal* pulse before and after splinting.

10.12. D, The popliteal pulse is posterior to (behind) the knee.

10.13. D, A femur fracture may cause up to 1000 mL of blood loss.

10.14. A, The hip is a ball and socket joint. The elbow and finger joints are examples of hinge joints. The joint in the forearm that allows the radius to rotate around the ulna is a pivot joint. The wrist is a gliding joint.

10.15. C, The best way to evaluate circulation distal to this injury is to check distal skin color and temperature. Movement and sensation could be affected by direct injury to nerves and therefore would not provide information about circulation that would be as accurate as skin color and temperature. The femoral pulse is proximal to the injury and therefore would not provide information about distal circulation.

10.16. A, This patient most likely has a fracture of the femur. A hip fracture would cause lateral rotation of the leg. A hip dislocation would cause lateral or medial rotation of the leg, depending on the direction the head of the femur was displaced from the acetabulum. A fracture of the fibula would not produce swelling of the thigh.

10.17. A, Swelling in the thigh supports the diagnosis of a femur fracture. Shortening of the leg also could be associated with a hip injury.

10.18. B, The patient's femur being injured by her landing on her feet is an example of indirect force because the injury is located in a part of the body away from the original impact.

10.19. d, Connective tissue includes ligaments, tendons, bone, fat, and cartilage.

   a, Epithelial tissue comprises linings that cover internal and external body surfaces.

   b, Muscle tissue can contract, generating movement.

   c, Nervous tissue conducts electrical impulses that control and coordinate body functions.

10.20. c, Tendons attach muscles to bones.

   b, Cartilage is a firm but flexible tissue that cushions bone ends at joints and allows the bones to move smoothly.

   a, Bone is a hard, connective tissue that consists of living cells in a mineralized matrix.

   d, Ligaments attach bones to other bones.

10.21. Functions of the skeletal system include protecting vital organs from injury, providing a framework and support for the body, allowing for movement, producing blood cells, and storing minerals (e.g., calcium, phosphorus).

SCENARIO THREE (TAYLOR)

Plan of Action
1. BSI
2. Is the scene safe? Yes. Assess MOI, number of patients, and need for additional resources.
3. Manual stabilization of head and neck. Assess the mental status. Ensure open airway, assess breathing, apply oxygen 10-15 lpm, assess circulatory status, and control bleeding from right lower leg laceration.
4. Determine priority. Consider ALS, air transport.
5. Rapid trauma examination
6. Apply cervical collar, long spine board, and cervical immobilization device.
7. Baseline vital signs
8. SAMPLE
9. During transport do detailed physical examination if time permits and perform ongoing assessment.

Rationale
Taylor appears to have lacerated an artery in her lower leg. The bleeding should be controlled as quickly as possible using direct pressure. She is hypotensive and very tachycardic, indicating decompensated shock. High-concentration oxygen should be administered, and she should be placed supine on a spine board with her lower extremities elevated. Air transport should be considered. If air transport is not available, Taylor should be transported by ground ambulance immediately. An ALS ambulance could be called to meet you en route. However, there should be no delays in getting Taylor to definitive care.

SCENARIO THREE (JORDAN)

Plan of Action
1. BSI
2. Is the scene safe? Yes. Assess MOI, number of patients, and need for additional resources.
3. Manual stabilization of head and neck. Assess mental status. Ensure open airway, assess breathing, apply oxygen at 10-15 lpm, and assess circulatory status.

Continued

SCENARIO THREE (JORDAN)—cont'd

Plan of Action

4. Determine priority, consider ALS.

5. Rapid trauma examination

6. Apply cervical collar, long spine board, and cervical immobilization device.

7. Baseline vital signs

8. SAMPLE

9. Do a detailed physical examination if time permits and perform ongoing assessment en route.

Rationale

Jordan does not appear to be as seriously injured as Taylor. However, because Taylor has significant trauma from essentially the same event, you should perform a rapid trauma examination on Jordan rather than simply focusing on her extremity. Splint the injured extremity, and place her on a spine board with a cervical collar and cervical immobilization device. If air transport is not readily available, Jordan may have to be rapidly transported by ground along with Taylor.

10.22. **D,** Place a pressure dressing on the laceration below Taylor's right knee. The most immediate problem is Taylor's external bleeding because children have small blood volumes and can easily develop hypovolemic shock.

10.23. **B,** Preventing further nerve, blood vessel, or soft tissue damage is the most important reason for splinting. Covering open soft tissue injuries is the purpose of bandaging rather than splinting. Although splinting will reduce pain, the patient should not be able to move a splinted extremity. Although effective splinting will make transporting the patient easier, this is not the most important reason to apply a splint.

10.24. **D,** Circulation, sensation, and motor response should be checked before and after splinting. Although a fracture may have to be realigned for effective splinting, bone ends should *not* be pulled back under the skin because this increases the risk of infection. If a patient's airway, breathing, or circulation is impaired by his or her injuries, the need for rapid transport for surgery may make splinting of all injuries impossible. Adequate padding increases rather than decreases the effectiveness of splinting by allowing the splint to conform to the extremity.

10.25. **B,** A properly applied splint will immobilize the injury site, the joint above, and the joint below.

10.26. A, Your first priority when treating an extremity injury is to ensure the patient's airway, breathing, and circulation are adequate. Evaluation of the extremity or application of splints should not be initiated until all potentially life-threatening problems are identified and corrected. Although correction of life-threatening external bleeding is a priority in the initial assessment, small amounts of external bleeding may have a lower priority than stabilizing a major long bone fracture that is producing significant internal blood loss.

10.27. D, A bicycle accident is not necessarily a significant MOI in a pediatric patient.

10.28. D, Because Taylor has what reasonably appears to be a life-threatening injury and her parents are not available, their consent to treat her is implied.

10.29. C, The elbow is proximal to the hand because it lies closer to the origin of the extremity (the shoulder) than the hand.

10.30. D, The tibia and fibula are located in the lower leg. The radius and ulna are found in the forearm.

10.31. B, Because the metacarpals are located in the hand, a serious injury here would be most likely to interfere with Jordan's ability to write.

10.32. D, The brachial artery is most likely to be injured by a humerus fracture. The subclavian artery is located in the chest just below the clavicle. The radial and ulnar arteries are located in the forearm.

SCENARIO FOUR

Plan of Action
1. BSI
2. Is the scene safe? Yes. Assess MOI, number of patients, and need for additional resources.
3. Assess the mental status. Ensure open airway, assess breathing, apply oxygen 10-15 lpm, and assess circulatory status.
4. Determine priority.
5. Focused trauma assessment of right upper extremity
6. Splint injury.
7. Baseline vital signs
8. SAMPLE
9. Transport, provide ongoing assessment.

Rationale
There is no significant MOI. The initial assessment identifies no life-threatening problems. The patient has no other complaints, is alert, and is oriented to person, place, time, and events. The examination can focus on the painful, swollen, and deformed right upper extremity.

10.33. **D,** Your first action would be to manually stabilize the right arm and apply a splint. The hand and forearm can be elevated, and an ice pack can be applied to the fracture site to reduce swelling after a splint is applied. Because the patient is awake and oriented and appears to have only an isolated extremity injury, there is no reason to immediately obtain another set of vital signs.

10.34. **C,** Crepitation is the sound or sensation caused by broken bone ends rubbing together. Although crepitation may be found during an assessment, it should *never* be actively sought.

10.35. **B,** A dislocation is the disruption or separation of bones at a joint.

10.36. **A,** When a closed fracture is present, the bone is broken, but the overlying skin is intact.

10.37. **B,** Distal circulation, motion, and sensation should be checked before manual stabilization is applied. You also would check after the splint is applied to determine whether any changes have occurred.

10.38. **D,** Traction splints are used to immobilize femur fractures.

10.39. **A,** Because the patient has a fracture of the wrist and forearm, the best splint would be a padded short board splint, sling, and swathe. A long board splint would extend from the shoulder to the fingertips, making it difficult for the patient to sit up or move. An air splint could be used to stabilize the forearm, but a sling and swathe would be necessary to adequately immobilize the elbow after the air splint was in place. Also, air splints may change pressure when they are moved from a cold environment to a hot environment. A pillow splint would be more useful for an ankle injury.

10.40. **D,** You would *not* expect to find a full range of motion in an injured extremity.

10.41. **B,** The anatomic position is standing, facing forward with the palms facing forward.

10.42. **B,** The femoral artery is the main artery in the thigh. The posterior tibial artery is located behind the medial malleolus (medial ankle). The popliteal artery is located behind the knee. The dorsal pedal artery is on the dorsal (top) surface of the foot.

SCENARIO FIVE

Plan of Action

1. BSI

2. Is the scene safe? Yes. Assess MOI, number of patients, and need for additional resources.

3. Manual stabilization of head and neck. Assess mental status. Ensure open airway, assess breathing, apply oxygen at 10-15 lpm, and assess circulatory status.

4. Determine priority, consider ALS.

Continued

SCENARIO FIVE—cont'd

Plan of Action

5. Rapid trauma examination

6. Baseline vital signs

7. SAMPLE

8. Apply traction splint to femur fracture.

9. Apply cervical collar, long spine board, and cervical immobilization device.

10. Transport. Perform detailed assessment if time allows and provide ongoing assessment.

Rationale

The initial assessment reveals no immediate life-threatening injuries. However, there is a significant MOI, and sufficient force was involved to produce a femur fracture. A rapid trauma examination should be performed to identify any undetected potentially life-threatening problems. A traction splint should be applied to the fractured femur, and the patient should be secured to a long spine board with a cervical collar and cervical immobilization device. ALS should be considered because of the potential for significant internal blood loss at the fracture site.

10.43. **B,** A femur fracture is best splinted with a traction splint. The traction will help overcome spasms in the thigh's large muscles, stabilizing the bone ends, lessening pain, and reducing soft tissue damage.

10.44. **A,** Ecchymosis (bruising) near the injury site suggests bleeding underneath the skin surface. A pale, cool distal extremity with weak or absent pulses suggests impaired distal circulation. Absent or altered sensation or movement indicates nerve involvement. Although infection is unlikely in this situation, the indicators of infection at an injury site are redness, warmth, pain, swelling, and the presence of pus.

10.45. **A,** Distal means farther from the point of origin of a structure. Because the point of origin of the femur is the hip joint, the end closer to the knee is the distal end.

10.46. **C,** Manual traction is applied until mechanical traction has been applied and all straps are secured.

SCENARIO SIX

Plan of Action

1. BSI

2. Is the scene safe? Yes. Assess MOI, number of patients, and need for additional resources.

3. Manual stabilization of head and neck. Assess mental status. Ensure open airway, assess breathing, apply oxygen at 10-15 lpm, and assess circulatory status.

4. Determine priority.

5. Rapid trauma assessment

6. Baseline vital signs

7. SAMPLE

8. Use long spine board to immobilize the hip. Consider full spinal motion restriction based on evaluation of MOI and results of rapid trauma examination.

9. Transport.

Rationale

The initial assessment reveals no immediately life-threatening problems. Normally, a fall out of bed would not be a significant MOI. However, older patients—particularly older females—may suffer from osteoporosis. MOIs unlikely to produce significant injuries in younger people may lead to multiple fractures. This patient should receive a rapid trauma assessment to identify injuries that may be present in addition to her fractured hip. Padding should be placed between her legs; her legs should be secured together; and she should be placed on a long spine board to stabilize her fractured hip. Based on the results of the rapid trauma assessment, application of a cervical collar and cervical immobilization device should be considered.

10.47. **B,** Shortening and lateral rotation of the leg suggest a hip fracture.

10.48. **D,** This patient should be placed on a long spine board for full body immobilization. Geriatric patients—particularly older females—tend to have fragile bones that break with minimal force. Because this patient fell out of bed, she may have suffered other fractures, including possible spinal injuries.

10.49. **B,** An open fracture is a break in the continuity of a bone associated with a break in the continuity of the overlying soft tissues.

10.50. **D,** The next step after completing the initial assessment is to determine the patient's priority for transport. Does the patient need immediate transport to the hospital for definitive care, or can she be stabilized more completely on the scene before being moved?

10.51. **D,** Bones of the lower extremity include the femur, tibia, fibula, tarsals, and metatarsals. The acetabulum is the depression in the pelvis that articulates with the head of the femur. The ulna is located in the upper extremity.

11

Head and Spinal Injuries

ANATOMY

- Skull—Bony box that surrounds and protects brain. Composed of:
  - Cranium (brain case)
    - Frontal bone
    - Parietal bones
    - Temporal bones
    - Occipital bone
  - Face
    - Orbits—Eye sockets
    - Nasal bones—Proximal ⅓ of bridge of nose
    - Mandible—Lower jaw
    - Maxilla—Upper jaw
    - Zygoma—Cheek bones
- Spine—Extends from base of skull to pelvis. Surrounds, protects spinal cord
  - 33 vertebrae
  - Five sections
    - Cervical spine—Seven vertebrae
    - Thoracic spine—12 vertebrae
    - Lumbar spine—Five vertebrae
    - Sacral spine—Five fused vertebrae. Joins spine to pelvis
    - Coccygeal spine—Three to five fused vertebrae. "Tail bone"
- Meninges—Protective membranes enclosing brain and spinal cord
  - Dura mater—Tough, fibrous outer layer
  - Arachnoid—Middle layer. Resembles a spider (arachnid) web
  - Pia mater—Thin, vascular inner layer
- Meningeal spaces
  - Epidural space—Between bone and dura mater
  - Subdural space—Between dura mater and arachnoid
  - Subarachnoid space—Between arachnoid and pia mater
- Central nervous system (CNS)
  - Brain
    - Cerebrum—Conscious sensation and movement, thought, and memory
    - Cerebellum—Posture, balance, and equilibrium; coordination of complex movements
    - Brain stem—Autonomic functions. Breathing, heart rate, and peripheral vascular resistance
  - Spinal cord
    - Carries nerve impulses between brain and body
    - Reflexes

TYPES OF SKULL FRACTURES

- Linear
  - Straight line crack in skull
  - Diagnosed with x-rays
  - Can be suspected after hard blows to head, especially with overlying soft tissue damage
  - No out-of-hospital treatment
  - Consider possible presence of cervical spine injury
- Stellate
  - Starlike fracture with multiple cracks radiating from central point

- ○ Diagnosed with x-rays
- ○ Can be suspected after hard blows to head, especially with overlying soft tissue damage
- ○ No out-of-hospital treatment
- ○ Consider possible presence of cervical spine injury
- Depressed
  - ○ Segment of bone is detached, moved below level of rest of skull
  - ○ Deformity in skull felt, seen
  - ○ Major concern is damage to brain
  - ○ Consider possible presence of cervical spine injury
- Basilar
  - ○ Fracture through floor of cranial cavity (brain case)
  - ○ Difficult to detect on x-ray
  - ○ Blood or clear fluid (cerebrospinal fluid [CSF]) from nose, ears
  - ○ Bruising around both eyes (periorbital ecchymosis, raccoon's eyes)
  - ○ Bruising over mastoid process behind ear (Battle's sign)
- Open
  - ○ Skull, overlying scalp opened
  - ○ Brain exposed
  - ○ Manage as evisceration, cover with moist, sterile dressings

TYPES OF INTRACRANIAL INJURIES

- Concussion
  - ○ Sudden movement of brain within skull disrupts nerve impulse movement
  - ○ Brief loss of consciousness (<5 minutes)
  - ○ Patient cannot remember injury event or immediately preceding events (retrograde amnesia)
  - ○ No neurologic deficits remain after patient awakens
  - ○ With severe concussion some patients experience persistent irritability, depression, and headaches (postconcussion syndrome)
- Cerebral contusion
  - ○ Impact of brain against skull bruises brain tissue
    - ■ Coup—Injury on side of initial blow or impact
    - ■ Contrecoup—Injury opposite side of initial blow or impact
  - ○ Prolonged loss of consciousness (>5 minutes)
  - ○ Some may experience coma lasting for months
  - ○ Neurologic deficits related to location of contusion
  - ○ Associated edema may cause increased intracranial pressure
- Cerebral laceration
  - ○ Penetrating trauma or movement of brain across projections on floor of skull during sudden decelerations
  - ○ Neurologic deficits related to location of lacerations
  - ○ Associated edema may cause increased intracranial pressure
- Epidural hematoma
  - ○ Impact to head tears arteries between skull and dura mater
  - ○ Bleeding occurs in epidural space, causing increased intracranial pressure
  - ○ Patient unconscious initially, then awakens and appears uninjured (lucid interval), followed by rapid deterioration
  - ○ Headache

  ○ Nausea, vomiting
  ○ Weakness or paralysis of one side of body
  ○ Altered mental status
  ○ Unequal pupils (dilated pupil is on side of hematoma)
  ○ Cushing's triad (slowing pulse, increasing blood pressure [BP], and altered respiratory pattern)
- Subdural hematoma
  ○ Impact to head tears veins between dura mater and arachnoid
  ○ Bleeding occurs in subdural space, causing increased intracranial pressure
  ○ Signs, symptoms resemble those of epidural hematoma but have slower onset (hours to days)
  ○ Common in older persons after blows to head; may mimic stroke
- Intracerebral hematoma
  ○ Bleeding within brain itself
  ○ Penetrating trauma, sudden decelerations leading to vessel tearing
  ○ Neurologic deficits related to location of hematomas
  ○ Hematomas cause increased intracranial pressure

SPINAL AND SPINAL CORD INJURY

- Injury to the spinal cord can cause:
  ○ Death from respiratory failure
  ○ Neurogenic (spinal) shock
  ○ Permanent disability (paraplegia or quadriplegia)
- Not all spinal injuries initially result in spinal cord injury
- Twenty-five percent of spinal cord injuries result from improper handling or spinal motion restriction techniques
- Indicators of possible spinal and spinal cord injury
  ○ Mechanism of injury (MOI)—Any mechanism that causes abnormal motion of the spine—hyperflexion, hyperextension, lateral bending, rotation, compression, and distraction
  ○ Altered mental status—Unresponsive patients should be assumed to have a spinal injury
  ○ Blunt trauma above the level of the clavicles
  ○ Pain in or adjacent to the spine
  ○ Tenderness of the spine
  ○ Paralysis or weakness
  ○ Abnormal sensation (tingling, numbness)
  ○ Impaired breathing caused by chest wall paralysis
  ○ Hypotension associated with normal or low heart rate and dry skin
  ○ Loss of bladder, bowel control
  ○ Priapism (persistent, nonsexual erection)

BRIEF NEUROLOGIC EXAMINATION

- Apply manual stabilization to head and neck
- Ask patient to move fingers and toes
- Ask the patient to grip your hands and squeeze both simultaneously. Compare the strength. Is it equal in both hands?
- Ask the patient to push with his or her feet against your hands. Compare the strength. Is it equal in both feet?
- Ask the patient if he or she can feel you touching his or her fingers or toes

SPINAL MOTION RESTRICTION
Devices
- Cervical collars (rigid collars limit approximately 50% of movement of cervical spine)
  - Stiff-neck collar
  - Philadelphia collar
  - Nec-loc collar
- Long spine board
- Short spine board
- Full body immobilizer
- Vest-type immobilizers

Seated Patient
- Body substance isolation procedures
- Place, maintain head in neutral in-line position
- Maintain manual stabilization of head and neck
- Reassess motor, sensory, and circulatory function in each extremity
- Apply appropriately sized extrication collar
- Position immobilization device behind patient
- Secure device to patient's torso
- Evaluate torso fixation, adjust as necessary
- Evaluate, pad behind patient's head as necessary
- Secure patient's head to device
- Move patient to long board
- Reassess motor, sensory, and circulatory function in each extremity

Supine Patient
- Body substance isolation procedures
- Place, maintain head in neutral in-line position
- Maintain manual stabilization of head and neck
- Reassess motor, sensory, and circulatory function in each extremity
- Apply appropriately sized extrication collar
- Position immobilization device appropriately
- Move patient to device without compromising integrity of spine
- Apply padding to voids between torso and board as necessary
- Immobilize patient's torso to device
- Pad behind head as necessary
- Immobilize patient's head to device
- Secure patient's legs to device
- Secure patient's arms to device
- Reassess motor, sensory, and circulatory function in each extremity

REVIEW QUESTIONS
Scenario One

A 19-y.o. female was involved a two-car motor vehicle collision (MVC). She was not wearing a seat belt. The patient is conscious and is c/o a headache, left arm pain, and right lower leg pain. She says she did not lose consciousness, but she repeatedly asks you where she is and what happened. The driver of the other vehicle tells you the patient suddenly veered into his lane, and they hit head-on at approximately 40 mph. The patient reports no significant past medical history. Vital signs are BP—102/50; pulse (P)—96, strong, regular; respiration (R)—22, shallow, regular; and SaO_2—97%.

Your Plan of Action

Fill in the blank lines with your treatment plan for this patient. Then compare your plan with the questions, answers, and rationale.

1. _____
2. _____
3. _____
4. _____
5. _____
6. _____
7. _____
8. _____
9. _____

Multiple Choice

11.1. When you made contact with the patient your *first* action should have been to:
   a. restrict motion of the cervical spine using a hard cervical collar.
   b. obtain a set of vital signs.
   c. assess mental status, airway, breathing, and circulation.
   d. perform a rapid head-to-toe trauma examination.

11.2. When patients are oriented × 4, this means they know:
   a. where they are, how they arrived there, who their family is, and what their past medical history is.
   b. who they are, where they are, what happened, and who the President of the United States is.
   c. who they are, where they are, what day it is, and what happened.
   d. who they are, where they are, what day it is, and if they had anyone riding with them.

11.3. The brain and spinal cord also are known as the:
   a. autonomic nervous system.
   b. voluntary nervous system.
   c. peripheral nervous system.
   d. central nervous system.

11.4. How many vertebrae are found in the thoracic spine?
   a. Three to five
   b. Five
   c. Seven
   d. 12

11.5. An open head injury is a:
   a. scalp laceration with the underlying skull bones remaining intact.
   b. skull fracture with no laceration of or break in the scalp.
   c. skull fracture with an overlying open soft tissue injury of the scalp.
   d. break in the continuity of any of the bones of the skull.

11.6. En route to the hospital, the patient in Scenario One suddenly loses consciousness. Your *immediate* response should be to:
   a. notify the hospital because you now suspect a serious head injury.
   b. quickly recheck the vital signs.
   c. increase the flow of oxygen.
   d. reevaluate airway, breathing, and circulation.

11.7. Swelling of the brain associated with a head injury can increase resistance to blood flow, leading to:
   a. low oxygen levels and low carbon dioxide levels in brain tissue.
   b. high carbon dioxide levels and low oxygen levels in brain tissue.
   c. high carbon dioxide levels and high oxygen levels in brain tissue.
   d. low carbon dioxide levels and high oxygen levels in brain tissue.

11.8. Bruising around both eyes resulting from a basilar skull fracture is called:
   a. raccoon's eyes or periorbital ecchymosis.
   b. Battle's sign.
   c. panda sign or periocular ecchymosis.
   d. Cushing's sign.

11.9. What bones comprise the cranium (brain case)?
   a. Frontal, occipital, zygomatic, and temporal
   b. Frontal, occipital, mandible, and temporal
   c. Frontal, occipital, ethmoid, and temporal
   d. Frontal, occipital, parietal, and temporal

Scenario Two

You respond to an "unknown injury." The patient is a 42-y.o. male who was working in the hayloft of the barn when he lost his footing and fell approximately 20 feet, landing on the cement below. The men he was working with tell you he initially was responsive to verbal stimuli. His speech was disoriented, and he said his vision was blurred. After approximately 5 minutes he became unconscious and unresponsive. Pupils are unequal and sluggish to react. He has a deformed right wrist and bruising on the right hip, right shoulder, and behind the ears. No one knows if he has any past medical history or allergies. Vital signs are BP—174/90; P—55, strong, regular; and R—14, shallow, regular.

Your Plan of Action

Fill in the blank lines with your treatment plan for this patient. Then compare your plan with the questions, answers, and rationale.

1. _____

2. _____

3. _____

4. _____

5. _____

6. _____

7. _____

8. _____

9. _____

Multiple Choice

11.10. Which of the following is the largest part of the human brain?
  a. Cerebrum
  b. Cerebellum
  c. Medulla oblongata
  d. Pons

11.11. Bruising behind the ears associated with a basilar skull fracture is:
  a. Battle's sign.
  b. raccoon's eyes.
  c. Cushing's sign.
  d. Beck's sign.

11.12. To determine the patient's Glasgow Coma Score, you would evaluate:
  a. alertness, response to verbal stimuli, and response to painful stimuli.
  b. eye opening, verbal response, and motor response.
  c. responsiveness to verbal and painful stimuli, pupil response, and respirations.
  d. pupil response, verbal response, and motor response.

11.13. When immobilizing a patient on a long spine board, you should check sensation, movement, and circulation in all four extremities:
  a. before you place the patient on the board to obtain a baseline.
  b. after you have placed the patient on the board to ensure there has been no further neurologic damage.
  c. before you place the patient on the board and as you arrive at the hospital.
  d. before placing the patient on a board, after the patient is immobilized, and during transport to the hospital.

Scenario Three

A 27-y.o. was driving at approximately 20 mph when her vehicle skidded on a patch of ice, going off the road into a ditch. The car did not roll over completely but did end up resting on its side. The patient is alert and oriented to person, place, and time but does not remember the MVC. She is c/o neck and back pain and a headache. She was wearing a seat belt. She has no significant past medical history and no known allergies. Vital signs are BP—140/90; P—68, strong, regular; and R—16, regular, unlabored.

Your Plan of Action

Fill in the blank lines with your treatment plan for this patient. Then compare your plan with the questions, answers, and rationale.

1. _____
2. _____
3. _____
4. _____
5. _____
6. _____
7. _____
8. _____
9. _____

Multiple Choice

11.14. The *best* way to extricate this patient from the vehicle would be to:
   a. apply a cervical collar and rapidly extricate her to a long spine board.
   b. apply a cervical collar and Kendrick extrication device (KED), then extricate her to a long spine board.
   c. apply a cervical collar and KED, then extricate her directly to the ambulance stretcher.
   d. determine whether she has motor and sensory function in all four extremities, and if she does, have her self-extricate and then lie down on the stretcher.

11.15. All of the following statements about concussions are correct *except:*
   a. the patient experiences a brief loss of consciousness.
   b. there is no obvious structural damage to the brain.
   c. a fracture of the skull usually is present.
   d. the patient will not remember the incident or the events immediately before it.

11.16. When you care for a patient with a head injury, you should:
   a. not give too much oxygen because it may increase the intracranial pressure.
   b. constantly monitor the blood pressure for hypotension.
   c. also suspect a potential neck injury.
   d. keep the patient supine to avoid elevating the intracranial pressure.

Scenario Four

You respond to a report of an injured person at the community swimming pool. The patient is a 17-y.o. male lying beside the pool. Bystanders say he dove off the high board, and one minute later was seen floating on the top of the water. His friends pulled him out of the pool. The patient is awake and alert. He tells you he cannot move his arms and legs. Vital signs are BP—106 /66; P—90, weak, regular; and R—16, shallow, unlabored.

Your Plan of Action

Fill in the blank lines with your treatment plan for this patient. Then compare your plan with the questions, answers, and rationale.

1. _____

2. _____

3. _____

4. _____

5. _____

6. _____

7. _____

8. _____

9. _____

Multiple Choice

11.17. Based on the MOI and symptoms, you should suspect the patient:

    a. struck his head on the bottom of the pool and has a closed head injury.

    b. became hypoxic while submerged and suffered a brain injury.

    c. became hypoxic while submerged and suffered a spinal cord injury.

    d. struck his head on the bottom of the pool and has a spinal injury.

11.18. Where is this patient's injury most likely located?

    a. In the lower part of the cervical spine (C6 to C7)

    b. In the motor cortex of the frontal lobe of the brain

    c. In the cerebellum

    d. In the upper part of the cervical spine (C1 to C2)

11.19. Movement of this patient to a long spine board should be directed by the EMT:

    a. in charge.

    b. with the most experience.

    c. manually stabilizing the patient's head.

    d. moving the patient's torso.

11.20. What is the percentage of spinal cord injuries believed to result from improper handling and spinal motion restriction techniques?

    a. 5%

    b. 10%

    c. 25%

    d. 35%

11.21. How many vertebrae are found in the cervical spine?

    a. Four

    b. Five

    c. Seven

    d. Twelve

11.22. The innermost layer of the meninges is the:

    a. dura mater.

    b. pia mater.

    c. arachnoid layer.

    d. vascular layer.

11.23. Which of the following statements about cervical motion restriction is *correct*?

    a. A collar that is the wrong size may do the patient more harm than good.

    b. It would be better to have the collar too big rather than too small.

    c. If the proper size of collar is not available, inform the hospital, and do not attempt to immobilize the patient.

    d. Never use a rolled towel or blanket to maintain stabilization.

Scenario Five

A 31-y.o. female is c/o of a headache, nausea, vomiting, and weakness in her right arm and right leg. She tells you this is the "worst headache she has ever had." The pain began approximately 3 hours ago and is getting worse. She denies any recent trauma. There is no significant past medical history. The patient does not take any medications and has no known allergies. Vital signs are BP—156/100; P—64, bounding, regular; and R—22, regular, unlabored.

> **Your Plan of Action**
>
> *Fill in the blank lines with your treatment plan for this patient. Then compare your plan with the questions, answers, and rationale.*
>
> 1. _____
> 2. _____
> 3. _____
> 4. _____
> 5. _____
> 6. _____
> 7. _____
> 8. _____
> 9. _____

Multiple Choice

11.24. You should immediately suspect what problem?

    a. A possible migraine headache

    b. A possible subarachnoid hemorrhage

    c. A possible headache caused by severe high blood pressure

    d. Possible meningitis

11.25. What change in the vital signs would be expected with increasing intracranial pressure?

    a. High blood pressure, rapid pulse

    b. Low blood pressure, rapid pulse

    c. High blood pressure, slow pulse

    d. Low blood pressure, slow pulse

11.26. The *most important* treatment you can give this patient is to:
    a. gather any medication bottles so the hospital personnel will know what she may have already taken.
    b. immobilize the cervical spine because she may have had trauma she has forgotten about.
    c. call for advanced life support (ALS) because of the possibility of impending shock.
    d. keep the patient in a semi-Fowler's position and give 15 liters of oxygen.

11.27. A classic indicator of a subarachnoid hemorrhage is:
    a. weakness in both arms.
    b. the worst headache the patient has ever had.
    c. a combination of headache, nausea, vomiting, and weakness.
    d. a decreasing blood pressure.

True/False

11.28. This patient's problem is not an emergency because it takes weeks or months to develop.
    a. True
    b. False

Scenario Six

A drunk driver crossed the center line of a highway and struck an approaching vehicle head-on. The drunk driver is dead on the scene. The driver of the other vehicle is a 28-y.o. male who was not restrained. On the AVPU scale he responds to pain only. There is a "star" in the windshield. The patient has facial lacerations, blood in his ears, bruising behind the ears, a hematoma on his forehead, bruising under the eyes, and a deformed, swollen left upper arm. Vital signs are BP—158/100; P—48, bounding, regular; and R—16, regular, unlabored.

Your Plan of Action

Fill in the blank lines with your treatment plan for this patient. Then compare your plan with the questions, answers, and rationale.

1. _____
2. _____
3. _____
4. _____
5. _____
6. _____
7. _____
8. _____
9. _____

Multiple Choice

11.29. The bruising under the eyes and behind the ears indicates a:
    a. neck injury.
    b. basilar skull fracture.
    c. severe concussion.
    d. ruptured tympanic membrane.

11.30. The MOI of this crash indicates the patient most likely went:
   a. down-and-under.
   b. side-to-side.
   c. up-and-over.
   d. top-to-bottom.

11.31. Blood or clear fluid in the ear canal of a trauma patient indicates:
   a. a basilar skull fracture.
   b. intracranial bleeding.
   c. eardrum injury.
   d. a cervical spine injury.

11.32. All of the following statements about CSF are correct *except:*
   a. it is a clear fluid that surrounds the brain and spinal cord.
   b. it is manufactured in the ventricles of the brain.
   c. an infection such as meningitis probably is present if the fluid is cloudy.
   d. it must be suctioned out to avoid hearing loss if it is present in the ear canal.

Scenario Seven

You respond to a report of a "bicycle accident." The patient is an 8-y.o female who was found lying on the sidewalk. There were no witnesses to what happened. The patient opens her eyes spontaneously but is quiet. She cannot remember her last name and responds to all other questions by saying, "I don't know." She is able to follow commands slowly. She has multiple abrasions on her arms and legs, a contusion on her forehead, and a deformed left ankle. Her Glasgow Coma Score is 14. Vital signs are BP—102/66; P—90, strong, regular; and R—28, shallow, unlabored.

Your Plan of Action

Fill in the blank lines with your treatment plan for this patient. Then compare your plan with the questions, answers, and rationale.

1. _____
2. _____
3. _____
4. _____
5. _____
6. _____
7. _____
8. _____
9. _____

Multiple Choice

11.33. When you perform your neurologic examination, the patient tells you she cannot feel you touching her toes. What is the significance of this finding?

    a. it is nothing to be concerned about because the patient is only 8 and is not completely oriented.

    b. it indicates a possible injury to the brain.

    c. it probably is because of the injury of the left ankle.

    d. it indicates a possible spinal cord injury.

11.34. What two portions of the spine are most commonly injured?

    a. Cervical, thoracic

    b. Cervical, lumbar

    c. Thoracic, lumbar

    d. Thoracic, sacral

11.35. Absence of feeling in the lower extremities associated with feeling in the upper extremities and complete function and sensation in the chest wall indicates spinal cord injury has occurred:

    a. below C5 to C6.

    b. below T4.

    c. below T10.

    d. below S1.

11.36. Which of the following is the *most* reliable sign of a potential spinal cord injury in this patient?

    a. The abrasions on her arms and legs

    b. The Glasgow Coma Scale of 14

    c. The decreased sensation in her lower extremities

    d. The contusion on her forehead

11.37. When you secure this patient to the long spine board in what order do you apply the straps?

    a. Torso, legs, head

    b. Torso, head, legs

    c. Head, torso, legs

    d. Legs, head, torso

SCENARIO ONE

Plan of Action

1. Body Substance Isolation (BSI)
2. Is the scene safe? Yes. Assess MOI, number of patients, and need for additional resources.
3. Manually stabilize head and neck, assess mental status. Ensure open airway, assess breathing, apply oxygen 10-15 lpm, and assess circulatory status.
4. Determine priority, consider ALS.
5. Rapid trauma examination
6. Baseline vital signs
7. SAMPLE
8. Apply cervical collar and KED, stabilize left arm and right lower leg, and extricate patient to long spine board.
9. En route to the hospital, do a detailed physical examination if time permits and perform ongoing assessment.

Rationale

The initial assessment reveals no immediate life-threatening problems. However, the MOI was significant because of the amount of kinetic energy involved. The patient should be given a head-to-toe rapid trauma examination to identify any injuries that could develop into life-threatening problems or that would affect your ability to move her easily. Vital signs and a SAMPLE history also should be obtained. Because the patient is stable, she should be placed in a cervical collar and KED. Her extremity injuries should be stabilized, and she should then be extricated to a long spine board. En route, she should be reassessed repeatedly with emphasis on identifying any early signs of increasing intracranial pressure.

11.1. C, The first action taken whenever contact is made with a patient is to perform an initial assessment of airway, breathing, and circulation. If the presence of spinal trauma is suspected, the head and neck should be manually stabilized. However, a cervical collar should *not* be applied until the initial assessment has been completed. The initial assessment must be completed and any immediate life-threatening problems corrected before the rapid trauma examination is performed or the vital signs are taken.

11.2. C, Patients who are oriented × 4 know who they are, where they are, what day it is, and what happened to them. Remember that people who are traveling through an area may not know exact locations or street names. Also, some patients, particularly the elderly, may not know what day of the week it is. If the patient is unsure about the day of the week, ask what year it is.

11.3. D, The brain and spinal cord also are known as the CNS. The rest of the structures in the nervous system make up the peripheral nervous system.

11.4. D, There are 12 vertebrae in the thoracic spine. The cervical spine contains seven vertebrae. The lumbar spine consists of five vertebrae. The sacral spine (sacrum) is composed of five fused vertebrae. There are three or five fused vertebrae in the coccyx (tail bone).

11.5. C, A head injury is open when an open soft tissue injury of the scalp overlies a skull fracture.

11.6. D, When a patient loses consciousness, you should repeat the initial assessment by evaluating airway, breathing, and circulation.

11.7. B, Cerebral edema (brain swelling) caused by a head injury can cause high carbon dioxide and low oxygen levels in the brain by interfering with normal blood flow. High carbon dioxide and low oxygen levels in turn will increase cerebral edema, further interfering with normal blood flow.

11.8. A, Bruising around the eyes ("raccoon's eyes" or periorbital ecchymosis) is caused by a basilar skull fracture. Battle's sign is bruising behind the ears caused by a basilar skull fracture. The doll's eyes maneuver is used to assess for brain injury for unconscious patients who do *not* have a neck injury.

11.9. D, The cranium consists of the frontal, occipital, parietal, and temporal bones.

SCENARIO TWO

Plan of Action

1. BSI

2. Is the scene safe? Yes. Assess MOI, number of patients, and need for additional resources.

3. Manually stabilize head and neck. Assess mental status. Ensure open airway, assess breathing, apply oxygen 10-15 lpm, consider assisted ventilations, and assess circulatory status.

Continued

SCENARIO TWO—cont'd

Plan of Action

4. Determine priority, consider ALS.

5. Apply cervical collar, secure patient to long spine board, and apply cervical immobilization device.

6. Transport.

7. Rapid trauma examination en route to hospital

8. Baseline vital signs

9. SAMPLE

10. En route to the hospital, do a detailed physical examination if time permits and perform ongoing assessment.

Rationale

The initial assessment suggests this patient has a significant closed head injury with a possible intracranial hematoma. The baseline vital signs are consistent with increased intracranial pressure. The patient should be secured to a long spine board with a cervical collar and a cervical immobilization device in place and transported as soon as possible to a hospital with neurosurgical capabilities. A head-to-toe rapid trauma assessment can be completed en route, and his right wrist fracture can be splinted if time allows. En route, he should be given high-concentration oxygen. Controlled hyperventilation at 20 breaths/min should be considered to reduce the intracranial pressure.

11.10. A, The cerebrum is the largest part of the human brain. The cerebellum is located below and behind the cerebrum and controls posture, balance, and equilibrium. The pons and medulla oblongata are parts of the brain stem and are involved in regulation of involuntary functions.

11.11. A, Battle's sign is bruising behind the ears in the mastoid region caused by a basilar skull fracture. It may not be present until 10 to 12 hours after the fracture has occurred.

11.12. B, The components of the Glasgow Coma Score are eye opening, verbal response, and motor response.

11.13. D, You should assess movement, sensation, and circulation in all four extremities of a patient with possible spinal injuries to establish a baseline before placing the patient on a board, after the patient is immobilized to document that no damage was done, en route to the hospital to detect any changes that might be caused by swelling of the spinal cord, and on arrival at the hospital during report to the emergency department staff.

SCENARIO THREE

Plan of Action

1. BSI

2. Is the scene safe? Yes. Evaluate MOI, number of patients, and need for additional resources.

3. Manually stabilize head and neck. Assess mental status. Ensure open airway, assess breathing, apply oxygen 10-15 lpm, and assess circulatory status.

4. Determine priority, consider ALS.

5. Focused trauma assessment

6. Baseline vital signs

7. SAMPLE

8. Apply cervical collar, extricate patient to long spine board, and apply cervical immobilization device.

9. Transport, perform ongoing assessment en route.

Rationale

The initial assessment reveals no problems with the patient's mental status, airway, breathing, or circulation. The vehicle was traveling at a low speed and did not roll over completely. Also, the patient was restrained. Therefore, the examination probably can focus on the areas where she is experiencing pain and her neurologic function. Because she is stable, she should be packaged as thoroughly as possible before being extricated. Given the location of the vehicle, the best strategy to remove the patient may be to have the fire department cut away the roof so the patient can be slid directly to a long board.

11.14. **B,** This patient has no problems with her ABCs, and her vital signs are stable. However, she is complaining of neck and back pain. After a cervical collar is applied, she should be placed in a KED. She can then be extricated to a long spine board. Because she is stable she does not need to be rapidly extricated from the vehicle.

11.15. **C,** A skull fracture usually does *not* accompany a concussion. The patient will have experienced a brief loss of consciousness. There will be no obvious structural damage to the brain. The patient usually will not remember the incident that caused the concussion or events immediately before it.

11.16. **C,** A patient with a head injury should always be suspected of also having a neck injury. Keeping the patient well oxygenated will decrease the risk of cerebral edema. Increasing intracranial pressure will cause hypertension rather than hypotension. Placing the patient in a supine position may increase intracranial pressure.

SCENARIO FOUR

Plan of Action

1. BSI
2. Is the scene safe? Yes. Assess MOI, number of patients, and need for additional resources.
3. Manually stabilize head and neck. Assess mental status. Ensure open airway, assess breathing, apply oxygen 10-15 lpm, consider assisted ventilations, and assess circulatory status.
4. Determine priority, consider ALS.
5. Rapid trauma examination
6. Baseline vital signs
7. SAMPLE
8. Apply cervical collar, secure patient to long spine board, and apply cervical immobilization device.
9. En route, do a detailed physical examination if time permits and perform ongoing assessment.

Rationale

The patient's initial assessment suggests no immediate problems with airway, breathing, or circulation. However, the absence of movement and sensation in all four extremities indicates an injury of the cervical spinal cord has occurred. The patient should be given high-concentration oxygen, and his ventilations should be monitored carefully. Because his respiratory effort is coming entirely from his diaphragm, he may require assistance if he begins to tire. A head-to-toe rapid trauma examination should be performed to identify any other injuries. The patient should be secured to a long spine board with a cervical collar and cervical immobilization device in place. Because of the MOI he should be reassessed repeatedly en route for a possible head injury. The motor and sensory function in his extremities also should be evaluated repeatedly.

11.17. D, Because the patient cannot move his arms or legs and dove off the high board, he most likely struck his head on the bottom of the pool, causing a cervical spine injury.

11.18. A, The patient cannot move his arms and legs but is still able to breathe using his diaphragm; therefore, he probably has injured his spinal cord in the lower part of the cervical spine. An injury in the motor cortex of the brain would be more likely to produce paralysis or weakness of the arm and leg on one side of the body (hemiplegia). Injury to the cerebellum would interfere with coordination of the movement of muscle groups and with balance and equilibrium. An injury at C1 or C2 would interrupt the nerve impulses to the diaphragm and cause apnea.

11.19. C, The EMT manually stabilizing the patient's head directs all movements.

11.20. C, Approximately 25% of spinal cord injuries result from improper handling and spinal motion restriction technique.

11.21. C, The cervical spine contains seven vertebrae.

11.22. B, The innermost layer of the meninges is the pia mater. The dura mater is the tough outer layer. The arachnoid membrane is the middle layer that resembles a spider's (arachnid's) web. CSF circulates in the space between the arachnoid and the pia mater, the subarachnoid space.

11.23. A, A cervical collar that is too big or too small may do the patient more harm than good. If the proper size of cervical collar is not available, the patient should still have motion of the cervical spine limited by using a rolled towel or blanket as a substitute.

SCENARIO FIVE

Plan of Action

1. BSI

2. Is the scene safe? Yes. Assess nature of illness, number of patients, and need for additional resources.

3. Assess mental status. Ensure an open airway, assess breathing, apply oxygen 10-15 lpm, and assess circulatory status.

4. Determine priority, consider ALS.

5. Transport.

6. HPI, SAMPLE

7. Focused physical examination

8. Baseline vital signs

9. Perform ongoing assessment.

Rationale

The patient's chief complaint of the worst headache she has ever had combined with weakness of one side of the body (hemiplegia) suggests a cerebrovascular accident (stroke) involving a subarachnoid hemorrhage. The vital signs include an elevated BP and decreased pulse rate. These changes indicate increasing intracranial pressure. The patient needs to be transported to a facility with neurosurgical capabilities as soon as possible. During transport she should receive high-concentration oxygen and be placed in a semi-sitting position. If her mental status continues to deteriorate, controlled hyperventilation at 20 breaths/min can be used to temporarily decrease intracranial pressure.

11.24. B, This patient has a combination of a severe headache, a loss of motor function on one side of the body, elevated blood pressure, and a slowing pulse that suggests a subarachnoid hemorrhage. Subarachnoid hemorrhage is a common form of stroke in younger people and is associated with small weaknesses in the walls of the cerebral arteries called berry aneurysms. Patients with a subarachnoid bleed typically complain of the worst headache of their lives. Although migraine headaches can be severe, they are not associated with altered motor or sensory function in the extremities. The patient's past medical history and medications do not indicate she has a history of hypertension that could account for a stroke. This patient's high blood pressure and low pulse are part of the body's attempt to compensate for increasing intracranial pressure. Meningitis can cause headache, nausea, and vomiting. However, it is accompanied by a fever and usually does not cause hemiplegia. A stiff neck also probably would accompany meningitis.

11.25. C, Increasing intracranial pressure causes high BP and a slow pulse. As pressure increases within the cranial cavity, the circulatory system compensates by constricting the peripheral blood vessels and increasing the blood pressure to force blood into the cranial cavity against the increasing pressure. The heart rate decreases in response to the increasing blood pressure.

11.26. D, The patient should be given oxygen and transported in a semi-Fowler's (semi-sitting) position. Giving oxygen will increase oxygen delivery to the brain, decreasing the risk of edema, which would further increase intracranial pressure. Placing the patient in a semi-sitting position improves blood return from the head and helps decrease intracranial pressure. Any patient with suspected intracranial pressure must be transported as quickly as possible to a facility where neurosurgery can be performed.

11.27. B, The classic indicator of subarachnoid hemorrhage is a complaint of the worst headache the patient has ever had. The losses of motor and sensory function associated with subarachnoid hemorrhage and other types of stroke tend to affect the arm and the leg on one side of the body rather than both arms or both legs. Hemorrhage into the cranial cavity will produce an increasing BP, not a decreasing one.

11.28. B, A subarachnoid hemorrhage is a life-threatening emergency. Because one of the cerebral arteries has burst, blood flow to an area of the brain has been interrupted. Also, as the vessel continues to bleed, the pressure in the cranial cavity increases, decreasing blood flow to the brain as a whole.

SCENARIO SIX

Plan of Action

1. BSI
2. Is the scene safe? Yes. Assess MOI, number of patients, and need for additional resources.
3. Manually stabilize head and neck. Assess mental status. Ensure open airway, assess breathing, apply oxygen 10-15 lpm, and assess circulatory status.
4. Determine priority, consider ALS.

Continued

SCENARIO SIX—cont'd

Plan of Action

5. Apply cervical collar. Rapidly extricate to long spine board. Apply cervical immobilization device.

6. Transport.

7. Rapid trauma examination

8. Baseline vital signs

9. SAMPLE

10. En route, perform detailed physical examination if time permits and provide ongoing assessment.

Rationale

The MOI indicates the potential for severe trauma. Because the patient is unresponsive a significant head injury should be suspected. The patient should be rapidly extricated to a long spine board and transported as soon as possible to a facility equipped to care for patients with multiple systems trauma, including neurosurgery. The patient's elevated BP and slow pulse suggest increasing intracranial pressure. If the patient's condition continues to deteriorate, controlled hyperventilation at 20 breaths/min can be used to temporarily decrease the intracranial pressure. Injuries such as the upper extremity fracture can be splinted en route if time allows.

11.29. **B,** Bruising under the eyes (raccoon's eyes) or behind the ears (Battle's sign) suggests a basilar skull fracture. The bruising in these areas may not become obvious until 10 to 12 hours after the injury has occurred.

11.30. **C,** The frontal impact and the "starring" of the windshield indicate the patient went up-and-over the steering wheel, striking his head on the windshield.

11.31. **A,** Blood or clear fluid in the ear canal of a patient who has been injured indicates a possible basilar skull fracture. Intracerebral bleeding is contained within the cranium. An injury to the eardrum may produce bleeding but not clear fluid. A cervical spine injury would not produce fluid drainage from the ears.

11.32. **D,** CSF should *not* be suctioned from the ear canal. Because CSF provides a protective cushion for the brain and spinal cord, suctioning it out can increase the damage associated with a head injury. CSF normally is clear and is produced within two cavities in the cerebral hemispheres called cerebral ventricles. Cloudy CSF suggests an infection such as meningitis.

SCENARIO SEVEN

Plan of Action

1. BSI
2. Is the scene safe? Yes. Assess MOI, number of patients, and need for additional resources.
3. Manually stabilize head and neck. Assess mental status. Ensure open airway, assess breathing, apply oxygen 10-15 lpm, and assess circulatory status.
4. Determine priority, consider ALS.
5. Rapid trauma examination
6. Baseline vital signs
7. SAMPLE
8. Splint injured ankle with pillow splint.
9. Apply cervical collar, long spine board, and cervical immobilization device.
10. En route, perform detailed physical examination if time permits and provide ongoing assessment.

Rationale

The initial assessment reveals no immediate problems with airway, breathing, or circulation. However, the patient's inability to respond to questions appropriately indicates a possible head injury. Because there were no witnesses, it is impossible to determine the MOI. The possibility that the patient was struck by a motor vehicle should be considered. A rapid head-to-toe trauma examination should be performed to identify any injuries that are not immediately obvious. The injured ankle can be splinted with a pillow, and the patient should be placed on a long spine board with a cervical collar and cervical immobilization device in place. En route to the hospital, a detailed physical examination should be performed. Ongoing assessment should focus on the patient's mental status and other neurologic signs.

11.33. D, Absence of sensation in both lower extremities indicates presence of a spinal cord injury. An injury to the brain would be more likely to cause loss of sensation on one side of the body rather than of both legs. Injury to the left ankle could affect sensation in the left foot but not in the right foot. A report of absent or decreased motor sensory function should always be taken seriously regardless of the patient's age.

11.34. B, Because they are more mobile, the cervical and lumbar spine are the most frequently injured parts of the spinal column. The thoracic spine is braced by its attachment to the ribs and therefore is less frequently injured. The sacrum is a solid mass of bone that joins the pelvis. Because of its dense construction and location, it also is less frequently injured.

11.35. C, Absence of feeling in the lower extremities associated with feeling in the upper extremities and with complete function and sensation of the chest wall would be associated with an injury below T10. An injury below C5 or C6 would cause loss of sensation and function over the entire chest wall. An injury at T4 would produce loss of chest wall function and sensation below the nipple line. Injuries of the sacral spine would spare motor and sensory function over most of the lower extremities but would cause loss of sensation along the lateral surface of the foot and over the buttocks.

11.36. **C,** The most reliable sign of a potential spinal cord injury in this patient is the decreased sensation in her lower extremities. Abrasions on the arms and legs do not suggest the presence of a spinal cord injury. Altered mental status (Glasgow Coma Score of 12) and the contusion on the forehead indicate the probable presence of a head injury.

11.37. **A,** The torso should be secured to the board first, then the lower extremities, and finally the head. The head should be secured last to ensure the patient could be rolled as a unit if vomiting occurs. If the head were secured first, it would not be possible to keep the head in line with the body if vomiting occurs and the patient must be rolled. Manual stabilization of the head and neck should be maintained until the body, extremities, and head are secured.

12

Soft Tissue Injuries and Bleeding Control

ANATOMY OF SKIN

- Epidermis
  - Outer, thinner layer
  - Surface consists of dead, cornified (hardened) cells
  - Provides bacteria-proof, watertight barrier
- Dermis
  - Inner, thicker layer
  - Contains sweat glands, sebaceous glands, hair follicles, blood vessels, and nerve endings
- Subcutaneous layer
  - Contains fat
  - Helps conserve body heat

ASSOCIATED STRUCTURES OF SKIN

- Sweat glands
- Sebaceous (oil) glands
- Hair follicles
- Nerve endings (touch, pressure, heat, cold, and pain)
- Nails

FUNCTIONS OF SKIN

- Protects against bacteria and other pathogens
- Prevents loss of water from body tissues
- Regulates body temperature
  - Sweating
  - Control of heat loss by vasoconstriction and vasodilation
- Transmits sensations of touch, heat, cold, pressure, and pain to brain

SOFT TISSUE INJURIES

- Closed
  - Damage to skin and underlying tissues with no break in skin surface
  - Consider possibility of damage to underlying blood vessels and organs
  - Remember the force that caused the contusion did not stop at the skin
  - Contusion
    - Also called a bruise
    - Skin intact
    - Underlying tissues, blood vessels damaged
    - Ecchymosis (discoloration from blood under skin) present
  - Hematoma
    - More tissue damage than with contusion
    - Larger blood vessels may be damaged
    - Blood collects in a lump under skin ("goose egg")
    - Fist-sized hematoma—10% blood loss
  - Crush injury
    - Blow to or pressure against body surface crushes underlying tissue, whereas skin remains intact
    - Force may be great enough to damage internal organs
    - Contents of damaged organs (urine, blood, and food) may leak into surrounding tissue

- Materials leaking into blood from damaged tissue (e.g., myoglobin, potassium) may depress heart or damage kidneys
- Open
  - ○ Abrasion
    - "Carpet burn," "road rash"
    - Epidermis scraped, rubbed, or sheared away, but underlying layers remain intact
    - Minimal bleeding
    - High potential for infection
  - ○ Lacerations
    - Wound passes through epidermis and dermis
    - Wound is longer than it is deep
    - Edges may be smooth or jagged
    - Underlying blood vessels, organs may be damaged
  - ○ Punctures
    - Wound passes through epidermis and dermis
    - Wound is deeper than it is long
    - Underlying blood vessels, organs may be damaged
    - Severity of underlying injury is difficult to determine from size of wound
  - ○ Penetrating chest injuries
    - Apply occlusive dressing to prevent air entry when patient inhales
    - Tape three sides, leave fourth open to allow air to escape when patient exhales
  - ○ Eviscerations
    - Internal organs protruding through wound
    - Do not touch or try to replace exposed organs
    - Cover exposed organs with large sterile dressing moistened with saline solution
    - Cover moist dressing with bulky, dry dressing to prevent heat loss and evaporation
    - Do *not* apply pneumatic antishock garment (PASG) with abdominal eviscerations
  - ○ Impaled objects
    - Do *not* remove unless object:
      - Compromises airway
      - Interferes with chest compressions
      - Is through cheek
      - Interferes with extrication or transport and cannot otherwise be shortened or immobilized
    - Secure object to prevent movement
    - Control any bleeding around object
  - ○ Avulsions
    - Skin, tissue flaps torn loose or completely pulled off
    - Reposition flaps into normal position before bandaging
    - Treat completely avulsed tissue like an amputation
  - ○ Amputations
    - Extremities or parts of extremities completely severed or torn off
    - Bleeding may range from minor to very severe
    - Wrap amputated part in sterile dressing (follow local protocol regarding use of wet or dry dressing)
    - Place dressing-wrapped amputated part in plastic bag, keep cool with ice
    - Do *not* place amputated part directly on ice (damage from freezing may occur)

- Do *not* use dry ice
- Transport amputated part with patient
  ○ Large, open neck wounds
    - May cause air embolism
    - Apply an occlusive dressing
    - Cover occlusive dressing with a bulky dressing

Dressings and Bandages

- Dressings
  ○ Any material that covers a wound
  ○ Help to stop bleeding, protect wound from contamination, further damage
  ○ Should be sterile whenever possible
  ○ Types
    - Universal (multitrauma)
    - Gauze (2 × 2s, 4 × 4s, and 5 × 9s)
    - Adhesive dressings
    - Occlusive dressings (Vaseline gauze, plastic wrap, and aluminum foil)
- Bandages
  ○ Any material used to hold or secure dressings in place
  ○ Should be tight enough to control bleeding but not so tight that they impair distal circulation
  ○ Types
    - Gauze roller bandages
    - Triangular bandages
    - Self-adherent bandages
    - Elastic bandages
    - Adhesive tape

EXTERNAL BLEEDING

- Normal blood volume
  ○ Adult—5000 to 6000 mL
  ○ Child—Approximately 80 mL/kg of body weight
- Blood loss is severe when:
  ○ An adult loses 1000 mL.
  ○ A child loses 500 mL.
  ○ An infant loses 100 to 200 mL.
- Types of bleeding
  ○ Arterial
    - Bright red blood (oxygen enriched)
    - Spurts from wound
    - Sometimes difficult to control depending on the size of artery
  ○ Venous
    - Dark red or maroon blood (oxygen poor)
    - Steady flow
    - Easier to control than arterial bleeding
  ○ Capillary
    - Dark red blood
    - Oozes from wound
    - Easier to control than venous bleeding

Methods to Control Bleeding

- Direct pressure
  - Slows bleeding, allows clotting to take place
  - Apply pressure with hand over sterile dressing
  - Always wear gloves, and take appropriate body substance isolation precautions
- Elevation
  - Elevate the extremity above level of heart
  - If swelling or deformity present, splint before elevating
- Pressure point
  - Apply pressure to femoral or brachial artery
  - Slows blood flow to distal extremity
- Tourniquet
  - Use only as last resort
  - May damage nerves, blood vessels, and muscles
  - To apply:
    - Use wide bandage
    - Wrap around extremity at least twice
    - Tie one knot in bandage
    - Place rod or stick on top of knot
    - Tie ends of bandage over rod or stick
    - Twist rod or stick until bleeding stops
    - Secure rod or stick in place
    - Record time tourniquet was applied

INTERNAL BLEEDING

- Bleeding inside body
- Causes include:
  - Blunt trauma
  - Fractures—Especially pelvis, femur
  - Rupture of blood vessels
  - Clotting disorders
  - Medical problems such as ulcers in the gastrointestinal tract
- Signs and symptoms of internal bleeding
  - Body surface injuries indicating underlying trauma
  - Bruising, swelling, or pain over vital organs
  - Painful, swollen, or deformed extremities
  - Bleeding from the mouth, rectum, vagina, or other body orifices
  - Abdominal distension, tenderness, or rigidity
  - Vomiting bright red blood or coffee ground–like material
  - Dark, tarry stools or bright red blood in the stool
  - Signs and symptoms of shock

Management of Internal Bleeding

  - Support the ABCs
  - Give high-concentration oxygen by non-rebreather mask or bag valve mask
  - Control any external bleeding
  - Rapid transport to a facility equipped to perform surgical control of internal bleeding

SHOCK—HYPOPERFUSION

- Failure of cardiovascular system to deliver adequate amount of oxygenated blood to body tissues
- Types of shock
  - Cardiogenic—Hypoperfusion caused by heart not pumping adequately
  - Hypovolemic—Hypoperfusion resulting from inadequate blood volume. Causes include bleeding, vomiting, diarrhea, heavy sweating, excessive urination, and fluid loss from burns.
  - Hemorrhagic—Hypovolemic shock resulting from bleeding
  - Neurogenic—Hypoperfusion caused by dilation of peripheral blood vessels after spinal cord injury
  - Septic—Hypoperfusion caused by blood vessel dilation and leakage of fluid from vessels resulting from bloodstream infection (sepsis)
  - Anaphylactic—Hypoperfusion caused by blood vessel dilation and leakage of fluid from vessels resulting from severe allergic reaction
- Signs and symptoms of shock
  - Restlessness and anxiety
  - Altered mental status
  - Pale, cool clammy skin
  - Weak, thready, or absent peripheral pulses
  - Nausea, vomiting
  - Thirst
  - Rapid breathing
  - Dilated, sluggish pupils
  - Low blood pressure (BP) late sign
- Management of shock
  - Maintain an open airway
  - Administer oxygen by non-rebreather mask; assist ventilations as needed
  - Control any external bleeding
  - Apply and inflate the PASG as approved by local medical direction
  - Elevate the lower extremities 8 to 12 inches if PASG is not applied
    - The lower extremities should *not* be elevated in cases of cardiogenic shock because of the increase in cardiac work
  - Splint any suspected bone and joint injuries
  - Cover the patient with a blanket to prevent loss of body heat
  - Transport immediately
  - Reassure the patient during transport

REVIEW QUESTIONS

Scenario One

A 38-y.o. male was cutting wood when he slipped and lacerated his right forearm. Large amounts of bright red blood are coming from a jagged 4-inch laceration on the medial aspect of the right forearm. The patient is alert and oriented to person, place, time, and events, but he is very anxious and keeps telling you to "hurry up." He has no significant past medical history, takes no medications, and has no known allergies. Vital signs are BP—102 /66; pulse (P)—118, weak, regular; respiration (R)—22, shallow, regular; and SaO$_2$—96%.

Your Plan of Action

Fill in the blank lines with your treatment plan for this patient. Then compare your plan with the questions, answers, and rationale.

1. _____
2. _____
3. _____
4. _____
5. _____
6. _____
7. _____
8. _____
9. _____

Multiple Choice

12.1. The bright red bleeding indicates:
    a. venous bleeding, a minor concern.
    b. arterial bleeding, a minor concern.
    c. venous bleeding, a major concern.
    d. arterial bleeding, a major concern.

12.2. Arterial bleeding is:
    a. rapid and spurting.
    b. slow and steadily flowing.
    c. slow and oozing.
    d. rapid and steadily flowing.

12.3. All of the following statements about skin are correct *except:*
    a. skin is the body's largest organ.
    b. skin provides support for the body against gravity.
    c. skin consists of three layers: the epidermis, dermis, and subcutaneous layers.
    d. skin contains blood vessels, oil glands, sweat glands, and nerve endings.

12.4. Treatment for the patient in Scenario One would include:
    a. doing an initial assessment and then a rapid trauma examination.
    b. giving oxygen at 15 lpm and splinting the injured extremity.
    c. splinting the injured extremity and calling for advanced life support (ALS).
    d. applying direct pressure to the wound and giving oxygen at 15 lpm.

12.5. If the actions taken in question 12.4 do not control the bleeding, your *next* step would be to:
    a. elevate the injured extremity.
    b. use a pressure point to control bleeding.
    c. apply a tourniquet.
    d. remove the initial dressing, add a new pressure dressing, and elevate.

12.6. Which of the following statements about arteries is *correct?*
  a. They carry unoxygenated blood back to the heart and bleed dark red blood profusely.
  b. They carry oxygenated blood back to the heart and bleed bright red blood profusely.
  c. They carry oxygenated blood away from the heart and ooze either bright red or dark red blood.
  d. They carry oxygenated blood away from the heart and bleed bright red blood profusely.

12.7. An *early* indication of hypovolemic shock is:
  a. low BP.
  b. a pulse rate >150.
  c. restlessness and anxiety.
  d. vomiting.

Scenario Two

You have been called to a report of a pipe bomb explosion at a sandwich shop where a group of teenagers usually hangs out. The police have secured the scene. Back-up ambulances have an ETA of approximately 5 minutes. There are four patients.

- Patient #1 is an 18-y.o. male who is unable to walk. Respirations are 24 breaths/min; radial pulses are present; and he can follow directions. The right upper quadrant of his abdomen is bruised and tender. Vital signs are BP—104/84; P—124, weak, regular at the carotid; and R—24, shallow, regular.

- Patient #2 is a 16-y.o. female. She is able to walk, is breathing 22 breaths/min, and has radial pulses. She can follow directions. She appears uninjured, but she is very quiet. Vital signs are BP—98 /60; P—116, weak, regular; and R—22, shallow, regular.

- Patient #3 is a 13-y.o. male with an amputated right forearm, who is unable to walk, is breathing 20 breaths/min, has a radial pulse in his left arm, and can follow directions. Bleeding is minimal. Vital signs are BP—106/78; P—124, weak, regular; and R—20, shallow, regular.

- Patient #4 is a 12-y.o. female who is unable to walk. Her respirations are labored at 32 breaths/min. Radial pulses are present, and she can follow directions. She has multiple abrasions and contusions on her abdomen and chest and minor lacerations on her upper extremities. Vital signs are BP—90/62; P—132, weak, regular; and R—32, labored, regular.

Your Plan of Action
Fill in the blank lines with your treatment plan for this patient. Then compare your plan with the questions, answers, and rationale.

1. _____
2. _____
3. _____
4. _____
5. _____
6. _____
7. _____
8. _____
9. _____

Multiple Choice

12.8. The START (Simple Triage and Rapid Treatment) method of triage includes evaluating all of the following *except:*
   a. level of responsiveness.
   b. airway and breathing.
   c. extremity motor or sensory deficits.
   d. perfusion.

12.9. The highest priority patient is:
   a. Patient #1.
   b. Patient #2.
   c. Patient #3.
   d. Patient #4.

12.10. Normal capillary refill time is:
   a. >2 seconds.
   b. >4 seconds.
   c. <2 seconds.
   d. <4 seconds.

12.11. Patient #4's difficult breathing is *most likely* because of:
   a. hyperventilation caused by anxiety.
   b. hypovolemic shock.
   c. pneumothorax or hemothorax.
   d. a chest wall contusion.

12.12. The pressure point you would use to control Patient #3's bleeding would be the:
   a. axillary artery.
   b. radial artery.
   c. brachial artery.
   d. subclavian artery.

12.13. If you had to apply a tourniquet to Patient #3, you would use it:
   a. before applying direct pressure.
   b. only as a last resort.
   c. with a dressing over the wound to prevent infection.
   d. in conjunction with a pressure point.

12.14. All of the following statements about hemorrhage control are correct *except:*
   a. once a tourniquet has been applied, it should not be removed.
   b. direct pressure to the wound is the first measure used to control bleeding.
   c. large, open wounds may require direct pressure and use of a pressure point.
   d. tourniquets should be narrow to reduce underlying tissue damage.

12.15. The care of any of the patients in Scenario Two should begin with:
   a. full spinal immobilization.
   b. assessing for and controlling major bleeding.
   c. assessing breathing and giving oxygen by non-rebreather mask.
   d. assessing and opening the airway.

Scenario Three

A 34-y.o. female's car skidded on a patch of ice, left the road, and rolled over twice. When you arrive, the fire department already has secured the scene and stabilized the vehicle. The patient is pinned by a crushed dashboard. She is alert and oriented to person, place, time, and events. She complains of abdominal pain and severe left wrist pain. She also has several minor lacerations on her arms and face from broken glass. The patient was wearing a seat belt and does not think she lost consciousness. She has no significant past medical history and no known allergies. Vital signs are BP—100/54; P—128, weak, regular; R—18, shallow, regular; and SaO_2—95%.

Your Plan of Action

Fill in the blank lines with your treatment plan for this patient. Then compare your plan with the questions, answers, and rationale.

1. _____

2. _____

3. _____

4. _____

5. _____

6. _____

7. _____

8. _____

9. _____

Multiple Choice

12.16. Which of the following is an open soft tissue injury?

    a. A hematoma

    b. A contusion

    c. An abrasion

    d. A crush injury

12.17. Your *first* action should be to:

    a. hold manual cervical spine stabilization, open the airway, and give oxygen.

    b. listen to lung sounds.

    c. palpate the abdomen for tenderness and auscultate for bowel sounds.

    d. place a dressing over the abrasions.

12.18. Because the patient has a pulse rate of 128 beats/min, she has:

    a. bradycardia.

    b. tachypnea.

    c. bradypnea.

    d. tachycardia.

Scenario Four

You are called to the local high school where a 16-y.o. male cut himself in wood shop. There is a large pool of blood on the floor. The patient has a 4-inch laceration across his left forearm with heavy bright red bleeding. He is conscious, alert, and oriented to person, place, time, and events. He has no significant past medical history, takes no medications, and has no known drug allergies. Vital signs are BP—106/72; P—114, weak, regular; R—20; and SaO$_2$—98%.

Your Plan of Action

Fill in the blank lines with your treatment plan for this patient. Then compare your plan with the questions, answers, and rationale.

1. _____
2. _____
3. _____
4. _____
5. _____
6. _____
7. _____
8. _____
9. _____

Multiple Choice

12.19. Blood loss in an adult becomes serious if it exceeds:
   a. 500 mL.
   b. 1000 mL.
   c. 2000 mL.
   d. 3000 mL.

12.20. Your *first* action after determining there are no dangers to you or your patient should be to:
   a. put on gloves and other personal protective equipment.
   b. give the patient high-concentration oxygen.
   c. begin an initial assessment for life-threatening problems.
   d. obtain consent to treat the patient because he is a minor.

12.21. All of the following statements about lacerations are correct *except:*
   a. they are deeper than abrasions, involving all three layers of the skin.
   b. they are caused by shearing forces that damage the epidermis.
   c. they may be regular (linear) or irregular in shape.
   d. they may involve large blood vessels and nerves.

12.22. Because the bleeding is bright red, you should be concerned the patient:
   a. cut a group of veins in the lower forearm.
   b. is going into shock.
   c. has injured the motor and sensory nerves supplying his hand.
   d. has cut an artery.

12.23. The body's normal response to a laceration is to:
   a. minimize circulation to the extremity.
   b. dilate collateral vessels to shift blood away from the injured vessel.
   c. constrict the injured vessel to reduce blood loss.
   d. shunt blood toward the heart to allow the clotting process to begin.

12.24. Because the patient shows signs of early hypovolemic shock, you should:
   a. give high-concentration oxygen, and apply the PASG.
   b. keep the patient from losing heat, and give high-concentration oxygen.
   c. give high-concentration oxygen, keep the patient from losing heat, and give oral fluids to replace blood loss.
   d. give high-concentration oxygen, keep the patient from losing heat, and elevate the feet.

12.25. Which statement about dressings and bandages is *correct?*
   a. Dressings are placed directly over the wound, and bandages then are placed over the dressing.
   b. Bandages are placed on the wound with dressings over them.
   c. Bandages are various sizes of gauze pads, and dressings are usually self-adherent.
   d. A dressing is considered occlusive if a bandage does not cover it.

12.26. Which of the following is a contraindication to using the PASG?
   a. Patients aged less than 16 years
   b. Anaphylactic shock
   c. Pulmonary edema
   d. Abdominal trauma

12.27. The PASG is inflated until the:
   a. BP reaches 120 mm Hg systolic.
   b. Velcro starts to crackle.
   c. bleeding is controlled.
   d. pressure gauge on the PASG reads 90 mm Hg.

12.28. Increased pulse rate; increased respiratory rate; cool, pale, and moist skin; and a normal BP are signs of what type of shock?
   a. Compensated
   b. Decompensated
   c. Irreversible
   d. Neurogenic

Scenario Four—cont'd

The patient is becoming irritable and restless. Vitals signs now are BP—90/54; P—146, thready, regular; and R—22, shallow, regular. Because the hospital is 30 minutes away, you are transporting to meet an ALS unit.

12.29. As shock worsens which of the following groups of signs and symptoms would you be *most* likely to find?
   a. Altered mental status; thirst; nausea and vomiting; and warm, moist skin
   b. Increased pulse; decreased BP; and warm, moist skin
   c. Altered mental status; increased pulse; decreased BP; and warm, moist skin
   d. Altered mental status; increased pulse; decreased BP; thirst; and nausea and vomiting

Scenario Five

A 28-y.o. female who was involved in a motor vehicle collision (MVC) has a deep laceration to the right side of her neck. A moderate amount of dark red blood is flowing from the injury. The patient is alert and oriented to person, place, time, and events. She complains of pain in her right thigh, which is swollen and deformed. She was wearing a seat belt, has no significant past medical history, takes no medications, and is allergic to penicillin. Vital signs are BP—110/62; P—114, weak, regular; and R—18, shallow, regular.

Your Plan of Action

Fill in the blank lines with your treatment plan for this patient. Then compare your plan with the questions, answers, and rationale.

1. _____
2. _____
3. _____
4. _____
5. _____
6. _____
7. _____
8. _____
9. _____

Multiple Choice

12.30. Your *first* action to care for this patient should be to:
   a. perform a focused assessment.
   b. rapidly extricate her from the vehicle.
   c. apply oxygen and perform a rapid trauma examination.
   d. do an initial assessment while applying pressure to the neck laceration.

12.31. Your *most immediate* concern is:
   a. preventing additional blood loss at the site of the femur fracture.
   b. rapidly extricating the patient to a long spine board.
   c. controlling the bleeding from the neck laceration.
   d. beginning treatment for hypovolemic shock.

12.32. All of the following statements about open soft tissue injuries to the neck are correct *except:*
   a. air may enter a lacerated vein and travel to the brain, causing a stroke.
   b. air may enter an injured vein, causing a pulmonary embolism.
   c. frothy blood or subcutaneous emphysema indicate the trachea may be injured.
   d. bleeding may be difficult to control because there are no pressure points.

12.33. An injury to a large neck vein should be covered with:
   a. an occlusive dressing.
   b. a multitrauma dressing.
   c. multiple layers of gauze roller bandage.
   d. a dressing taped only on three sides.

Scenario Six

A 28-y.o. male working on a construction site fell from a 3-foot ladder. He has a 6-inch nail impaled in the lower right abdominal quadrant. Approximately 3½ inches of the nail are visible. A moderate amount of bleeding is present. The patient is alert and oriented to person, place, time, and events. He has no significant past medical history and no known drug allergies. Vital signs are BP—128/88; P—102, weak, regular; and R—18, regular, unlabored.

Your Plan of Action

Fill in the blank lines with your treatment plan for this patient. Then compare your plan with the questions, answers, and rationale.

1. _____
2. _____
3. _____
4. _____
5. _____
6. _____
7. _____
8. _____
9. _____

Multiple Choice

12.34. To control the bleeding, you should:
   a. apply direct pressure after removing the object.
   b. use a pressure point so you do not dislodge the object.
   c. place a dressing on injury and stabilize the object underneath it.
   d. apply a bulky dressing around the nail after stabilizing it.

12.35. Your treatment of this patient would include:
   a. performing an initial assessment and focused examination and stabilizing the object.
   b. performing an initial assessment and a rapid trauma assessment.
   c. performing a rapid trauma assessment and stabilizing the object.
   d. forming a general impression, checking circulatory status, and controlling bleeding with a bulky dressing.

Scenario Seven

A 62-y.o. farmer was gored by a bull. He is lying on the floor of the barn, bleeding from a large wound in the anterior abdominal wall. A loop of small intestine is outside the abdominal cavity. The patient is alert and oriented to person, place, time, and events. He has a history of "heart problems." He takes digoxin and has no known allergies. Vital signs are BP—108/58; P—110, weak, regular; and R—20, regular, labored.

Your Plan of Action

Fill in the blank lines with your treatment plan for this patient. Then compare your plan with the questions, answers, and rationale.

1. _____

2. _____

3. _____

4. _____

5. _____

6. _____

7. _____

8. _____

9. _____

Multiple Choice

12.36. In this case, which of the following problems would *most* concern you?

    a. Large, open abdominal wounds can cause rapid loss of body heat.

    b. Because the patient was injured in a barn there is a high infection risk.

    c. The patient may have involvement of the nerve supply to the lower extremities.

    d. There may be considerable damage to abdominal organs with bleeding and spillage of contents.

12.37. Your treatment of this patient would include:

    a. giving high-concentration oxygen, applying PASG, and transporting.

    b. applying oxygen; covering the wound with a bulky, moistened sterile dressing; and transporting.

    c. giving high-concentration oxygen; covering the wound with a bulky, moistened dressing; and then applying PASG.

    d. giving oxygen, applying an occlusive dry sterile dressing, and performing spinal motion restriction.

12.38. All of the following statements about eviscerations are correct *except:*

    a. immediately replace the organs into the body to prevent drying.

    b. cover the exposed organs with a moistened sterile dressing.

    c. avoid touching the exposed organs.

    d. cover the moistened sterile dressing with a dry or occlusive dressing to prevent loss of heat and moisture.

Scenario Eight

Your next call is for "a man down in the woods." It is November, and deer hunting season opened 3 days ago. On arrival you find a 20-y.o. male with an arrow embedded in the upper right chest. A moderate amount of bleeding is present around the base of the arrow. The patient is alert and oriented to person, place, time, and events. Vital signs are BP—110/66; P—96, weak, regular; R—22, shallow, unlabored; and SaO_2—96%.

Your Plan of Action

Fill in the blank lines with your treatment plan for this patient. Then compare your plan with the questions, answers, and rationale.

1. _____
2. _____
3. _____
4. _____
5. _____
6. _____
7. _____
8. _____
9. _____

Multiple Choice

12.39. Your initial management should focus on:

    a. treating for shock because the patient's aorta probably has been injured.

    b. ensuring adequate oxygenation and ventilation because the patient probably has a pneumothorax.

    c. manually stabilizing the head and neck and beginning spinal motion restriction because the spine probably is injured.

    d. removing the arrow and applying an occlusive dressing because the patient probably has a sucking chest wound.

12.40. Your care of this patient should include:

    a. giving oxygen, stabilizing the object, and transporting.

    b. ventilating the patient, applying an occlusive dressing, and transporting.

    c. giving oxygen, stabilizing the object, applying PASG, and transporting.

    d. giving oxygen, applying an occlusive dressing, stabilizing the object, and transporting.

12.41. En route to the hospital, the patient develops increasing respiratory distress. He is restless and anxious. His skin is pale, cool, and moist with cyanosis around the mouth. Radial pulses are absent. Carotid pulses are rapid and weak. You should:

    a. increase the rate at which oxygen is being given.

    b. forcefully ventilate the patient with a bag-valve mask and oxygen.

    c. temporarily lift or remove the occlusive dressing.

    d. ensure the occlusive dressing is tightly sealed, and increase the flow of oxygen.

Scenario Nine

A call comes in for an "attempted suicide." On arrival you find a 14-y.o. female who has cut her wrists with a razor blade. She is oriented to person, place, and time but not to events. There is a considerable amount of bright red bleeding from both wrists. Vital signs are BP—92/58; P—126, weak, regular; and R—24, regular, unlabored.

Your Plan of Action

Fill in the blank lines with your treatment plan for this patient. Then compare your plan with the questions, answers, and rationale.

1. _____
2. _____
3. _____
4. _____
5. _____
6. _____
7. _____
8. _____
9. _____

Multiple Choice

12.42. Your *first* action should be to:
   a. do an initial assessment.
   b. apply direct pressure to both wrists.
   c. get the PASG ready in case BP decreases.
   d. do an initial assessment, and call for an ALS ambulance.

12.43. Which of these statements about using pressure points is *correct?*
   a. Pressure points are always used as a last resort.
   b. Using a pressure point may result in permanent nerve damage.
   c. The correct sequence would be direct pressure, elevation, and pressure point.
   d. Pressure points are used when tourniquets have failed to control bleeding.

12.44. Which of the following blood components starts the clotting process?
   a. Leukocytes
   b. Erythrocytes
   c. Plasma
   d. Platelets

Answer Key—Chapter 12

SCENARIO ONE

Plan of Action

1. <u>Body Substance Isolation (BSI)</u>
2. <u>Is the scene safe? Yes. Assess MOI, number of patients, and need for additional resources.</u>
3. <u>Assess mental status. Ensure open airway, assess breathing, apply oxygen 10-15 lpm, assess circulation, and control bleeding from laceration</u>
4. <u>Determine priority, consider ALS.</u>
5. <u>Focused trauma assessment of injured extremity</u>
6. <u>Baseline vital signs</u>
7. <u>SAMPLE</u>
8. <u>Transport, perform ongoing assessment, and meet ALS unit.</u>

Rationale

The initial assessment reveals an immediately life-threatening problem—arterial bleeding from the laceration on the patient's thigh. The bleeding should be controlled as quickly as possible using a combination of direct pressure, elevation, and if necessary a pressure point. A tourniquet should be applied if bleeding cannot be controlled by other means. Once bleeding is controlled, the extremity's distal circulation, sensation, and movement should be assessed. Baseline vital signs should be obtained, and treatment for hypovolemic shock continued. If a significant amount of blood has been lost, an ALS unit should be requested.

12.1. D, Bright red bleeding indicates arterial bleeding. Hemorrhage from an artery is a major concern because the high pressure in arteries can cause rapid blood loss.

12.2. A, Arterial bleeding usually is rapid and spurting because blood in the arteries is moving under high pressure generated by the heart's contractions. Venous bleeding usually is slower and flows steadily. Blood oozes from damaged capillaries.

12.3. B, The skin does *not* provide support for the body against gravity. The musculoskeletal system provides the body's support and a framework. The skin is the largest body organ. It consists of the dermis, the epidermis, and the subcutaneous tissues. Skin contains blood vessels, oil glands, sweat glands, and nerve endings.

12.4. **D,** This patient's treatment would include giving high-concentration oxygen and applying direct pressure to the laceration. Because the patient has an isolated soft tissue injury, a rapid head-to-toe trauma examination is not necessary. Splinting of the injured extremity may not be necessary and should not be considered until the bleeding is controlled.

12.5. **A,** If direct pressure does not control bleeding, the injured extremity should be elevated above the level of the heart. Gravity will slow the flow of blood into the injured area, giving the blood an opportunity to clot. If direct pressure and elevation do not stop the bleeding, a pressure point can be used to further restrict blood flow. A tourniquet is used only as a last resort when all other methods of hemorrhage control have failed.

12.6. **D,** Arteries carry oxygenated blood and nutrients away from the heart. Because arteries carry blood that is moving under high pressure, they spurt blood profusely when injured.

12.7. **C,** The earliest indicator of shock is restlessness and anxiety. Shock is failure of the circulatory system to deliver adequate amounts of oxygenated blood to the body's tissues. Because the brain is the body organ with the highest need for oxygen, it feels the effects of shock first. The result is restlessness and anxiety. As volume is lost from the circulatory system, the heart rate will increase steadily in an attempt to maintain adequate blood flow. However, during the early stages of shock the pulse rate may be only slightly above normal. A decreasing BP is a late sign of shock that indicates failure of the body's attempts to compensate.

SCENARIO TWO

Plan of Action

1. BSI

2. Is the scene safe to enter? Based on the initial assessment by the police, yes. However, appropriate protective equipment (helmet, gloves, boots, and turnout coat) should be worn. Extreme caution should be exercised because a secondary explosive device might be present.

3. Establish a command post in cooperation with ranking on-scene law enforcement and fire officers.

4. Begin triage of patients using the START method. Assess MOI(s), number of patients, and need for additional resources.

Continued

SCENARIO TWO—cont'd

5. <u>Establish a staging area for additional ambulances.</u>

6. <u>Begin establishing a treatment area for casualties.</u>

Rationale

In a mass casualty incident, the responsibility of the first-arriving EMS unit is to establish a command structure that will allow effective, efficient management of the incident. One member of the crew should serve as initial EMS commander. The EMS commander should request a response by additional ambulances, establish a command post in cooperation with law enforcement and fire officials, designate a staging area for additional ambulances, and establish a treatment area for casualties. Another crewmember from the first-arriving EMS unit should initiate triage, which is the sorting of casualties for treatment based on the severity of their injuries. The START system is a simple method to quickly evaluate large numbers of casualties. Because Patient #2 is able to walk, she initially will be tagged green (walking wounded). Patient #1 will be tagged yellow (delayed) because he cannot walk, but his respiratory rate is <30 breaths/min, he has radial pulses, and he can follow directions. After the bleeding from his arm injury is controlled, Patient #3 also will be tagged yellow because he cannot walk, but his respiratory rate is <30 breaths/min, he has a radial pulse in his uninjured arm, and he can follow directions. Patient #4 will be tagged red (immediate) because her respiratory rate is >30 breaths/min.

12.8. **C,** The START method of triage includes evaluation of mental status, airway, breathing, and circulation. An assessment for extremity motor or sensory deficits is not performed during START triage.

12.9. **D,** Patient #4 has the highest priority because she has a respiratory rate of 32 breaths/min and is experiencing difficulty breathing.

12.10. **C,** Normal capillary refill time is less than 2 seconds. Anything longer than 2 seconds indicates decreased perfusion to the tissues. Capillary refill is most reliable in infants and children aged less than 6 years. Capillary refill may be prolonged in cold environments.

12.11. **C,** Patient #4's difficulty breathing associated with the abrasions and contusions on her chest wall suggests she may have a pneumothorax or hemothorax. Hypovolemic shock causes rapid, unlabored breathing (quiet tachypnea). Hyperventilation associated with anxiety typically is unlabored and is associated with an elevated BP and strong pulse. A chest wall contusion would not by itself account for this patient's difficulty breathing and the signs of shock that are present.

12.12. **C,** Pressure on the brachial artery can be used to control bleeding from injuries of the upper extremity.

12.13. **B,** A tourniquet should be used as the last resort when all other methods of controlling bleeding have failed. Direct pressure or use of a pressure point is unnecessary once a tourniquet is in place because the tourniquet shuts off all distal blood flow.

12.14. **D,** Tourniquets should be wide to reduce damage to underlying blood vessels and nerves. A BP cuff makes an excellent tourniquet because it uniformly compresses underlying structures.

12.15. D, Ensuring an open airway is the first step in patient care. Without an airway, a patient cannot breathe. Without breathing, oxygenated blood is unavailable to perfuse the tissues.

SCENARIO THREE

Plan of Action
1. BSI
2. Is the scene safe? Yes. Assess MOI, number of patients, and need for additional resources.
3. Manually stabilize head and neck. Assess mental status. Ensure open airway, assess breathing, apply oxygen 10-15 lpm, and assess circulation.
4. Determine priority. Consider ALS.
5. Rapid trauma assessment
6. Baseline vital signs
7. SAMPLE
8. Apply cervical collar, rapidly extricate to long spine board, and apply cervical immobilization device.
9. Transport. Perform detailed physical examination and ongoing assessment en route. Meet ALS unit.

Rationale
The initial assessment reveals no immediate life-threatening problems. However, a rapid trauma assessment should be performed because of the significant MOI. The rapid trauma examination and baseline vital signs indicate early hypovolemic shock, probably from bleeding into the abdominal cavity. A response by an ALS unit should be requested. A cervical collar should be applied, and the patient should be rapidly extricated to a long spine board. Transport should be begun immediately after extrication is complete. Splinting of the wrist can be completed en route to meet the ALS unit. If the patient's BP continues to decrease, PASG could be applied and inflated. The patient should reach a facility with surgical capabilities as quickly as possible.

12.16. C, Abrasions are open soft tissue injuries. Hematomas, contusions, and crush injuries are closed soft tissue injuries because the overlying skin is intact.

12.17. A, Because of the mechanism of injury (MOI), the patient may have a spinal injury. Your first step should be to manually stabilize her head and neck. She can then be given high-concentration oxygen.

12.18. D, Tachycardia is a rapid heart rate, >100 beats/min. Bradycardia is a heart rate <60 beats/min. Tachypnea is breathing >20 breaths/min. Bradypnea is breathing <12 breaths/min.

12.19. B, Usually blood loss >1000 mL in an average-sized adult is cause for concern. It is important to remember that smaller adults may become inadequately perfused after smaller amounts of blood loss.

SCENARIO FOUR

Plan of Action

1. BSI
2. Is the scene safe? Yes. Assess MOI, number of patients, and need for additional resources.
3. Assess mental status. Ensure open airway, assess breathing, apply oxygen 10-15 lpm, assess circulation, and control bleeding from arm laceration.
4. Determine priority. Consider ALS.
5. Focused assessment of circulation, sensation, and movement distal to injury
6. Baseline vital signs
7. SAMPLE
8. Transport, perform ongoing assessment, and meet ALS unit.

Rationale

The initial assessment reveals an immediately life-threatening problem—arterial bleeding from the forearm laceration. The bleeding should be controlled using direct pressure, elevation, and then a pressure point. A tourniquet should be applied if all other attempts to control bleeding fail. After bleeding is controlled, treatment for shock should be continued. A focused assessment of circulation, sensation, and movement in the injured extremity should be performed. If significant blood loss has occurred, a meeting with an ALS unit should be arranged so IVs can be started for volume replacement.

12.20. A, The scene is secure, but you still must ensure your own safety. Gloves should be worn on every call because of the possibility of touching blood or other body fluids.

12.21. B, Abrasions, not lacerations, are caused by shearing forces that damage the epidermis.

12.22. D, The patient may have lacerated an artery because the blood appears bright red. Arterial blood appears bright red because it is oxygenated. Venous blood is dark red because it is unoxygenated.

12.23. C, When a blood vessel is injured it constricts to reduce blood flow and allow clotting to take place.

12.24. D, It would be appropriate to give this patient high-concentration oxygen, prevent loss of body heat, and elevate the feet to promote blood return from the lower extremities. Giving oral fluids is not appropriate because the patient may vomit. Use of PASG in this patient is contraindicated because the site of bleeding is above the level of the suit. Increasing the patient's BP with the PASG may restart bleeding at the injury site. Also, PASG is usually indicated only when the systolic BP is <80 mm Hg.

12.25. A, A dressing is a sterile material that is placed directly on the wound. The dressing may be used to aid application of direct pressure while not contaminating the wound or yourself. Bandages are materials that are placed over the dressing to help hold it in place.

12.26. C, Pulmonary edema is a contraindication to using the PASG. PASG increases the amount of blood available to be pumped by the heart. If the patient already has pulmonary edema because the heart is not pumping adequately, increasing the volume of blood the heart must pump can worsen the edema. Pediatric PASGs are available to use with children. PASG may be useful to manage the decreased peripheral vascular resistance and leakage of fluid from the vascular space that cause anaphylaxis. PASG is useful for abdominal trauma because it applies direct pressure to bleeding within the abdominal cavity and increases the amount of blood available for the heart to pump.

12.27. B, PASG is inflated until the Velcro (loop and hook tape) starts to crackle. A good target for the BP when PASG is applied is 90 to 100 mm Hg systolic. Attempting to increase BP into the "normal" range may worsen bleeding. Some older versions of PASG include gauges to measure pressure in the suit. This information is of little value when treating the patient or determining whether the suit is adequately inflated.

12.28. A, A patient with a rapid pulse; cool, pale, and moist skin; and a normal BP would have compensated shock. Shock is decompensated when the BP begins to decrease.

12.29. D, As shock worsens mental status will become altered because of decreased blood flow to the brain. The heart rate will increase in an attempt to maintain adequate perfusion of the vital organs. The BP will decrease as the mechanisms for maintaining adequate blood flow fail. Thirst will be present as part of the body's attempt to increase blood volume to compensate for inadequate perfusion. The skin will become cool, pale, and moist as the body shifts blood toward the vital organs.

SCENARIO FIVE

Plan of Action

1. BSI
2. Is the scene safe? Yes. Assess MOI, number of patients, and need for additional resources.
3. Manually stabilize head and neck. Assess the mental status. Ensure open airway, assess breathing, apply oxygen 10-15 lpm, assess circulation, control bleeding from neck laceration, and apply occlusive dressing.
4. Determine priority. Consider ALS.

Continued

SCENARIO FIVE—cont'd

5. Rapid trauma assessment

6. Baseline vital signs

7. SAMPLE

8. Apply cervical collar and Kendrick extrication device (KED), extricate patient from vehicle to long spine board, apply cervical immobilization device, and apply traction splint to right thigh.

9. Transport, perform detailed examination and ongoing assessment en route if time allows, and meet ALS unit.

Rationale

The initial examination reveals an immediately life-threatening injury—a laceration to a large neck vein. Bleeding should be controlled with direct pressure, and an occlusive dressing should be placed over the wound to help prevent air embolism. If bleeding is controlled easily and there are no obvious signs of shock, a rapid trauma assessment should be performed and vital signs obtained. Because the patient's condition appears to be stable, a KED can be applied, and she can be extricated to a long spine board. A traction splint can be applied to help stabilize the femur fracture. A meeting with an ALS unit should be arranged so IVs can be started for volume replacement while the patient is transported for surgical management of the neck wound and femur fracture.

12.30. **D,** Because the scene is secure and the patient has an open airway with adequate breathing, you should apply direct pressure to the neck laceration to control bleeding.

12.31. **C,** Your most immediate concern is to control the bleeding from the neck laceration.

12.32. **A,** Air entering a lacerated neck vein is unlikely to move to the brain and cause a stroke because the blood flow in the veins is away from the brain. An injury to a large neck vein can cause a pulmonary embolism if air entering the vein returns to the heart and is pumped out into the lungs. Presence of subcutaneous emphysema or frothy blood near a neck laceration suggests involvement of the trachea. Bleeding from neck wounds is difficult to control because of the size of the vessels involved and the absence of pressure points.

12.33. **A,** A laceration of a large neck vein should be covered with an occlusive dressing to prevent air from entering the vein, returning to the heart, and being pumped into the lungs, causing a pulmonary embolism.

SCENARIO SIX

Plan of Action

1. BSI

2. Is the scene safe? Yes. Assess MOI, number of patients, and need for additional resources.

3. Assess mental status. Ensure open airway, assess breathing, apply oxygen 10-15 lpm, assess circulation, and apply bulky dressing around object to help control bleeding.

4. Determine priority. Consider ALS.

5. Focused trauma assessment of abdomen

6. Baseline vital signs

7. SAMPLE

8. Stabilize impaled object. Transport. Perform ongoing assessment en route.

Rationale

The initial assessment reveals no immediately life-threatening problems, although internal bleeding into the abdominal cavity is a concern. A bulky dressing can be placed around the object to help control external bleeding. A quick, focused examination of the abdomen should be performed, and baseline vital signs should be obtained. Spinal motion restriction is not necessary in this case because the patient fell only 3 feet. The impaled object should be left in place and stabilized to avoid causing additional injuries during transport.

12.34. D, The impaled object should be stabilized, and a bulky dressing should be placed around it. Removing the object may worsen bleeding inside the abdomen. Applying pressure over the object may worsen internal injuries.

12.35. A, Your management would include performing an initial assessment and a focused examination, then stabilizing the object. The MOI suggests this patient has a local injury (the impaled object); therefore, the examination can be focused on that problem. The initial assessment should include an evaluation of mental status, airway, breathing, and circulation.

Scenario Seven

Plan of Action

1. BSI

2. Is the scene safe? Possibly not. Where is the bull? Once scene is secure, assess MOI, number of patients, and need for additional resources.

3. Manually stabilize head and neck, Assess mental status. Ensure open airway, assess breathing, apply oxygen 10-15 lpm, and assess circulation.

4. Determine priority. Consider ALS.

5. Rapid trauma examination

6. Baseline vital signs

7. SAMPLE

8. Cover eviscerated bowel with moist, sterile dressing. Do not replace into abdomen.

9. Apply cervical collar, secure patient to long spine board with cervical immobilization device.

10. Detailed physical examination and ongoing assessing en route if time permits. Meet ALS unit or consider air transport.

Rationale

The MOI suggests the patient may have injuries other than the evisceration. The head and neck should be manually stabilized, and a rapid trauma assessment should be performed to identify any other injuries. The eviscerated bowel should be protected with a moistened sterile dressing. Because of the forces involved in the incident, a cervical collar should be applied, and the patient should be secured to a long spine board. A meeting should be arranged with an ALS unit so fluid replacement can be started. Depending on transport times, a request for a helicopter may be appropriate.

12.36. **D,** The major concern is possible damage to the abdominal organs. Infection is a concern, but it is not as immediate a problem as the risk of hypovolemic shock from the abdominal trauma. Although large, open wounds of the chest or abdomen can cause loss of body heat, bleeding from the injury is a more immediate concern.

12.37. **B,** The patient should be given high-concentration oxygen to help manage shock. The exposed organs should be covered with a moist, sterile dressing to prevent them from drying out. PASG should *not* be applied because pressure on the abdomen could worsen the evisceration. Placing a dry dressing directly on the exposed organs could damage them.

12.38. **A,** The exposed organs should *not* be replaced into the abdominal cavity because they might be damaged or might not be returned to the correct location. The organs should be covered with a moist, sterile dressing to prevent drying. A dry or occlusive dressing can be placed on top of the moist dressing to slow heat and moisture loss. Contact with the organs should be avoided to reduce the chance of infection.

SCENARIO EIGHT

Plan of Action

1. BSI
2. Is the scene safe? Yes. Assess MOI, number of patients, and need for additional resources.
3. Assess mental status. Ensure open airway, assess breathing, apply oxygen 10-15 lpm, and assess circulation.
4. Determine priority. Consider ALS.
5. Focused assessment of chest
6. Baseline vital signs
7. SAMPLE
8. Apply occlusive dressing around base of arrow, stabilize arrow with bulky dressing.
9. Transport. Perform ongoing assessment. Consider air transport.

Rationale

There is no immediate evidence of difficulty breathing or shock. However, because the chest wall has been penetrated, the patient probably has a pneumothorax. An occlusive dressing should be placed around the base of the arrow, and it should be stabilized with a bulky dressing. Depending on the location and transport time, use of a helicopter should be considered.

12.39. **B,** Your initial management should focus on ensuring adequate oxygenation and ventilation because the patient probably has a pneumothorax. Given the location of the injury, it is unlikely that the aorta or spine is injured. Attempting to remove the arrow could worsen the internal injuries.

12.40. **D,** You should apply oxygen, place an occlusive dressing around the base of the arrow, stabilize the arrow so it will not move during transport, and transport carefully. PASG is contraindicated with penetrating chest injuries because increasing the BP can increase the rate of bleeding into the chest cavity.

12.41. **C,** If a patient with penetrating chest trauma develops increasing respiratory distress accompanied by signs of shock, a tension pneumothorax may be present. The occlusive dressing should be temporarily lifted or removed to allow air to escape from the pleural space. If removing the occlusive dressing does not correct the problem, an ALS unit should be called so a paramedic can perform a needle decompression of the tension pneumothorax.

SCENARIO NINE

Plan of Action

1. BSI
2. Is the scene safe? Possibly not. Request a response by the police, and check carefully for any weapons that could be used against you, like the razor blade. After the scene is secure, assess MOI, number of patients, and need for additional resources.
3. Assess mental status. Ensure open airway, assess breathing, apply oxygen 10-15 lpm, and assess circulation. Control bleeding from wrists.
4. Determine priority. Consider ALS.
5. Focused assessment of circulation, sensation, and movement in hands
6. Baseline vital signs
7. SAMPLE
8. Transport. Perform ongoing assessment en route.

Rationale

Although this patient has an immediately life-threatening arterial bleeding from the wrist lacerations, caution should be used in approaching her. Persons who attempt suicide frequently object to the efforts of other to help them. A response by the police should be requested, and the scene should be checked carefully for any weapons—like the razor blade. The bleeding from the patient's wrist lacerations should be controlled with direct pressure and elevation. Once the bleeding has been controlled, a focused assessment of circulation, movement, and sensation in each of the hands should be performed. The patient should be transported to a facility where the wounds can be closed and where she can receive an appropriate psychiatric evaluation.

12.42. **B,** Your first action should be to apply direct pressure to the patient's wrists to control the bleeding.

12.43. **C,** The correct sequence to control bleeding is direct pressure, elevation, and pressure point. Tourniquets are used as a last resort when all other methods have failed.

12.44. **D,** Platelets (thrombocytes) are the blood component that starts the clotting process.

13

Shock Management

PHYSIOLOGY

- Shock—Failure of circulatory system to maintain adequate tissue perfusion
- Maintaining adequate perfusion depends on:
  - Pump—Heart
  - Volume—Blood
  - Container—Blood vessels
- Failure to maintain adequate tissue perfusion results in:
  - Inadequate tissue oxygenation
  - Inadequate waste product removal
  - Cellular damage, leading to tissue damage, leading to organ and organ system failure
  - Death

TYPES OF SHOCK

- Hypovolemic—Volume loss
  - External or internal bleeding (hemorrhagic shock)
  - Burns
  - Vomiting
  - Diarrhea
  - Sweating
  - Leakage into body cavities (peritonitis)
- Cardiogenic—Pump failure
  - Acute myocardial infarction
  - Severe congestive heart failure
  - Abnormally slow heart rates
  - Abnormally fast heart rates
- Neurogenic—Container failure
  - Vasodilation, loss of peripheral resistance from spinal cord injury
  - Vasodilation, loss of peripheral resistance from central nervous system (CNS) depressant toxicity
- Anaphylactic—Container failure + volume loss
  - Vasodilation, leakage of fluid from vascular space caused by histamine release during severe allergic reaction
- Septic—Container failure + volume loss
  - Vasodilation, leakage of fluid from vascular space caused by systemic inflammatory response in severe infection

CLASSES OF HEMORRHAGIC SHOCK

- Class I—750 to 1500 mL blood loss
  - Restlessness and anxiety
  - Tachycardia
  - Cool skin
  - Delayed capillary refill
- Class II—1500 to 2000 mL blood loss
  - Altered mental status
  - Tachycardia
  - Tachypnea
  - Pale, cool, and moist skin
  - Hypotension

- Class III—>2000 mL blood loss
  - Unresponsive
  - Extreme tachycardia progressing to bradycardia and loss of pulse
  - Shallow, agonal respirations
  - Cold, mottled, or cyanotic skin

STAGES OF SHOCK

- Compensated shock—Blood pressure (BP) remains within normal limits.
  - Restlessness, anxiety, confusion, and combativeness
  - Tachycardia
  - Tachypnea
  - Pale, cool, and moist skin
  - Delayed capillary refill
  - Thirst
  - Weakness
  - Nausea
- Decompensated shock—BP begins to decrease.
  - Increasing confusion, possibly unconsciousness
  - Increasing tachycardia
  - Very cool extremities
  - Delayed capillary refill
  - Nausea and vomiting
  - Decreased urinary output
  - Hypotension
- Irreversible shock—Cell damage occurs; organ systems fail.
  - Coma
  - Bradycardia
  - Cold, mottled, or cyanotic skin
  - Severe hypotension
  - Failure of kidneys, liver
  - Death

MANAGEMENT OF SHOCK

- Maintain open airway
- Oxygen by non-rebreather mask at 15 lpm; assist ventilations as needed
- Control external bleeding
  - Direct pressure
  - Elevation
  - Pressure point
  - Tourniquet if other methods fail to control bleeding
- Apply pneumatic antishock garment (PASG) to control internal bleeding, immobilize pelvic fracture, or support BP as specified by local medical direction
- Consider request for advanced life support (ALS) unit to begin fluid replacement or drug therapy
- Keep patient from losing body heat
- Keep patient flat
  - Promote blood return to heart by elevating lower extremities if shock is caused by volume loss or container failure (hypovolemic, neurogenic, septic, or anaphylactic)

- Assess for lower extremity fractures before elevating legs of trauma patients
- Elevation of lower extremities should be avoided for patients with possible spinal injuries. However, venous return may be improved by elevating the lower (foot) end of the spine board.
  ○ Do *not* elevate lower extremities of patients with cardiogenic shock because increased blood return will overwork failing heart
- Provide emotional support
- Rapid transport

PNEUMATIC ANTISHOCK GARMENT

- Indications
  ○ To stabilize fractures of pelvis and proximal femur
  ○ To control significant internal bleeding
  ○ To control massive soft tissue bleeding from lower extremities
  ○ To support BP as specified by local medical direction
- Contraindications
  ○ Congestive heart failure
  ○ Cardiogenic shock
  ○ Pulmonary edema
  ○ Chest trauma
  ○ Pregnancy—Inflate legs only
  ○ Abdominal eviscerations or impaled objects

REVIEW QUESTIONS

Scenario One

A 39-y.o. male was cutting a board when he slipped on an oily area of the garage floor and fell into the saw, lacerating his leg. A friend who was with the patient wrapped his shirt around the wound and then called for help. Blood has completely saturated the patient's pants. There is a jagged 4-inch laceration extending from just superior to the knee onto the inner aspect of the thigh. Bright red blood is spurting from the wound. Distal sensation is present. The patient's skin is cool and very pale. Vital signs are BP—104/72; pulse (P)—128, thready, regular; and respiration (R)—24, regular, nonlabored.

Your Plan of Action

Fill in the blank lines with your treatment plan for this patient. Then compare your plan with the questions, answers, and rationale.

1. _____
2. _____
3. _____
4. _____
5. _____
6. _____
7. _____
8. _____
9. _____

Multiple Choice

13.1. Because the patient is awake and talking without difficulty, your *next* step should be to:
  a. take vital signs.
  b. apply oxygen at 10 to 15 lpm.
  c. bandage the extremity.
  d. apply direct pressure and elevate the extremity.

13.2. Which of the following should be your *most immediate* concern?
  a. The size of the laceration because there may be considerable nerve and muscle damage.
  b. The bright red bleeding because this is an indication of arterial bleeding.
  c. The patient's pale skin because this is an early sign of shock.
  d. The BP of 104/72 because this is abnormally low.

13.3. The *most important* aspect of treating this patient is to:
  a. control the bleeding.
  b. keep the wound as clean as possible to reduce the possibility of infection.
  c. call for an ALS unit so the patient may have fluid replacement.
  d. elevate the patient's feet, and keep him warm in an attempt to increase the BP.

13.4. At this point the patient is in which of the following states?
  a. Cardiovascular collapse
  b. A vasodilated state
  c. Compensated shock
  d. Uncompensated shock

Scenario Two

A 56-y.o. male is c/o left upper quadrant abdominal pain, which has been present for 2 days. Nausea, vomiting, and tarry, black stools have accompanied the pain. The patient has a past medical history of "stomach problems" and high BP diagnosed by "that machine at the drug store." However, he has never seen a doctor for either problem. He has smoked approximately 1 pack of cigarettes per day for 35 years and takes no prescription medications. However, he has been taking over-the-counter medications for his "stomach problems." The emesis in a basin beside him has specks of dark red blood in it. He is very pale, and his skin is cool and moist. Vital signs are BP—94/50; P—136, weak, regular; and R—24, regular, slightly labored.

Your Plan of Action

Fill in the blank lines with your treatment plan for this patient. Then compare your plan with the questions, answers, and rationale.

1. _____

2. _____

3. _____

4. _____

5. _____

6. _____

7. _____

8. _____

9. _____

Multiple Choice

13.5. Which of the following should be your *most immediate* concern?

    a. He smokes, may have emphysema, and is having difficulty breathing.

    b. He has been vomiting and has a potential for airway obstruction.

    c. His skin is cool and moist, and his pulse is 136, weak, regular.

    d. He is vomiting blood and may have internal bleeding.

13.6. The *first* action you should take is:

    a. calling for an ALS unit because the patient may need a breathing treatment.

    b. having suction ready in case the patient vomits again.

    c. placing the patient on oxygen, keeping him warm, and elevating his lower extremities.

    d. placing pressure on the abdomen to help control any internal bleeding.

13.7. The *most important* aspect of treating this patient is:

    a. controlling the bleeding.

    b. assessing the abdomen for rigidity.

    c. calling for a paramedic because he may need fluid replacement.

    d. placing him on oxygen, keeping him warm, and elevating his feet.

13.8. The tarry, black stools indicate:

    a. liver disease.

    b. bleeding in the gastrointestinal (GI) tract.

    c. gallstones.

    d. a disorder of blood clotting.

Scenario Three

You are dispatched to the local drug store for "a child stung by a bee." The patient is a 16-y.o. male who is extremely diaphoretic and pale. He is vomiting, and hives are visible on his face, neck, and upper chest. The patient tells you he was at home on the farm when he was stung. He could not find his epinephrine autoinjector, so he drove approximately 6 miles to the drug store. The pharmacist says, "I can't give him anything." Vital signs are BP—78/56; P—too weak to count; and R—26, regular, labored with wheezing. Your ambulance carries epinephrine autoinjectors, and you are authorized by protocol to use them when appropriate.

Your Plan of Action

Fill in the blank lines with your treatment plan for this patient. Then compare your plan with the questions, answers, and rationale.

1. _____

2. _____

3. _____

4. _____

5. _____

6. _____

7. _____

8. _____

9. _____

Multiple Choice

13.9. This patient has:
   a. anaphylactic shock.
   b. cardiogenic shock.
   c. neurogenic shock.
   d. septic shock.

13.10. This type of shock results from:
   a. vascular dilation caused by histamine release.
   b. pump failure caused by histamine release.
   c. vascular dilation caused by spinal cord injury.
   d. vascular dilation caused by systemic infection.

13.11. All of the following statements about anaphylactic shock are correct *except:*
   a. it may be caused by insect bites and stings, medications, or foods.
   b. urticaria, wheezing, and hypotension are common signs and symptoms.
   c. some reactions may be fatal if not treated within minutes.
   d. allergens are substances that may be given to reverse anaphylactic shock.

13.12. The *most appropriate* treatment for this patient would be:
   a. using an epinephrine autoinjector and calling for an ALS unit to meet you.
   b. applying oxygen 10 lpm via non-rebreather mask.
   c. administering nebulized albuterol for the wheezing, then giving oxygen at 10 lpm by non-rebreather mask.
   d. using the epinephrine autoinjector and then seeing if you can locate the patient's parents.

True/False

13.13. Allergens may enter the body by absorption, inhalation, injection, or ingestion.
   a. True
   b. False

Scenario Four

You are called to see a 56-y.o. male who is having difficulty breathing. As you question him, you discover he also has dull, aching pain in his left shoulder and left arm. When the pain began approximately 4 hours ago, he experienced an episode of weakness and almost passed out. The patient's skin is pale, cool, and diaphoretic with cyanosis around the lips. He says he also is nauseated. The patient has no significant past medical history and no known allergies. Vital signs are BP—86/54; P—132, weak, regular; and R—26, regular, labored.

Your Plan of Action

Fill in the blank lines with your treatment plan for this patient. Then compare your plan with the questions, answers, and rationale.

1. _____
2. _____
3. _____
4. _____
5. _____
6. _____
7. _____
8. _____
9. _____

Multiple Choice

13.14. This patient has:
   a. anaphylactic shock.
   b. cardiogenic shock.
   c. neurogenic shock.
   d. psychogenic shock.

13.15. This type of shock results from:
   a. vascular dilation caused by histamine release.
   b. pump failure caused by damage to the myocardium.
   c. vascular dilation caused by injury to the spinal cord.
   d. vascular dilation caused by a stress reaction to pain.

13.16. You would treat this patient by:
   a. applying oxygen at 4 lpm via nasal cannula.
   b. giving oxygen at 15 lpm, keeping the patient warm, and elevating the feet.
   c. assisting the patient to take nitroglycerin.
   d. applying oxygen at 15 lpm, keeping the patient warm, and calling for an ALS unit.

13.17. The patient's condition was *most likely* caused by:
   a. an allergic reaction to something he may have eaten.
   b. a blood disorder resulting in dilation of the arteries.
   c. a possible heart attack resulting in pump failure.
   d. inability of the lungs to complete oxygen and carbon dioxide exchange, resulting in heart failure.

Scenario Five

You are dispatched to a local nursing home for an "episode of syncope." The patient is an 89-y.o. female who is lying in bed. The nurse tells you the patient has had a urinary tract infection for the past 2 weeks, and the doctor is treating her with antibiotics. She has a past history of angina, a cerebrovascular accident (CVA) 10 years ago from which she partially recovered, hypertension, and ulcers. She has a long list of medications but no known allergies. Because of the past stroke it is difficult to tell if she is alert and oriented. Vital signs are BP—94/50; P—124, weak; R—26, slightly labored; and temperature—102° F. Her skin is pale, very warm, and moist.

Your Plan of Action

Fill in the blank lines with your treatment plan for this patient. Then compare your plan with the questions, answers, and rationale.

1. _____
2. _____
3. _____
4. _____
5. _____
6. _____
7. _____
8. _____
9. _____

Multiple Choice

13.18. This patient's problem is:
   a. hypovolemic shock from bleeding ulcers.
   b. septic shock from a urinary tract infection.
   c. a new CVA caused by hypertension.
   d. cardiogenic shock caused by atherosclerosis.

13.19. The sign or symptom you should be *most* concerned with is the:
   a. respiratory rate of 26 and slightly labored.
   b. pale but warm, moist skin.
   c. BP of 94 systolic.
   d. pulse of 124 and weak.

13.20. A severe infection causing toxin release into the bloodstream is associated with:
   a. septic shock.
   b. hypovolemic shock.
   c. neurogenic shock.
   d. anaphylactic shock.

13.21. Your treatment of this patient would include:
   a. applying oxygen and keeping her warm.
   b. elevating her head and shoulders to help her breathe more easily.
   c. applying cold packs to attempt to reduce her body temperature.
   d. applying oxygen and calling for an ALS unit.

13.22. An *early* indicator of shock is:
   a. an increase or decrease in the pulse rate.
   b. constricted pupils.
   c. confusion, restlessness, and anxiety.
   d. pale, dry skin.

13.23. All of the following statements about shock's signs and symptoms are true *except:*
   a. initially there is an increase in the pulse and an increase in the BP.
   b. a late sign is a decrease in the pulse rate and BP.
   c. nausea, vomiting, and thirst are early signs of shock.
   d. tachycardia and tachypnea usually occur before hypotension.

Scenario Six

The patient is a 13-y.o. female who is lying unresponsive on a sofa. Her sister tells you the patient has a history of diabetes mellitus. She has had an upper respiratory infection with a fever for approximately 5 days. Earlier today she began complaining of a headache and nausea. During the past 2 hours she has become progressively less responsive. She has been taking her insulin and has been eating normally. During the rapid physical examination, you smell a fruity odor on the patient's breath. Vital signs are BP—92/68; P—130, weak, regular; and R—24, regular, unlabored.

Your Plan of Action

Fill in the blank lines with your treatment plan for this patient. Then compare your plan with the questions, answers, and rationale.

1. _____
2. _____
3. _____
4. _____
5. _____
6. _____
7. _____
8. _____
9. _____

Multiple Choice

13.24. This patient *most likely* has:
   a. an insulin overdose.
   b. hypovolemic shock.
   c. low blood sugar.
   d. septic shock.

13.25. How should you treat this patient?
   a. Give high-concentration oxygen, elevate her lower extremities, and request an ALS unit so the paramedics can give intravenous (IV) glucose.
   b. Give high-concentration oxygen, elevate her lower extremities, and request an ALS unit so the paramedics can give IV fluid for hypovolemia.
   c. Give the patient a glass of orange juice with sugar.
   d. Give oxygen at 4 lpm by nasal cannula, roll the patient on her left side to protect the airway, and call for an ALS unit so the paramedics can give insulin.

13.26. This patient's problem was caused by:
- **a.** increased urine output caused by high blood sugar.
- **b.** increased water loss from rapid respirations.
- **c.** pump failure caused by inadequate blood glucose.
- **d.** vasodilation caused by high blood sugar.

Scenario Seven

You respond to a report of an "injured person" at a factory. The patient is a 24-y.o. male who is lying on the floor. His right arm has been amputated at the elbow. The extremity is still bleeding even though other workers have applied pressure to the stump with a bandage. There is a pool of blood, which you estimate to be approximately 800 mL. The patient is anxious but is oriented to person, place, time, and event. His skin is pale, cool, and moist. Capillary refill is 2 seconds. Pupils are slightly dilated but are equal and react to light. Vital signs are BP—102/84; P—118, weak, regular; and R—20, regular, unlabored.

Your Plan of Action

Fill in the blank lines with your treatment plan for this patient. Then compare your plan with the questions, answers, and rationale.

1. _____
2. _____
3. _____
4. _____
5. _____
6. _____
7. _____
8. _____
9. _____

Multiple Choice

13.27. This patient has suffered what class of hemorrhage?
- **a.** I
- **b.** II
- **c.** III
- **d.** IV

13.28. The *best* choice to control bleeding at this time would be a:
- **a.** pressure point.
- **b.** tourniquet.
- **c.** gloved hand.
- **d.** vacuum splint.

13.29. The pressure point to use for this injury would be the:
   a. brachial artery.
   b. radial artery.
   c. femoral artery.
   d. subclavian artery.

13.30. If you decide to use a tourniquet, you should:
   a. not loosen it until the patient has been evaluated at the hospital.
   b. loosen it every 30 to 60 minutes to resupply the area below it with oxygenated blood.
   c. ensure it is less than 1 inch wide.
   d. loosen it every 20 minutes to resupply the area below with oxygenated blood.

13.31. The tourniquet should be tightened:
   a. until the pain is relieved.
   b. as much as possible.
   c. until venous bleeding stops.
   d. until arterial bleeding stops.

13.32. The *most important* point to remember about using a tourniquet is to:
   a. cover the wound with sterile dressings.
   b. document the time it was applied.
   c. keep the extremity above the level of the heart.
   d. make sure it is a narrow constrictive band.

Scenario Eight

An 18-y.o. female attempted suicide by cutting both wrists. You estimate the pool of blood on the floor to be approximately 2000 mL. The patient is unresponsive. Her skin is pale, cool, and very moist with cyanosis around the lips. Vital signs are BP—60/30; P—144, thready at the carotid; and R—38, very shallow.

Your Plan of Action

Fill in the blank lines with your treatment plan for this patient. Then compare your plan with the questions, answers, and rationale.

1. _____
2. _____
3. _____
4. _____
5. _____
6. _____
7. _____
8. _____
9. _____

Multiple Choice

13.33. Blood loss of 2000 mL is equal to approximately:
  a. 1 pint.
  b. 2 pints.
  c. 1 quart.
  d. 2 quarts.

13.34. Your treatment of this patient would *most likely* include:
  a. oxygen 10 lpm and rapid transport.
  b. rapid transport and a request for an ALS unit to meet you.
  c. oxygen at 15 lpm, application of the PASG, and a request for an ALS unit to meet you.
  d. oxygen at 15 lpm and a request for an ALS unit to meet you.

13.35. What stage of shock is this patient in?
  a. Compensated shock
  b. Decompensated shock
  c. Irreversible shock
  d. Complex shock

13.36. The type of shock this patient has is:
  a. hypovolemic shock.
  b. cardiogenic shock.
  c. neurogenic shock.
  d. distributive shock.

Scenario Nine

The patient is a 31-y.o. male who lost his footing while working in a tree and fell approximately 15 feet to the ground. The patient is c/o of left shoulder pain and lower back pain. He patient has no motor or sensory function in his lower extremities. He has a history of hypertension for which he takes a diuretic once a day. Vital signs are BP—90/56; P—62, weak, regular; and R—22, regular, unlabored.

Your Plan of Action

Fill in the blank lines with your treatment plan for this patient. Then compare your plan with the questions, answers, and rationale.

1. _____
2. _____
3. _____
4. _____
5. _____
6. _____
7. _____
8. _____
9. _____

Multiple Choice

13.37. This patient *most likely* has:
  a. hypovolemic shock.
  b. cardiogenic shock.
  c. neurogenic shock.
  d. hemorrhagic shock.

True/False

13.38. The vital signs indicate the patient has lost a considerable amount of fluid.
  a. True
  b. False

13.39. In this type of shock the blood vessels constrict, decreasing blood flow to the periphery.
  a. True
  b. False

Multiple Choice

13.40. Which stage of shock is this patient in?
  a. Compensated shock
  b. Decompensated shock
  c. Irreversible shock
  d. Complex shock

Scenario Ten

The patient is a 4-y.o. female who was riding her bike when she was struck by a car. The car was traveling at approximately 30 mph. The patient is lying in the street, unconscious. She was wearing a helmet. Her pupils are equal but are dilated and react sluggishly. Multiple abrasions and contusions are present on the trunk, arms, and legs. The right thigh appears swollen and deformed. Capillary refill is 3 seconds, and the skin is pale and cool. Vital signs are BP—86/40; P—130, weak, regular; and R—26, nonlabored.

Your Plan of Action

Fill in the blank lines with your treatment plan for this patient. Then compare your plan with the questions, answers, and rationale.

1. _____
2. _____
3. _____
4. _____
5. _____
6. _____
7. _____
8. _____
9. _____

Multiple Choice

13.41. The *first* step to treat this patient would be to:
  a. apply oxygen and call for an ALS ambulance.
  b. check the patient's mental status and her airway, breathing, and circulation.
  c. try to find the parents so consent to treat can be obtained.
  d. transport immediately if an ALS unit is available to meet you.

13.42. Which stage of shock is this patient in?
  a. Compensated shock
  b. Decompensated shock
  c. Irreversible shock
  d. Hypovolemic shock

13.43. This patient is *least* likely to have:
  a. cardiogenic shock.
  b. neurogenic shock.
  c. hypovolemic shock.
  d. septic shock.

13.44. Your management would include which of the following:
  a. maintaining the airway and applying oxygen at 10 to 15 lpm.
  b. restricting spinal motion and giving oxygen at 10 to 15 lpm.
  c. applying a traction splint and giving oxygen at 10 to 15 lpm.
  d. maintaining the airway, giving oxygen at 10 to 15 lpm, and restricting spinal motion.

13.45. All of the following statements about this patient are true *except:*
  a. she may have a serious head injury because she is unconscious.
  b. the pulse rate is tachycardic for a child of her age group.
  c. capillary refill for children is normally 2 to 4 seconds.
  d. she may have intraabdominal bleeding.

Scenario Eleven

A 2-y.o. male pulled a paring knife off the kitchen table, cutting his left forearm. The laceration is approximately 1 inch long, and there is a pool of blood on the floor, which you estimate to be approximately 50 mL. The patient is crying loudly. Capillary refill is 2 seconds. Vital signs are BP—98/50; P—128, strong, regular; and R—28, regular, unlabored.

Your Plan of Action

Fill in the blank lines with your treatment plan for this patient. Then compare your plan with the questions, answers, and rationale.

1. _____
2. _____
3. _____
4. _____
5. _____
6. _____
7. _____
8. _____
9. _____

Multiple Choice

13.46. All of the following statements about this patient are true *except:*

    a. his BP is within the normal range.

    b. the blood loss is serious, and he should be transported immediately.

    c. his heart rate is consistent with the circumstances and his other vital signs.

    d. respirations are within the normal range for a 2-y.o. child.

13.47. To control the bleeding, you should *first:*

    a. use the brachial artery pressure point.

    b. use the radial artery pressure point.

    c. apply direct pressure using a dressing.

    d. apply a bandage.

13.48. As an EMT-Basic, your *most important* function on this scene is to:

    a. control the bleeding, calm the child, and manage any potential shock.

    b. call for an ALS unit.

    c. do a rapid head-to-toe trauma examination.

    d. keep the wound clean to prevent infection.

SCENARIO ONE

Plan of Action

1. Body Substance Isolation (BSI)

2. Is the scene safe? Yes. Assess MOI, number of patients, and need for additional resources.

3. Assess mental status. Ensure open airway, assess breathing, apply direct pressure to wound and elevate extremity, use pressure point if direct pressure does not control bleeding, use tourniquet if pressure point does not control bleeding, apply oxygen at 10-15 lpm, and assess circulatory status for shock. Elevate lower extremities because spinal injuries are not suspected, and cover with blanket if needed to help patient maintain normal body temperature.

4. Determine priority, consider ALS.

5. Transport.

6. Focused trauma assessment of injured extremity, including distal circulation, sensation, and movement

7. Baseline vital signs

8. SAMPLE

9. Perform ongoing assessment, meet ALS unit.

Rationale

This patient has an arterial bleed that needs to be controlled as quickly as possible using direct pressure, elevation of the injured extremity, a pressure point, and (if necessary) a tourniquet. While bleeding is being controlled, high-concentration oxygen can be applied. After bleeding is controlled the patient's circulatory status should be evaluated, and treatment for shock should be initiated. A focused examination of the limb should be performed to evaluate distal neurologic and circulatory function. Baseline vital signs indicate the patient has compensated shock. Although his BP is within normal limits, it is lower than would be expected for a patient with a heart rate of 128. An ALS response should be considered so the paramedics can begin fluid therapy to help support the patient's BP and perfusion.

13.1. **D,** The immediately life-threatening arterial bleeding should be controlled by applying direct pressure to the wound and elevating the extremity. Vital signs would not be taken until the bleeding is controlled. A bandage can be placed over the dressing to hold it in place after bleeding is controlled. While direct pressure is being applied to control bleeding, another EMT can apply oxygen, but because there are no immediate problems with airway and breathing, the highest priority is to stop the bleeding.

13.2. **B,** The most immediate concern is the bright red bleeding, which suggests injury to an artery. Because blood moving through arteries is under high pressure, arterial injuries can cause rapid blood loss. The patient's pale skin is an early sign of shock, and his BP is much lower than would be expected with a heart rate of 128. However, the presence of rapid external blood loss is your first concern. Once bleeding is controlled, steps can be taken to manage hypovolemic shock.

13.3. **A,** The most important part of treating this patient is to control the bleeding. After the bleeding is controlled, apply oxygen, elevate the feet, keep the patient warm, and call for an ALS unit.

13.4. **C,** The patient has compensated shock because he still is maintaining a normal BP. A decreasing BP indicates decompensated shock.

SCENARIO TWO

Plan of Action

1. BSI
2. Is the scene safe? Yes. Assess nature of illness, number of patients, and need for additional resources.
3. Assess mental status. Ensure open airway, assess breathing, apply oxygen at 10-15 lpm, and assess circulatory status for shock. Elevate lower extremities, cover with blanket if needed to help patient maintain normal body temperature.
4. Determine priority, consider ALS.
5. Chief complaint, signs and symptoms (OPQRST)
6. SAMPLE
7. Focused examination of abdomen
8. Baseline vital signs
9. Transport.
10. Perform ongoing assessment, meet ALS unit.

Rationale

The history of abdominal pain accompanied by nausea, vomiting, and dark, tarry stools suggests this patient is bleeding into his GI tract. Because he is pale, cool, tachycardic, and tachypneic, you should suspect he has lost enough blood to cause hypovolemic shock and begin transport to the hospital immediately. The patient should be placed in a supine position with his lower extremities elevated 8 to 12 inches, given oxygen, covered with a blanket if needed to help him maintain a normal body temperature, and transported.

13.5. **C,** The patient's weak, rapid pulse and cool, moist skin are early signs of shock. Although you can begin treatment for shock in the field, you can do nothing to correct the internal bleeding. Although the patient has been vomiting, there is no evidence of airway obstruction.

13.6. **C,** The patient should be treated for shock by giving him oxygen, keeping him warm, and elevating his feet 8 to 12 inches. Pressure should not be applied to the abdomen unless it is with the PASG for serious shock.

13.7. **D,** The most important care an EMT-Basic can provide this patient is to give oxygen, keep him warm, and elevate his feet. An ALS unit can be called to begin fluid replacement, depending on transport time. However, the patient needs to reach the hospital quickly so the bleeding can be controlled. Assessing the abdomen for rigidity will not provide any information that would alter the patient's care in the field. Because this patient is hemorrhaging internally into his GI tract, the bleeding will have to be controlled in the hospital.

13.8. **B,** The black, tarry stools (melena) are an indication of bleeding in the GI tract. Melena results from blood being digested as it passes through the GI tract. Liver disease and gallstones can interfere with the flow of bile into the GI tract, resulting in stools that are almost white in color. Although bleeding into the GI tract and melena can result from blood-clotting disorders, other diseases can cause GI bleeding and dark, tarry stools in patients who do not have blood-clotting problems.

SCENARIO THREE

Plan of Action

1. BSI

2. Is the scene safe? Yes. Assess nature of illness, number of patients, and need for additional resources.

3. Assess mental status. Ensure open airway, assess breathing, apply oxygen at 10-15 lpm, and assess circulatory status. Elevate lower extremities, cover with blanket if needed to help patient maintain normal body temperature.

4. Determine priority, consider ALS.

5. Chief complaint

6. History of present illness, SAMPLE

7. Focused examination for signs of allergic reaction (e.g., edema, hives, stridor, or wheezing)

8. Administer epinephrine by autoinjector, if permitted by local protocol.

9. Baseline vital signs

Continued

SCENARIO THREE—cont'd

10. Transport.

11. Perform ongoing assessment, meet ALS unit.

Rationale

This patient has anaphylactic shock—hypoperfusion caused by a severe allergic reaction. Anaphylactic shock occurs because the body releases large amounts of histamine in response to the presence of an allergen. Histamine causes peripheral blood vessels to dilate and capillaries to leak, resulting in a decreased blood volume in an oversized container. Leakage of fluid from the blood vessels can cause swelling of the tongue and pharynx that can obstruct the airways. Additionally, histamine can cause spasms of the lower airways that interfere with breathing. Epinephrine, administered with an epinephrine autoinjector, causes the blood vessels to constrict and dilates the lower airways, countering the effects of histamine and reversing the anaphylactic reaction. In addition to being given high-concentration oxygen, the patient should be placed in a supine position with his lower extremities elevated to promote blood return to the heart. An ALS unit should be called to start an IV infusion, which can be used to help support the BP. The paramedics also can give diphenhydramine (Benadryl) and a steroid to counter the effects of histamine.

13.9.   **A,** This patient has anaphylactic shock—hypoperfusion caused by a severe, uncontrolled allergic reaction. Cardiogenic shock is hypoperfusion caused by failure of the heart to pump blood adequately. Neurogenic shock results from damage to the spinal cord that causes dilation of the blood vessels and loss of resistance to blood flow. Septic shock is caused by an infection of the bloodstream (sepsis) that causes the blood vessels to dilate and leak fluid.

13.10. **A,** Patients develop anaphylactic shock because their immune system releases excessive amounts of histamine and other chemicals that act on the blood vessels. Histamine causes blood vessels to dilate, decreasing resistance to blood flow, and to leak, decreasing the amount of fluid in the blood vessels. The combination of decreased resistance and decreased blood volume causes hypoperfusion.

13.11. **D,** Allergens are substances that cause allergic reactions and anaphylaxis. Insect bites and stings, medications, plants, and food can trigger anaphylaxis. Some reactions are fatal within minutes, particularly if swelling of the tongue or pharynx closes the airway. Urticaria (hives), wheezing, dyspnea, and hypotension can occur during an anaphylactic reaction.

13.12. **A,** This patient should receive epinephrine immediately using an epinephrine autoinjector. Epinephrine will constrict the peripheral blood vessels, increasing the BP, and dilate the airways, decreasing the patient's work of breathing. After the epinephrine autoinjector is used, an ALS unit should be called. The paramedics can give diphenhydramine (Benadryl) and a steroid to further decrease the severity of the allergic reaction. Oxygen alone will not reverse the life-threatening effects of an anaphylactic reaction. Nebulized bronchodilators may reverse bronchospasm, but they will not constrict peripheral blood vessels sufficiently to correct hypotension in anaphylactic shock.

13.13. A, Allergens may enter the body through ingestion, inhalation, injection, or absorption through the skin or mucous membranes.

SCENARIO FOUR

Plan of Action

1. BSI
2. Is the scene safe? Yes. Assess nature of illness, number of patients, and need for additional resources.
3. Assess mental status. Ensure open airway, assess breathing, apply oxygen at 10-15 lpm, and assess circulatory status. Place patient in supine position but do *not* elevate lower extremities, cover with blanket if needed to help patient maintain normal body temperature.
4. Determine priority, consider ALS.
5. Chief complaint
6. History of present illness, SAMPLE
7. Focused examination for signs of cardiac compromise
8. Baseline vital signs
9. Transport.
10. Perform ongoing assessment en route, meet ALS unit.

Rationale

This patient has cardiogenic shock caused by an acute myocardial infarction. During an acute myocardial infarction, part of the heart muscle dies. If a large area is affected, the heart's pumping capacity can be reduced to the point where adequate perfusion no longer is maintained. The patient should be kept supine, given oxygen, and assisted in maintaining a normal body temperature. Elevating the lower extremities is *not* indicated for cardiogenic shock because increasing blood return to the heart will increase the cardiac workload and worsen the damage from the myocardial infarction. An ALS unit should be called so the paramedics can begin drug therapy to improve the patient's cardiac output and perfusion. Cardiogenic shock is an extremely serious problem that causes death in >80% of its victims, even with treatment.

13.14. B, This patient has cardiogenic shock caused by an acute myocardial infarction. Cardiogenic shock is pump failure—inability of the heart to maintain sufficient blood flow in the cardiovascular system to meet tissue needs for oxygen and nutrients.

13.15. B, Cardiogenic shock is a result of pump failure caused by damage to the myocardium (heart muscle). Anaphylactic shock is a result of vascular dilation and leakage of fluid from the blood vessels caused by histamine release during a severe allergic reaction. Neurogenic shock is a result of vascular dilation caused by injury to the spinal cord. Septic shock is caused by vasodilation and leakage of fluid from the blood vessels caused by a severe infection that has spread to the bloodstream (sepsis).

13.16. D, The patient should be given oxygen at 15 lpm and kept warm. An ALS unit should be called to begin drug therapy to support the patient's BP and perfusion. Oxygen by nasal cannula at 4 lpm will not meet the patient's needs. Elevating the patient's feet will increase blood return to the heart, increase the heart's workload, and increase the size of the myocardial infarction. Nitroglycerin is not indicated at this time because the patient's BP is too low.

13.17. C, The presence of substernal chest pain radiating to the shoulder and arm, weakness, nausea, and heavy sweating (diaphoresis) suggests this patient's pump failure has been caused by an acute myocardial infarction (heart attack).

SCENARIO FIVE

Plan of Action
1. BSI
2. Is the scene safe? Yes. Assess nature of illness, number of patients, and need for additional resources.
3. Assess mental status. Ensure open airway, assess breathing, apply oxygen at 10-15 lpm, and assess circulatory status. Place patient in supine position, consider elevating her lower extremities. Avoid covering patient with a blanket until body temperature can be reevaluated.
4. Determine priority, consider ALS.
5. Rapid head-to-toe examination
6. Assess baseline vital signs.
7. History of present illness, SAMPLE
8. Transport.
9. Detailed physical examination
10. Perform ongoing assessment, meet ALS unit.

Rationale
This patient has septic shock, probably caused by the urinary tract infection. Septic shock occurs when bacteria spread into a patient's bloodstream. In an attempt to fight the infection, the leukocytes release chemicals that cause the blood vessels to dilate and the capillary beds to leak fluid. The decreased blood volume in an oversized vascular container is inadequate to maintain adequate perfusion. Sepsis is most common in elderly patients, infants, and young children because these patients have poorly functioning immune systems. This patient should be given high-concentration oxygen, kept in a supine position, and transported rapidly. An ALS response can be requested to establish an IV line that will be used to infuse fluid and fill the dilated blood vessels. Ultimately, the patient will need antibiotic therapy to kill the organism responsible for the infection.

13.18. **B,** This patient has septic shock caused by a urinary tract infection that has spread to the bloodstream.

13.19. **C,** You should be most concerned about the patient's low BP. A decreasing BP is a late sign of shock and indicates the patient is no longer able to compensate. Because this patient is "normally" hypertensive, she may be severely hypoperfused at a systolic BP of 94.

13.20. **A,** In septic shock a severe infection causes toxins to be released into the bloodstream. The blood vessels respond by dilating and leaking fluid. The decreased resistance to blood flow and the loss of fluid from the cardiovascular system cause decreased tissue perfusion.

13.21. **D,** The patient should be given oxygen, and an ALS unit should be called. There is no reason to keep this patient warm because she already has an elevated body temperature. Elevating her head and shoulders will decrease blood flow to her brain.

13.22. **C,** The earliest sign of shock is restlessness and anxiety caused by decreased blood flow and oxygen delivery to the brain.

13.23. **A,** In the early stages of shock, the pulse increases, and the BP remains unchanged.

Scenario Six

Plan of Action

1. BSI

2. Is the scene safe? Yes. Assess nature of illness, number of patients, and need for additional resources.

3. Assess mental status. Ensure open airway, assess breathing, apply oxygen at 10-15 lpm, and assess circulatory status. Place patient in supine position, and elevate lower extremities.

4. Determine priority, consider ALS.

5. Rapid head-to-toe medical examination

6. Assess baseline vital signs.

7. History of present illness, SAMPLE

8. Transport.

9. Detailed physical examination

10. Perform ongoing assessment, meet ALS unit.

Rationale

Diabetic patients with infections frequently have high blood sugar levels, even when they take insulin and eat properly. When the body releases stored sugar to help produce the extra heat needed to run a fever, a diabetic patient lacks the insulin needed to use this extra sugar, so the blood glucose increases. As blood glucose levels increase, the kidney begins to excrete excess sugar into the urine. The patient loses water to dilute the excess sugar in the urine and becomes hypovolemic. These patients need to be treated initially for hypovolemic shock. The patient should be given high-concentration oxygen, placed in a supine position with her lower extremities elevated, and assisted in maintaining a normal body temperature. An ALS unit should be called so IV replacement of lost fluid can be initiated. At the hospital, the patient will receive insulin to decrease her blood sugar levels back into a normal range and to stop her excess urine production.

13.24. B, This patient probably has hypovolemia caused by diabetic ketoacidosis (DKA). In DKA, the patient develops an elevated blood sugar (hyperglycemia). As excess sugar leaves the body in the urine, it takes large amounts of water with it, causing an increase in urine output (polyuria). Patients with DKA urinate themselves into hypovolemic shock.

13.25. B, The prehospital management of DKA focuses on managing hypovolemic shock and restoring adequate blood flow to the tissues. Once hypovolemia is corrected and the patient is adequately perfused, insulin therapy will be started at the hospital to decrease the blood sugar.

13.26. A, This patient's problem was caused by increased urine output caused by high blood sugar.

SCENARIO SEVEN

Plan of Action

1. BSI

2. Is the scene safe? Yes. Assess MOI, number of patients, and need for additional resources.

3. Assess mental status. Ensure open airway, assess breathing, apply direct pressure to and elevate stump, use pressure point if direct pressure does not control bleeding, use tourniquet if pressure point does not control bleeding, apply oxygen at 10-15 lpm, and assess circulatory status for shock. Elevate lower extremities, cover with blanket if needed to help patient maintain normal body temperature.

4. Determine priority, consider ALS.

5. Transport patient and amputated part.

6. Focused trauma assessment

7. Baseline vital signs

8. SAMPLE

9. Perform ongoing assessment, meet ALS unit.

Rationale

The patient has suffered significant blood loss. The bandage applied by the patient's coworkers should be reinforced with additional gauze, and the stump should be elevated. If this does not control the bleeding, pressure should be applied to the brachial artery. If bleeding continues, a tourniquet should be applied. Although a tourniquet should be applied as the last resort to control hemorrhage, waiting too long to use one may result in a patient developing irreversible shock. As bleeding is controlled, begin oxygen therapy and other supportive care for hypovolemic shock. If the severed arm is found, wrap it in sterile gauze, place it in a container with ice, and transport it with the patient for possible reattachment at the hospital. Do not allow ice to come into direct contact with the tissues because frostbite could result. Request a response by an ALS unit so fluid replacement can be started.

13.27. C, This patient has suffered a class I hemorrhage of between 750 and 1500 mL.

13.28. A, Because direct pressure has not stopped the bleeding, you should apply pressure to a pressure point while continuing to elevate the extremity and apply pressure to the wound.

13.29. A, The pressure point to use for this injury would be the brachial artery.

13.30. A, The tourniquet should be left in place until the patient has reached the hospital and has been evaluated by a physician. The part of an extremity distal to a tourniquet is hypoperfused, leading to a buildup of potentially toxic substances such as lactic acid and potassium. Sudden release of a tourniquet causes these toxins to be returned to the body where they can depress the heart's function and worsen shock.

13.31. D, A tourniquet would be tightened until the arterial bleeding is stopped.

13.32. B, The most important thing an EMT can do when applying a tourniquet is to document the time it was applied, even if it is written on the patient's forehead. This way the doctors have a better idea whether they can save the extremity.

Scenario Eight

Plan of Action

1. BSI

2. Is the scene safe? Yes. Assess MOI, number of patients, and need for additional resources.

3. Assess mental status. Ensure open airway, assess breathing, apply direct pressure to wounds and elevate extremity, use pressure point if direct pressure does not control bleeding, use tourniquet if pressure point does not control bleeding, apply oxygen at 10-15 lpm, and assess circulatory status for shock. Elevate lower extremities, cover with blanket if needed to help patient maintain normal body temperature. Consider PASG application.

4. Determine priority, consider ALS.

5. Transport.

6. Rapid head-to-toe trauma assessment

7. Baseline vital signs

8. SAMPLE

9. Perform detailed physical examination, ongoing assessment en route. Meet ALS unit.

Rationale

This patient is profoundly hypotensive from a massive amount of external blood loss. Direct pressure, elevation, pressure points, and (if necessary) tourniquets should be used to stop any bleeding. The patient should be placed in a supine position with her lower extremities elevated, given high-concentration oxygen by bag-valve mask, and assisted in maintaining a normal body temperature. For patients who are this severely hypotensive, the PASG should be applied to support perfusion of the vital organs even though the site of bleeding is above the level of the garment. En route, a rapid head-to-toe trauma examination should be performed for any unseen self-inflicted injuries. An ALS unit should be met so fluid therapy can be started.

13.33. D, One liter is approximately equal to a quart. Blood loss of 2000 mL is equal to 2 liters or approximately 2 quarts.

13.34. C, Treatment of this patient would include giving oxygen at 15 lpm, application of the PASG, and a request for an ALS unit to meet you during transport. This patient is profoundly hypotensive. Application of the PASG is indicated in an attempt to maintain blood flow to her vital organs. The paramedics on an ALS unit will be able to start IVs and infuse fluid to help increase the blood volume and restore perfusion.

13.35. B, This patient's BP is decreasing; therefore, she has decompensated shock.

13.36. A, This patient has hypovolemic shock caused by blood loss.

SCENARIO NINE

Plan of Action

1. BSI

2. Is the scene safe? Yes. Assess MOI, number of patients, and need for additional resources.

3. Assess mental status. Ensure open airway, assess breathing, apply oxygen at 10-15 lpm, and assess circulatory status. Cover with blanket if needed to help patient maintain normal body temperature. Place patient on long spine board with cervical collar and cervical immobilization device in place. Elevate foot end of long spine board to help promote blood return to heart.

4. Determine priority, consider ALS.

5. Transport.

6. Rapid head-to-toe trauma assessment

7. Baseline vital signs

8. SAMPLE

9. Perform detailed physical examination, ongoing assessment. Meet ALS unit.

Rationale

The loss of movement and sensation in this patient's lower extremities suggest he has a spinal cord injury that is causing neurogenic shock. In neurogenic shock, injury to the spinal cord causes interruption of the nerve signals that cause the blood vessels to constrict. Blood vessels below the level of the spinal cord injury dilate, causing the vascular container to be much larger than the blood volume it holds. The result is a decrease in BP and inadequate perfusion. Because the spinal cord injury also interrupts the signals that would cause the heart rate to increase, patients in neurogenic shock often have a low heart rate rather than tachycardia. Trauma patients with neurogenic shock may also have hypovolemic shock hidden by the interruption of nerve impulses a spinal cord injury produces.

13.37. C, This patient has neurogenic shock. Neurogenic shock is caused by a spinal cord injury that interrupts the nerve impulses that keep peripheral blood vessels constricted. The blood vessels below the injury dilate, causing a loss of resistance to blood flow and a decrease in BP.

13.38. B, Patients who have neurogenic shock have not lost fluid. The volume of the dilated blood vessels is much larger than the volume of blood available to fill them. Therefore, the pressure in the circulatory system decreases, and tissue perfusion becomes inadequate.

13.39. B, With neurogenic shock, the peripheral blood vessels dilate.

13.40. B, The patient has decompensated shock because he is not maintaining a BP within normal limits.

SCENARIO TEN

Plan of Action

1. BSI

2. Is the scene safe? Yes. Assess MOI, number of patients, and need for additional resources.

3. Assess mental status. Ensure open airway, assess breathing, apply oxygen at 10-15 lpm, and assess circulatory status. Elevate lower extremities, and cover with blanket if needed to help patient maintain normal body temperature. Place patient on long spine board with cervical collar and cervical immobilization device in place.

4. Determine priority, consider ALS.

5. Transport.

6. Rapid head-to-toe trauma assessment

7. Baseline vital signs

8. SAMPLE

9. Perform detailed physical examination, ongoing assessment. Meet ALS unit.

Rationale

This patient could have hypovolemic shock caused by blood loss, cardiogenic shock caused by a bruised heart muscle (myocardial contusion), and neurogenic shock caused by a spinal cord injury. Additionally, she may have a closed head injury because she is unresponsive. Because children usually have healthy cardiovascular systems they tend to compensate well when they are injured, and their BP only decreases when all compensating mechanisms are exhausted. The patient should be given high-concentration oxygen, secured to a spine board with a cervical collar and head blocks in place, and transported immediately. An ALS unit should be met en route to the hospital so the paramedics can start fluid therapy. However, this patient needs to reach the operating room as quickly as possible where a surgeon can stop any internal bleeding.

13.41. B, The first step in the treatment of this patient is to perform an initial assessment for life-threatening problems by checking mental status, airway, breathing, and circulation.

13.42. A, This patient has compensated shock because she is maintaining a BP within normal limits for her age. The lowest acceptable BP for a 4-y.o. child is 78 mm Hg. The patient's pale, cool skin and rapid heart rate indicate she is constricting her blood vessels and increasing her heart's output to compensate for loss of volume from the circulatory system.

13.43. D, This patient is *least* likely to have septic shock. The most probable cause of shock in this patient is hypovolemia from blood loss. Because she has bruises and abrasions on her chest, she may have suffered a bruise of the heart muscle (myocardial contusion) that could be producing pump failure. Because of the mechanism of injury (MOI), you also should consider a possible spinal cord injury that could cause neurogenic shock.

13.44. D, The most appropriate treatment would be maintaining the airway by using a jaw-thrust, giving oxygen at 10 to 15 lpm, and restricting spinal motion. PASG is not recommended for use with small children because it may push the abdominal contents under the diaphragm, interfering with ventilation. Although a traction splint is indicated for isolated femur fractures, it is not appropriate for a patient with multiple injuries who is in shock because it takes too long to apply.

13.45. C, Normal pediatric capillary refill time is <2 seconds.

SCENARIO ELEVEN

Plan of Action

1. BSI
2. Is the scene safe? Yes. Assess MOI, number of patients, and need for additional resources.
3. Assess mental status. Ensure open airway, assess breathing, apply direct pressure, and assess circulatory status.
4. Determine priority, consider ALS.
5. Focused trauma assessment
6. Baseline vital signs
7. SAMPLE
8. Transport.
9. Perform ongoing assessment en route.

Rationale

This patient has not lost a significant amount of blood. Control the bleeding, apply a dressing and bandage, and calm him down. The vital signs are within a normal range for a 2-y.o. child. Transport to the hospital with his mother on board so a physician can evaluate and if necessary suture the wound. Before and after bandaging the wound, check distal circulation, sensation, and motor function.

13.46. B, The patient's vital signs are within the normal range for his age. The amount of blood loss observed is *not* serious, and immediate transport is *not* indicated.

13.47. C, To control the bleeding you should first place a dressing over the wound and apply direct pressure.

13.48. A, Your most important function on this scene is to control the bleeding, calm the patient, and manage any potential shock.

14

Medical Assessment

SCENE SIZE-UP

- Body substance isolation (BSI)
- Safety
- Nature of illness/mechanism of injury (MOI)

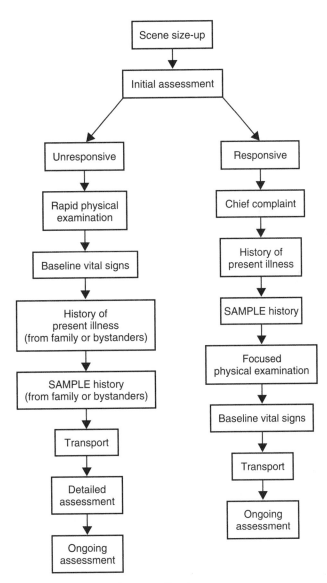

Figure 14-1   The medical assessment process.

INITIAL ASSESSMENT

- General impression (Figure 14-1)
- Level of responsiveness, airway, breathing, and circulation
- Priority

RESPONSIVE MEDICAL PATIENT

- History of present illness (HPI)
  - O—Onset of problem
  - P—Provoking factors. What triggered or caused onset of this pain or problem?
  - Q—Quality. Can you describe it? What does it feel like?
  - R—Radiation. Where is pain located? Does it radiate or travel anywhere else?
  - S—Severity. How severe is pain on a scale of 1 to 10, with 10 being worst?
  - T—Time of onset. When did pain or problem begin?
- SAMPLE history
  - S—Signs and symptoms (OPQRST part of HPI)
  - A—Allergies. Any allergies?
  - M—Medications. Does patient take any prescribed, over-the-counter, or recreational drugs?
  - P—Pertinent past medical history. Does the patient have any medical problems?
  - L—Last oral intake
  - E—Events leading up to present illness. What was patient doing just before this began?
- Focused physical examination
  - Focus examination based on chief complaint, HPI, and SAMPLE
- Baseline vital signs
  - Respirations (rate, depth, rhythm, effort, and abnormal patterns)
  - Pulse (rate, strength, and rhythm)
  - Blood pressure (BP)
  - Skin (color, temperature, and moisture)
  - Pupils (size, symmetry, and reactivity)
- Transport
- Ongoing assessment
  - Repeat initial assessment
    - General impression
    - Level of responsiveness, airway, breathing, and circulation
    - Reassess priority
  - Reassess vital signs
    - Every 5 minutes for unstable patient
    - Every 15 minutes for stable patient
  - Repeat focused assessment
  - Evaluate effectiveness of interventions

UNRESPONSIVE MEDICAL PATIENT

- Rapid physical examination
  - Head
    - Face—Symmetry. Does one side of the face droop? (Cerebrovascular accident [CVA])
    - Eyes—Color of sclera (yellow—liver disease)
    - Ears/nose—Any blood or clear fluid?
    - Pupils—Size, equality, and reactivity?
    - Mouth—Blood or vomitus present? Patient's breath odor unusual? (Ethanol, diabetes)
  - Neck
    - Jugular venous distension (JVD) present?
    - Stoma?
    - Using accessory muscles to breathe?

- Chest
  - Effort of respirations (accessory muscles)
  - Symmetrical? Does each side rise and fall equally?
  - Shape? (Barrel-shaped chest—chronic lung disease)
  - Breath sounds (wheezing, stridor, crackles, and rhonchi)
  - Abdomen—Inspect and palpate all four quadrants (bruising, swelling, tenderness, rigidity, masses, and pulsations)
  - Pelvis—Equal on both sides? Compress gently for potential fractures
  - Extremities
    - Any medical identification devices?
    - Assess pulses, sensation, motor function, capillary refill, and swelling of hands, feet, and ankles (fluid retention)
  - Posterior body—Swelling in sacral region (especially if patient is confined to bed)
- Baseline vital signs
- Consider requesting response by advanced life support (ALS)/paramedic unit
- History of present illness (OPQRST) from family or friends if present
- SAMPLE history from family or friends if present
- Transport
- Detailed physical examination
- Ongoing assessment
  - Repeat initial assessment
    - General impression
    - Level of responsiveness, airway, breathing, and circulation
    - Reassess priority
  - Reassess vital signs
    - Every 5 minutes for unstable patient
    - Every 15 minutes for stable patient
  - Repeat focused assessment
  - Evaluate effectiveness of interventions (i.e., oxygen, CPR)

REVIEW QUESTIONS
Scenario One

Your patient is a 58-y.o. female with a history of emphysema who is in moderate respiratory distress. She says the breathing difficulty began approximately 3 hours ago and is getting worse. The patient is using the muscles of her neck and upper chest to help her move air. She has used her Proventil inhaler three times during the past hour, but the relief only lasts a few minutes. Her skin is pink and dry. Vital signs are BP—140/90; pulse (P)—98, strong, regular; respiration (R)—26, regular, labored; and SaO$_2$—94%.

Your Plan of Action

Fill in the blank lines with your treatment plan for this patient. Then compare your plan with the questions, answers, and rationale.

1. _____
2. _____
3. _____
4. _____
5. _____
6. _____
7. _____
8. _____
9. _____

Multiple Choice

14.1. The normal respiratory rate for an adult is:
    a. 8 to 12 breaths/min.
    b. 12 to 15 breaths/min.
    c. 12 to 20 breaths/min.
    d. 12 to 30 breaths/minute.

14.2. You would perform a focused history and physical examination:
    a. after the initial assessment is completed.
    b. after the baseline set of vital signs is obtained.
    c. after the general impression is formed.
    d. while assessing the airway, breathing, and circulation.

14.3. Signs and symptoms that indicate the patient is experiencing acute respiratory distress include:
    a. jugular venous distension, clubbing of the fingers.
    b. shallow respirations, chest wall tenderness, and pursed lips during exhalation.
    c. use of accessory muscles, nasal flaring, and intercostal muscle retractions.
    d. peripheral edema, increased anterior-posterior chest diameter (barrel chest).

14.4. Which of the following would you perform during your assessment of this patient?
    a. Focused physical examination, vital signs
    b. Rapid physical examination, vital signs, and SAMPLE history
    c. Initial assessment, detailed physical examination
    d. SAMPLE history, focused physical examination, and vital signs

Scenario Two

Your patient is an 80-y.o. male who is lying in bed, apparently unconscious. His family tells you he was fine 2 hours ago when he went to take a nap. He has a past history of angina pectoris, coronary artery bypass surgery 4 years ago, hypertension, and colitis. His medications include nitroglycerin as needed, Catapres, and Librium. He has no known allergies.

Your Plan of Action

Fill in the blank lines with your treatment plan for this patient. Then compare your plan with the questions, answers, and rationale.

1. _____
2. _____
3. _____
4. _____
5. _____
6. _____
7. _____
8. _____
9. _____

Multiple Choice

14.5. Your *first* step to care for this patient would be to:
   a. perform a rapid physical examination.
   b. apply oxygen at 15 lpm.
   c. obtain a set of vital signs.
   d. assess his mental status and the status of his ABCs.

Scenario Two—cont'd

The patient does not respond to verbal stimuli or to being shaken gently. When you open his airway and check for breathing, he has shallow, regular respirations at 16 breaths/min. A strong radial pulse is present.

Multiple Choice

14.6. The *next* step would be to:
   a. perform a rapid physical examination.
   b. apply oxygen at 15 lpm.
   c. obtain a set of vital signs.
   d. get the SAMPLE history.

Scenario Two—cont'd

The patient's vital signs are BP—156/98; P—64, strong, regular; and R—16, shallow, regular. Breath sounds are present and equal bilaterally. The left pupil is dilated and does not react to light. The patient's left arm and leg withdraw from painful stimuli, but the right arm and leg do not. Capillary refill is <2 seconds.

Multiple Choice

14.7. The patient's problem is *most* likely:
- **a.** an episode of angina pectoris.
- **b.** a CVA (stroke).
- **c.** a head injury.
- **d.** an acute myocardial infarction (heart attack).

14.8. How would you treat this patient?
- **a.** Call medical control for orders to give sublingual nitroglycerin to decrease his BP.
- **b.** Manage his airway and breathing and transport rapidly to the hospital.
- **c.** Apply a cervical collar, long spine board, and cervical immobilization device.
- **d.** Place the patient supine and elevate his lower extremities 8 to 12 inches.

Scenario Three

Your patient is a 66-y.o. female whose family says she is "disoriented." They say the patient keeps asking the same question repeatedly. She has a past medical history of chronic obstructive pulmonary disease (COPD), an acute myocardial infarction 5 years ago, and hypertension. Her medications include Theo-Dur, Diazide, and nitroglycerin as needed. She has no known allergies. Vital signs are BP—162/88; P—88, bounding, regular; and R—24, regular, nonlabored. Pupils are equal and reactive; SaO_2—96%.

Your Plan of Action

Fill in the blank lines with your treatment plan for this patient. Then compare your plan with the questions, answers, and rationale.

1. _____
2. _____
3. _____
4. _____
5. _____
6. _____
7. _____
8. _____
9. _____

Multiple Choice

14.9. After you perform an initial assessment, your *next* step would be to:
- **a.** call for an ALS unit.
- **b.** begin transport.
- **c.** perform an HPI and SAMPLE history.
- **d.** perform a rapid physical examination.

14.10. You should suspect the patient is having:
   a. bronchoconstriction from the COPD leading to hypoxia.
   b. an episode of angina pectoris.
   c. a transient ischemic attack (TIA).
   d. a hypertensive crisis.

14.11. Your treatment of this patient should include:
   a. placing a nitroglycerin tablet under her tongue.
   b. giving oxygen, placing her in a semi-sitting position, and calling for ALS.
   c. keeping her supine, giving her oxygen at 10 to 15 lpm, and keeping her warm.
   d. giving oxygen via nasal cannula at 2 to 3 lpm and elevating her feet.

Scenario Four

You respond to the local baseball field for "an unknown medical problem." Your patient is a 35-y.o. female, who bystanders report had a syncopal episode. The patient now is responsive to verbal stimuli but appears confused and weak. She knows who she is and that she is at the baseball field. However, she does not remember what day it is or what happened. The patient's skin is pale, cool, and moist. She tells you she takes Orinase three times a day. Vital signs are BP—140/94; P—120, strong, regular; R—24, regular, unlabored; pupils are PEARRL; and SaO_2—97%.

Your Plan of Action

Fill in the blank lines with your treatment plan for this patient. Then compare your plan with the questions, answers, and rationale.

1. _____
2. _____
3. _____
4. _____
5. _____
6. _____
7. _____
8. _____
9. _____

Multiple Choice

14.12. You could describe this patient's mental status as being alert and oriented to:
   a. person and place, but not to time and events.
   b. person and events, but not to place and time.
   c. person, place, and events, but not to time.
   d. person, place, time, and events.

14.13. After obtaining a past medical history, you would next:
   a. recheck the mental status.
   b. perform a rapid physical examination.
   c. prepare to transport, and do ongoing assessment en route.
   d. obtain a baseline set of vital signs.

14.14. You should suspect the patient's problem is:
   a. an overdose of Orinase.
   b. hypovolemia caused by excessive sweating.
   c. low blood sugar.
   d. high blood sugar.

14.15. You would treat the patient by:
   a. giving oxygen and administering activated charcoal.
   b. administering oxygen, placing her in a supine position, and giving oral fluids.
   c. giving her a glass of orange juice with sugar added.
   d. giving oxygen and transporting for management of hyperglycemia.

Scenario Five

A 59-y.o. male was working outside approximately 2 hours ago when he slipped and fell, striking his left lateral chest on the edge of some concrete steps. He still has "sharp" pain in his left chest that he rates as a "5" on a 1 to 10 scale. The patient denies any weakness, dizziness, or shortness of breath. He has a past history of angina pectoris and arthritis. His medications include nitroglycerin as needed, Cardizem, and ibuprofen. He has no known allergies. Vital signs are BP—128/70; P—74, strong, regular; R—16, shallow, regular, and unlabored; and SaO_2—97%.

Your Plan of Action

Fill in the blank lines with your treatment plan for this patient. Then compare your plan with the questions, answers, and rationale.

1. _____
2. _____
3. _____
4. _____
5. _____
6. _____
7. _____
8. _____
9. _____

Multiple Choice

14.16. After performing the initial assessment, you should:
   a. do a detailed physical examination.
   b. obtain the vital signs.
   c. obtain a history and perform a focused physical examination.
   d. apply oxygen at 10 lpm.

14.17. Because of the patient's history, you would want to:
   a. focus on the chest examination but also ask the OPQRST questions.
   b. check motor and sensory function in all four extremities because he fell.
   c. consider a cervical collar and spinal immobilization.
   d. perform a rapid trauma examination.

14.18. One way to assess the pain's severity would be to:
    a. have the patient describe it in his own words.
    b. have the patient rate it on a 1 to 10 scale.
    c. have the patient describe whether the pain radiates to another part of the body.
    d. ask the patient if he has ever had this pain before.

14.19. The objective of the focused physical examination for this patient is to:
    a. determine the patient's chief complaint.
    b. determine the SAMPLE history.
    c. ensure there are no life-threatening problems and assess the chest pain.
    d. determine the need for a rapid physical examination.

14.20. Pertinent negative findings for this patient include all of the following *except:*
    a. shortness of breath is not present.
    b. he states the pain is 5 on 1 to 10 scale.
    c. he denies any weakness.
    d. he is not dizzy.

Scenario Six

You respond to a report of a "child with a fever." On arrival you find a 7-y.o. male with a temperature of 101° F. The patient's mother says he has been sick with fever, nausea, vomiting, and a headache for the past 2 to 3 days. He is lying very still and cries when you try to sit him up to examine him. He says his neck hurts. He has no significant past medical history, takes no medications, and is allergic to penicillin. Vital signs are BP—100/64; P—118, weak, regular; and R—24, shallow, regular, and unlabored.

Your Plan of Action

Fill in the blank lines with your treatment plan for this patient. Then compare your plan with the questions, answers, and rationale.

1. _____
2. _____
3. _____
4. _____
5. _____
6. _____
7. _____
8. _____
9. _____

Multiple Choice

14.21. The components of the focused physical examination are:
    a. not used with pediatric patients.
    b. guided by the chief complaint and the findings from the initial assessment.
    c. often guided by the medications the patient takes.
    d. always performed the same way for each patient.

14.22. This patient's BP is:
   a. normotensive.
   b. profoundly hypotensive.
   c. slightly hypotensive.
   d. hypertensive.

14.23. You should suspect this child has:
   a. flu with hypovolemia from vomiting.
   b. measles.
   c. meningitis.
   d. mumps.

14.24. The presence of neck pain in this patient is:
   a. a positive finding.
   b. a pertinent negative finding.
   c. part of the ongoing assessment.
   d. information that is nice to know but not necessary.

14.25. Treatment for this patient would include:
   a. taking BSI precautions and covering the patient with a blanket because he may be in septic shock.
   b. assisting ventilations with a BVM and oxygen.
   c. calling for an ALS unit and transporting with oxygen by non-rebreather mask.
   d. taking spinal precautions because neck pain is present.

Scenario Seven

A 68-y.o. male called EMS for his wife. The patient is a very frightened 62-y.o. female, who is sitting in a chair in her living room. Her husband tells you she slumped to the floor while she was walking across the room. When he helped her up, her left side was noticeably weak, and she could not speak. He says she has no significant past medical history, takes no medications, and has no known allergies.

Your Plan of Action

Fill in the blank lines with your treatment plan for this patient. Then compare your plan with the questions, answers, and rationale.

1. _____
2. _____
3. _____
4. _____
5. _____
6. _____
7. _____
8. _____
9. _____

Multiple Choice

14.26. When you examine the patient, you should perform a:

    a. detailed physical examination.

    b. focused physical examination.

    c. rapid physical examination.

    d. rapid trauma examination.

14.27. You should suspect that this patient has:

    a. a medical problem, a possible heart attack.

    b. trauma with damage to the cervical spine.

    c. trauma, a possible stroke.

    d. a medical problem, a possible stroke.

14.28. Treatment for this patient would include:

    a. basic life support transport with oxygen.

    b. ALS transport with spinal immobilization.

    c. performing a focused physical examination and calling for ALS.

    d. performing a rapid physical examination and taking spinal precautions.

14.29. After performing the focused physical examination, you would *next*:

    a. obtain a set of vital signs.

    b. prepare for transport.

    c. take SAMPLE history.

    d. reassess the patient's mental status.

14.30. Signs and symptoms of a CVA include:

    a. weakness on one side of the body and chest pain.

    b. headache, weakness in all four extremities, and stiff neck.

    c. paralysis of both upper extremities and visual disturbances.

    d. weakness of one side of the body, drooping of the mouth, and slurred speech.

Scenario Eight

You respond to a report of a "woman down" at a local grocery store. The patient is a 59-y.o. female who bystanders say suddenly "passed out." The patient does not remember what happened. There is no evidence of any trauma. The patient seems dazed but is oriented to person, place, and time. She says she has high BP for which she takes furosemide once a day. She has no known allergies. Vital signs are BP—138/90; P—98, strong, regular; and R—14, regular, nonlabored.

Your Plan of Action

Fill in the blank lines with your treatment plan for this patient. Then compare your plan with the questions, answers, and rationale.

1. _____
2. _____
3. _____
4. _____
5. _____
6. _____
7. _____
8. _____
9. _____

Multiple Choice

14.31. You would begin your examination with:

    a. the history and a focused physical examination.

    b. a baseline set of vital signs.

    c. a rapid physical examination.

    d. an initial assessment.

14.32. Your examination should focus on the:

    a. cardiovascular system.

    b. neurologic system.

    c. respiratory system.

    d. musculoskeletal system.

14.33. Syncope is another word for:

    a. blurred vision.

    b. weakness.

    c. fainting.

    d. dizziness.

14.34. This patient's problem could have been caused by:

    a. a reaction to her BP medication.

    b. a TIA.

    c. a decrease in her heart's output caused by an arrhythmia.

    d. either a TIA or an arrhythmia.

Scenario Nine

You respond to a possible "seizure." On arrival you find a 10-y.o. female actively seizing. Her mother says the seizure began approximately 3 minutes ago. The patient has a history of seizures but has not had one in several years. You attempt to ensure an open airway and adequate breathing, but the seizure makes this almost impossible.

Your Plan of Action

Fill in the blank lines with your treatment plan for this patient. Then compare your plan with the questions, answers, and rationale.

1. _____
2. _____
3. _____
4. _____
5. _____
6. _____
7. _____
8. _____
9. _____

Multiple Choice

14.35. Your *first* concern should be to:
  a. protect the airway.
  b. ensure a pulse.
  c. protect the extremities from injury.
  d. place padding under the head.

14.36. When the seizure ends, other care you should provide would include:
  a. immobilizing the patient's spine.
  b. calling for an ALS unit to transport.
  c. applying oxygen at 15 lpm.
  d. ensuring the airway is open by inserting an oropharyngeal airway.

14.37. Because the patient is unconscious, you would do an initial assessment followed by a:
  a. history and focused physical examination.
  b. HPI and SAMPLE.
  c. rapid physical examination.
  d. rapid trauma examination.

14.38. After the seizure is over, you would expect the patient to be:
  a. conscious but drowsy.
  b. conscious and alert.
  c. lethargic for at least 1 hour.
  d. unresponsive for at least 30 minutes.

14.39. Which of the following mnemonics represents "taking a patient's history"?
  a. DCAP-BTLS
  b. SAMPLE
  c. OPQRST
  d. AEIOU-TIPS

14.40. A visual examination of part of the body is:
   a. auscultation.
   b. inspection.
   c. palpation.
   d. percussion.

14.41. When you strike an area to elicit sounds or vibrations, it is known as:
   a. auscultation.
   b. inspection.
   c. palpation.
   d. percussion.

14.42. Listening with your stethoscope is called:
   a. auscultation.
   b. inspection.
   c. palpation.
   d. percussion.

14.43. The width of a correctly sized BP cuff should be:
   a. one-quarter the length of the upper arm.
   b. one-third the length of the upper arm.
   c. one-half the length of the upper arm.
   d. two-thirds the length of the upper arm.

SCENARIO ONE

Plan of Action

1. Body Substance Isolation (BSI)
2. Is the scene safe? Yes. Assess nature of illness, number of patients, and need for additional resources.
3. Assess mental status. Ensure open airway, assess breathing, apply oxygen 10-15 lpm by non-rebreather mask, and assess circulation.
4. Determine priority, consider ALS.
5. HPI, SAMPLE
6. Focused physical examination
7. Baseline vital signs
8. Transport, provide ongoing assessment.

Rationale

The initial assessment reveals difficulty breathing. The patient should be given high-concentration oxygen immediately. Because the patient has a chief complaint of shortness of breath and a past history of emphysema, the physical examination can focus initially on the respiratory system and the chest. If your local protocols allow administration of nebulized bronchodilators, you could consider treating the patient with Proventil or with an alternative bronchodilator such as Alupent or Bronkosol. If you cannot administer nebulized bronchodilators, you may consider calling for an ALS unit. The patient should receive high-concentration oxygen during transport. Ongoing assessment should be performed with an emphasis on breathing. If the patient's respirations slow or become shallow because she is tired, you should assist her breathing with a BVM.

14.1. **C,** The normal adult respiratory rate is 12 to 20 breaths/min.

14.2. **A,** The focused history and physical examination would be performed after the initial assessment is completed. A focused history and physical examination are performed when the initial assessment reveals no immediate life-threatening problems and the patient's chief complaint and history indicate the specific body region or system where the problem is located.

14.3. **C,** Signs and symptoms of respiratory distress would include accessory muscle use, nasal flaring, and intercostal retractions. Clubbing of the fingers develops in patients with COPD, but it is not a sign of respiratory distress. Pursing of the lips on exhalation is a common finding in patients with emphysema, but it does not indicate respiratory distress. The presence of peripheral edema or a barrel chest may indicate the presence of a chronic disease that can cause episodes of respiratory distress. However, their presence does not mean that the patient has acute difficulty breathing.

14.4. **D,** The examination of this patient would include a SAMPLE history, a focused physical examination, and vital signs. The rapid and detailed physical examinations are not indicated because the patient's complaint and history allow the examination to be focused on the respiratory system.

Scenario Two

Plan of Action

1. BSI

2. Is the scene safe? Yes. Assess nature of illness, number of patients, and need for additional resources.

3. Assess mental status. Ensure an open airway, assess breathing, apply oxygen 10-15 lpm by non-rebreather mask, and assess circulatory status.

4. Determine priority, consider ALS.

5. Rapid physical examination

6. Baseline vital signs

7. HPI, SAMPLE

8. Transport, provide ongoing assessment.

Rationale

An initial assessment should be performed to identify any immediately life-threatening problems. Because the patient is unconscious, his airway should be opened, and he should receive high-concentration oxygen. If the patient's breathing is inadequate, it should be assisted with a BVM. Because the patient is unconscious, a rapid physical examination should be performed to identify the problem. Because the patient has unequal pupils and no motor response on one side of his body, he has most probably had a cerebrovascular accident (CVA or stroke). The patient should be transported immediately to a facility with neurosurgical capability. The slow heart rate and elevated BP suggest increased intracranial pressure. If the patient continues to deteriorate, controlled hyperventilation at a rate of 20 breaths/min can be used to temporarily decrease the intracranial pressure.

14.5. **D,** Your first step to care for this patient would be to perform an initial assessment by checking his mental status and the status of his airway, breathing, and circulation. The rapid physical examination and vital signs are not performed until the initial assessment is completed. Giving oxygen by mask is not appropriate until the patient's breathing is assessed. If the breathing is inadequate, oxygen may have to be delivered using a bag-valve mask (BVM).

14.6. B, The patient's airway is open, and he seems to be ventilating adequately. However, he is unresponsive. Therefore, high-concentration oxygen should be given by non-rebreather mask before proceeding with the rest of the patient assessment. Problems identified during the initial assessment should be corrected as they are discovered.

14.7. B, The elevated BP, slow pulse, unequal pupils, and hemiplegia (one-sided paralysis) suggest the patient has had a CVA (stroke). An episode of angina pectoris can be associated with weakness or dizziness but is unlikely to cause unconsciousness. Unconsciousness after an acute myocardial infarction is likely to be associated with an irregularity in the heart's rhythm or a decrease in the heart's pumping action that causes poor perfusion. This patient's perfusion seems to be adequate. Nothing in the history or physical examination indicates possible presence of traumatic head injury.

14.8. B, The most appropriate care for this patient would be management of airway and breathing and rapid transport to the hospital. The elevated BP is part of the body's attempt to compensate for the stroke. Placing a nitroglycerin tablet under the tongue would interfere with this response and could result in the patient aspirating the tablet. Because there is no history or evidence of trauma, spinal motion restriction does not have to be performed. Elevating the patient's lower extremities is not indicated because the patient is not hypotensive and elevation of the legs could increase intracranial pressure.

SCENARIO THREE

Plan of Action
1. BSI
2. Is the scene safe? Yes. Assess nature of illness, number of patients, and need for additional resources.
3. Assess mental status. Ensure open airway, assess breathing, apply oxygen 10-15 lpm by non-rebreather mask, and assess circulation.
4. Determine priority, consider ALS.
5. HPI, SAMPLE
6. Focused physical examination
7. Baseline vital signs
8. Transport, perform ongoing assessment.

Rationale
No immediately life-threatening problems were identified during the initial assessment. Because the patient keeps asking the same questions repeatedly, she should be considered to have altered mental status and given high-concentration oxygen. Her chief complaint, HPI, and past history suggest that she may have had a TIA. A physical examination focusing on neurologic function should be performed. Because low blood glucose level can produce altered mental status, you should check her blood sugar level if your local protocols allow EMT-Basics to perform this procedure. Otherwise, you should request a response by an ALS unit. The patient should receive ongoing assessment during transport for other indicators of transient decreases in blood flow to her brain.

14.9. **C,** After the initial assessment, you should obtain a history of the present illness and pertinent past history (HPI and SAMPLE). The information obtained will help to focus the physical examination and determine whether a call for an ALS unit is necessary. The rapid physical examination is performed for unconscious medical patients when the information needed to focus the examination cannot be obtained.

14.10. **C,** The history and physical examination findings suggest a TIA. A TIA is an episode of altered brain function caused by a decreased blood flow. TIAs resolve themselves in a short time with no lasting effects, unlike CVAs (strokes), which produce lasting effects. This patient's TIA could be the result of atherosclerosis in her cerebral or carotid arteries. It also could have resulted from a temporary decrease in her heart's output. Because there is no history of chest pain, the patient did not suffer an episode of angina pectoris. The absence of wheezing and respiratory distress rules out bronchospasm from her COPD. Her BP is not sufficiently elevated to cause a hypertensive crisis.

14.11. **B,** Your treatment would include high-concentration oxygen, placing the patient in a semi-sitting position, and calling for an ALS unit. Placing a patient with a head injury or stroke in a supine position can increase intracranial pressure and worsen the problem. Because the patient is not experiencing cardiac chest pain, nitroglycerin is not indicated.

Scenario Four

Plan of Action

1. BSI
2. Is the scene safe? Yes. Assess nature of illness, number of patients, and need for additional resources.
3. Assess mental status. Ensure an open airway, assess breathing, apply oxygen 10-15 lpm by non-rebreather mask, and assess circulatory status.
4. Determine priority, consider ALS.
5. HPI, SAMPLE
6. Rapid physical examination
7. Baseline vital signs
8. Transport, perform ongoing assessment.

Rationale

The patient is confused and weak but seems to have no problems with airway, breathing, and circulation. The altered mental status; cool, moist skin; and history of diabetes suggest she has a low blood glucose level. The increased activity associated with playing baseball might have lowered her blood sugar level more rapidly than she had anticipated. The vital signs do not indicate any problem with volume loss from sweating and are consistent with the release of epinephrine (adrenaline) that occurs when the blood sugar level is too low. Because the patient is confused and has a history of syncope, it would be reasonable to perform a rapid physical examination to rule out other causes of altered mental status and to identify any injuries that might have occurred when she lost consciousness. If she is able to maintain her own airway and swallow, she can be given sugar in orange juice. If you are concerned about her ability to drink safely, an ALS unit should be called to confirm the presence of low blood sugar and to give glucose intravenously.

14.12. B, The patient knows who she is and where she is, but she cannot recall what day it is or what happened. Therefore, she is oriented to person and place but not to time and events.

14.13. B, After completing an initial assessment and obtaining the patient's past medical history you should perform a rapid physical examination. The patient and bystanders have not been able to provide enough information to allow the physical examination to be focused on a specific problem or body system.

14.14. C, The patient probably has low blood sugar. The circumstances under which she has presented suggest she took her Orinase and then exercised more heavily than normal while playing baseball, resulting in a rapid decrease in her blood sugar. If she was hypovolemic from sweating she would be expected to have a rapid, weak pulse and a BP lower than 140/94. Elevated blood sugars in diabetic patients are associated with an increase in urine output that leads to hypovolemic shock. If the patient had overdosed on Orinase, the decrease in her blood sugar would have been rapid, producing signs and symptoms much more dramatic than those seen in this case.

14.15. C, Because the patient is awake and alert enough to drink, she should be given a glass of orange juice with sugar added or some other source of glucose. In some systems, protocols may dictate checking the blood sugar level first.

SCENARIO FIVE

Plan of Action
1. BSI
2. Is the scene safe? Yes. Assess MOI and nature of illness, number of patients, and need for additional resources.
3. Assess mental status. Ensure an open airway, assess breathing, apply oxygen 10-15 lpm by non-rebreather mask, and assess circulation.
4. Determine priority, consider ALS.
5. HPI, SAMPLE
6. Focused physical examination
7. Baseline vital signs
8. Transport, perform ongoing assessment.

Rationale
The initial assessment reveals no immediately life-threatening problems. The patient should be given high-concentration oxygen because of his shallow respirations, the history of trauma to the chest wall, and the presence of chest pain. A focused examination of the chest accompanied by a careful history of the chest pain should be performed. Because the pain is "sharp" in quality and is located in the lateral chest wall rather than under the sternum, it probably is the result of the chest trauma instead of a cardiac problem. The physical examination should include auscultation of the chest to determine whether a pneumothorax caused by a rib fracture could be present. Securing the patient's injured arm over the injured area with cravats can splint the chest wall. He should receive high-concentration oxygen and be transported in a semi-sitting position.

14.16. C, You should obtain a history and perform a focused physical examination. The patient appears to have no immediate problems with his airway, breathing, and circulation. He is awake, alert, and oriented, so he will be able to provide information that will help focus the physical examination on the body system(s) that most likely are causing his problem.

14.17. A, The patient's signs and symptoms could be a result of his striking his chest or could be caused by a cardiac event. You should examine the chest for evidence of significant trauma and also explore the chief complaint of chest pain by asking the OPQRST questions. The MOI is unlikely to have produced spinal injuries, so performing a check of extremity motor and sensory function and spinal motion restriction are not indicated. The rapid trauma examination is performed in situations involving a significant MOI or when the patient is unable to provide information to help focus the examination.

14.18. B, The severity of the patient's pain can be assessed by asking him to rate it on a scale of 1 to 10, with 10 being the worst pain he has ever felt. The quality of the pain is described in the patient's own words but is unrelated to its severity. Whether the pain radiates to another area of the body also has nothing to do with its severity.

14.19. C, The purpose of the focused physical examination is to determine if there are any life-threatening problems and to identify possible causes of the patient's chest pain. The chief complaint and SAMPLE history are useful to guide the focused physical examination. A rapid physical examination is performed when a patient is unable to provide the information needed to focus the physical examination.

14.20. B, The patient's description of the severity of his pain is not a pertinent negative finding. A pertinent negative finding is one that you would expect a patient with a particular complaint to have that is *not* present. Because this patient has chest pain, the absence of shortness of breath, weakness, or dizziness are all pertinent.

SCENARIO SIX

Plan of Action

1. <u>BSI</u>

2. <u>Is the scene safe? Yes. Assess nature of illness, number of patients, and need for additional resources.</u>

3. <u>Assess mental status. Ensure open airway, assess breathing, apply oxygen 10-15 lpm by non-rebreather mask, and assess circulation.</u>

4. <u>Determine priority, consider ALS.</u>

5. <u>HPI, SAMPLE</u>

6. <u>Focused physical examination</u>

Continued

SCENARIO SIX—cont'd

7. <u>Baseline vital signs</u>

8. <u>Transport, provide ongoing assessment.</u>

Rationale

The complaints of fever, nausea, vomiting, and headache suggest the presence of an infectious disease. Immediate steps should be taken to reduce the risk of exposure for all responding personnel. In particular, face masks should be considered to reduce exposure to airborne pathogens. The stiff neck found during the focused examination strongly suggests that the patient has meningitis. The patient should be given high-concentration oxygen. All other personnel who might care for the patient should receive advanced warning to ensure they use appropriate protective equipment. During transport, this patient's perfusion should be monitored carefully. Although the BP is within normal limits for a 7-y.o. child, the weak, rapid pulse may indicate the patient is having difficulty maintaining adequate perfusion. Some types of bacterial meningitis frequently progress to septic shock.

14.21. B, The components of the focused examination are based on several factors: the presenting complaint, or the obvious injury; findings from the initial assessment; parts of the past medical history; and/or events that led up to the problem. Focused physical examinations can be performed on pediatric patients based on information provided by the patient and his or her parents. The focused examination is *not* performed the same way for each patient. The focus of the examination varies depending on the chief complaint, HPI, and past history.

14.22. A, For a 7-y.o. child a BP of 106/64 is within normal limits. Therefore, the patient is normotensive.

14.23. C, The combination of neck pain, headache, nausea, vomiting, and fever suggests meningitis.

14.24. A, Neck pain is a positive finding during this patient's physical examination because it is an observation related to the chief complaint that helps identify the underlying problem. In this patient, absence of neck pain would have been a pertinent negative finding because the other physical examination findings point to meningitis. The neck pain should be identified during the focused physical examination, not during the ongoing assessment.

14.25. C, You should request an ALS unit and begin transport with oxygen. The patient should be monitored closely because of increased risk of aspiration if vomiting occurs while an oxygen mask is in place. The ALS unit and the emergency department should be notified of your suspicions so they can be prepared with the proper isolation procedures. Covering the patient would not be appropriate because he is febrile. Spinal precautions are unnecessary because the neck pain is not the result of trauma. Because the patient's respiratory rate is within normal limits for his age and he shows no signs of difficulty breathing, he does not need to be ventilated with a bag-valve mask.

SCENARIO SEVEN

Plan of Action

1. BSI

2. Is the scene safe? Yes. Assess nature of illness, number of patients, and need for additional resources.

3. Assess mental status. Ensure open airway, assess breathing, apply oxygen 10-15 lpm by non-rebreather mask, and assess circulation.

4. Determine priority, consider ALS.

5. HPI, SAMPLE

6. Focused physical examination

7. Baseline vital signs

8. Transport, perform ongoing assessment.

Rationale

After an initial assessment is performed and any immediately life-threatening problems corrected, a focused physical examination should be performed based on the chief complaint and HPI. The patient should be given high-concentration oxygen because she has altered neurologic function. The physical examination findings suggest the patient has had a stroke. She should be transported rapidly to a facility that has the capability of performing a computed tomography (CAT) scan. If the patient's stroke is caused by obstruction of a blood vessel by a clot (rather than by a bleed), early use of thrombolytic agents (clot-dissolving drugs) may allow her to recover full function.

14.26. **B,** A focused physical examination of the neurologic system should be performed to help determine the cause of the patient's weakness and inability to speak. Because information is available to help focus the examination, the complete rapid physical examination or the detailed examination is not necessary. The mechanism does not suggest the presence of any significant injuries, so a rapid trauma examination is not necessary.

14.27. **D,** The history and physical examination findings indicate the presence of a stroke, a medical problem.

14.28. **C,** Treatment would include the focused physical examination and calling for an ALS unit. The ALS personnel will place the patient on an electrocardiographic (ECG) monitor because a cardiac problem may have triggered the stroke. They also will check the patient's blood glucose level and give glucose intravenously if necessary. Spinal immobilization is not necessary because the MOI does not indicate the presence of spinal trauma.

14.29. **A,** After completing the focused physical examination, you would obtain a set of vital signs.

14.30. **D,** Signs and symptoms of a stroke include weakness of one side of the body, drooping of one corner of the mouth, and slurred speech. Strokes usually produce signs and symptoms that affect only one side of the body. Weakness in all four extremities or in both upper extremities is unlikely to result from a stroke. Chest pain usually does not accompany a stroke.

SCENARIO EIGHT

Plan of Action

1. BSI

2. Is the scene safe? Yes. Assess nature of illness, number of patients, and need for additional resources.

3. Assess mental status. Ensure open airway, assess breathing, apply oxygen 10-15 lpm by non-rebreather mask, and assess circulation.

4. Determine priority, consider ALS.

5. HPI, SAMPLE

6. Focused physical examination

7. Baseline vital signs

8. Transport, perform ongoing assessment.

Rationale

The initial assessment reveals no immediately life-threatening problems involving airway, breathing, or circulation. The patient should be given high-concentration oxygen because she experienced a temporary loss of consciousness. A physical examination should be performed focusing initially on neurologic function and then on the cardiovascular system. The patient may have experienced a TIA. She also could have had an arrhythmia that led to a decrease in her cardiac output. An ALS unit should be requested for ECG monitoring. The patient's blood glucose level also should be checked. She should be transported with ongoing monitoring of her neurologic function and perfusion.

14.31. **D,** You would begin the physical examination by performing an initial assessment of mental status, airway, breathing, and circulation to identify and correct any immediately life-threatening problems.

14.32. **B,** Because she had a syncopal episode, the initial focus should be on the neurologic examination. She could have experienced a TIA. The vital signs and other physical findings do not indicate any problems with perfusion related to a cardiovascular problem. However, a temporary decrease in the heart's output because of an arrhythmia should be considered as an alternative cause.

14.33. **C,** Syncope is the medical term for fainting—a temporary loss of consciousness caused by a reduction in blood flow to the brain.

14.34. **D,** The patient's problem could have been caused by a TIA or by a decrease in cardiac output resulting from an arrhythmia. A patient who takes a diuretic such as furosemide may experience episodes of dizziness or syncope related to decreased blood volume. However, this patient's vital signs do not indicate a problem with her blood volume or perfusion.

SCENARIO NINE

Plan of Action

1. BSI

2. Is the scene safe? Yes. Assess nature of illness, number of patients, and need for additional resources.

3. Position patient to protect airway during seizure. Prevent injury by protecting patient's head and keeping it from striking the floor or nearby objects. Do *not* attempt to place anything in the patient's mouth.

4. When seizure stops, assess mental status. Ensure an open airway, assess breathing, apply oxygen at 10-15 lpm by non-rebreather mask, and assess circulation.

5. Determine priority, consider ALS.

6. Rapid physical examination

7. Baseline vital signs

8. HPI, SAMPLE

9. Transport, perform ongoing assessment.

Rationale

Because the patient was still seizing when you arrived, your priority is to keep her from injuring herself. Roll her on her side to prevent aspiration if she vomits. Never try to restrain a patient who is having a seizure. Never place anything in the patient's mouth. Place padding under the head and move any objects that may pose a danger. When the seizure ends, ensure an open airway and administer high-concentration oxygen. Perform a rapid physical examination for problems that may have caused the seizure or for injuries that could have occurred during it. Check the blood glucose level if EMT-Basics in your area are authorized to perform this procedure. The patient probably will be sleepy for a short period after the seizure ends. During this period give her high-concentration oxygen, and let her rest. Because the patient has not had seizures for several years, she will need to be transported for evaluation. You should consider requesting an ALS unit. The paramedics will be able to start an intravenous line and can give medications to stop any seizure activity that may recur.

14.35. **A,** Your first priority is to protect the patient's airway from aspiration by rolling her onto her side. Once the airway is protected, you should keep the patient from injuring herself by hitting her head or extremities against the floor or any nearby furniture.

14.36. **C,** When the seizure ends, the airway, breathing, and circulation should be assessed. Then the patient should be given oxygen at 15 lpm. Patients do not breathe during a seizure and therefore develop hypoxia. Early administration of oxygen will help the patient recover from the seizure more quickly. There is no need to immobilize the spine because the mechanism does not involve significant trauma. Inserting an oral airway could make the patient vomit.

14.37. C, Because the patient is unconscious, you would perform an initial assessment and then a rapid physical examination. The physical examination should include a check for any injuries that might have occurred during the seizure.

14.38. A, After a seizure, a patient usually experiences a brief period of drowsiness called the postictal phase.

14.39. B, SAMPLE represents taking a patient's history. DCAP-BTLS is a memory aid for common types of injuries found during a rapid trauma examination. OPQRST is a memory aid for questions to ask while evaluating pain. AEIOU-TIPS is a tool for recalling common causes of unconsciousness.

14.40. B, Inspection is a visual examination of part of a patient's body. Auscultation refers to listening with the stethoscope. Palpation means feeling. Percussion is performed by tapping part of the body with the tip of the finger and listening to the sound produced.

14.41. D, Percussion is an examination technique that consists of tapping with the fingertips to evaluate size and borders of some internal organs or to detect the presence of fluid or gas in a body cavity.

14.42. A, Listening with the stethoscope is auscultation.

14.43. D, A properly sized BP cuff should be approximately two-thirds the length of the upper arm.

15

Respiratory Diseases

RESPIRATORY SYSTEM FUNCTIONS

- Supply oxygen to cells and tissues of body
- Remove carbon dioxide from body

ANATOMY

- Upper airway
  - Nasal and oral cavities
  - Pharynx
    - Nasopharynx
    - Oropharynx
  - Laryngopharynx
  - Epiglottis
- Lower airway
  - Larynx
  - Trachea
  - Mainstem bronchi
  - Lobar, segmental, and subsegmental bronchi
  - Bronchioles
  - Alveoli
- Pleura
  - Visceral pleura—Covers lungs
  - Parietal pleura—Lies against inside of chest wall, superior surface of diaphragm
  - Pleural space—Potential space between visceral and parietal pleura. Contains only small amount of pleural fluid

PHYSIOLOGY

- Inspiration—Active phase of breathing; also known as inhalation
  - Intercostal muscles and diaphragm contract.
  - Ribs move upward and outward; diaphragm lowers.
  - Volume of chest cavity increases; intrathoracic pressure decreases.
  - Air flows into respiratory tract until pressure equalizes.
- Expiration—Passive phase of breathing; also known as exhalation
  - Intercostal muscles and diaphragm relax.
  - Elasticity of lungs pulls ribs downward and inward, diaphragm upward.
  - Volume of chest cavity decreases; intrathoracic pressure increases.
  - Air flows out of respiratory tract until pressure equalizes.

ASSESSMENT

- Scene size-up
  - Body substance isolation (BSI)
  - Is the scene safe?
  - How many patients?
  - Nature of illness/mechanism of injury
  - Any additional resources needed?
- Initial assessment
  - If trauma present or suspected, manually stabilize head, neck
  - Mental status

- Awake, alert, and oriented
- Restless, anxious? Possible hypoxia or shock
  - ○ Airway
    - Open with jaw-thrust if cervical spine injury suspected
    - Clear by suctioning and/or manual finger sweeps
    - Maintain by placing appropriate airway adjunct (oral or nasal airway)
  - ○ Breathing
    - Present?
    - Adequate air movement?
    - Rate too fast or too slow?
    - Labored or unlabored? Accessory muscle use? Retractions?
    - Equal chest expansion?
    - Abnormal respiratory sounds? Snoring, gurgling, stridor, wheezing, or crackles?
  - ○ Circulation
    - Pulses present? Location, rate, and quality?
    - Skin color, temperature?
  - ○ Determine priority, consider requesting advanced life support (ALS) unit
- Focused history and physical examination
  - ○ OPQRST
    - Onset gradual or sudden?
    - Provocation
      - What brought on the shortness of breath?
      - Does it appear at any particular time or with any particular activity?
    - Quality
      - What does it feel like?
      - Any associated pain? Where? What does the pain feel like?
    - Region, radiation
      - If pain is present, where is it felt?
      - Does it travel anywhere else?
    - Severity on a scale of 1 to 10, with 10 being most severe
    - Time
      - How long ago did it begin?
  - ○ Physical examination findings
    - Restlessness, anxiety, or confusion
    - Cough, hoarseness, or excessive sputum
    - Pallor, cyanosis
    - Nasal flaring, pursed lips
    - Use of accessory muscles
    - Retractions
    - Abdominal breathing
    - Barrel-shaped chest
    - Orthopnea (inability to lie down, must sit up to breathe)
    - Pleuritic chest pain (sharp or stabbing pain worsened by taking a deep breath)
    - Inability to speak full sentences because of breathing difficulty
    - Hemoptysis (coughing up blood)
    - Seesaw breathing (children)
    - Grunting (infants)

- Abnormal breath sounds
  - Snoring—Caused by tongue partially obstructing airway
  - Stridor—High-pitched, crowing sounds usually associated with upper airway obstruction; usually heard on inspiration
  - Gurgling—Caused by fluid in upper airway
  - Wheezes—High-pitched, whistling sounds caused by air moving through narrowed lower airways; usually heard on expiration
  - Rhonchi—Low-pitched, rattling sounds caused by fluid in the larger lower airways
  - Crackles—High-pitched sounds caused by air moving through fluid in the alveoli and small airways; sound like strands of hair being rolled between two fingers

COMMON RESPIRATORY PROBLEMS
Severe Foreign Body Airway Obstruction

- Conscious adult or child
  - Perform abdominal thrusts until relieved or patient becomes unresponsive
  - If patient is large or in late stages of pregnancy, perform chest thrusts
- Conscious infant
  - Alternate 5 back blows and 5 chest thrusts until obstruction relieved or patient becomes unresponsive
- Unconscious adult
  - Open airway, establish absence of breathing
  - Attempt to ventilate
  - Reposition head to ensure tongue is not blocking airway; look in mouth, remove object if seen
  - Attempt to ventilate again
  - Perform CPR—30 chest compressions
  - Look in mouth before attempting to ventilate, remove object if seen
  - Attempt to ventilate
  - If chest does not rise, perform 30 chest compressions, look in mouth, remove object if seen, attemt to ventilate
- Unconscious child
  - Open airway, establish absence of breathing
  - Attempt to ventilate
  - Reposition head to ensure tongue is not blocking airway; look in mouth, remove object if seen
  - Attempt to ventilate again
  - Perform CPR—30 compressions (1 rescuer) 15 compressions (2 rescuers)
  - Look in mouth before attempting to ventilate, remove object if seen
  - Attempt to ventilate
  - If chest does not rise, perform chest compressions, look in mouth; remove object if seen, attempt to ventilate
- Unconscious infant
  - Open airway, establish absence of breathing
  - Attempt to ventilate
  - Reposition head to ensure tongue is not blocking airway; look in mouth, remove object if seen
  - Attempt to ventilate again
  - Perform CPR—30 compressions (1 rescuer) 15 compressions (2 rescuers)
  - Look in mouth before attempting to ventilate, remove object if seen
  - Attempt to ventilate
  - If chest does not rise, perform chest compressions; look in mouth, remove object if seen, attempt to ventilate

Asthma

- Chronic disease involving the lower airways
- Most common in children but can occur at any age
- Family history of asthma frequently present
- Reversible episodes of bronchospasm, inflammatory swelling of lower airway walls, and increased production of thick mucus
- Attacks may be triggered by cold weather, allergens, respiratory infection, or vigorous exercise
- Wheezing, coughing, and shortness of breath
- A "silent chest" (absence of wheezing) during an asthma attack indicates impending respiratory arrest.
- Give high-concentration oxygen, encourage coughing to clear mucus plugs, and assist patients in using inhaler or give bronchodilator treatment if authorized

Chronic Bronchitis

- Increased mucus production in lower airway with a productive cough for at least 3 months a year for at least 2 consecutive years
- Caused by smoking or chronic exposure to pulmonary irritants
- Signs and symptoms
  - Productive cough
  - Labored breathing
  - Increased respiratory rate
  - Use of accessory muscles
  - Inability to speak in complete sentences
  - Cyanotic complexion
  - Peripheral edema
  - Sometimes referred to as a "blue bloater"
- Emergency care
  - Position of comfort
  - Oxygen at 10 to 15 lpm by non-rebreather mask or as per protocol
  - Ongoing assessment every 5 minutes
  - Encourage to cough deeply
  - As protocols allow, assist patient with prescribed inhaler or give nebulized bronchodilators
  - Call for ALS if needed

Emphysema

- Loss of lung elasticity and destruction of alveolar walls leading to decreased gas exchange
- Caused by smoking or, rarely, by inherited disease
- Loss of pulmonary elasticity causes trapping of air and a "barrel chest"
- Signs and symptoms
  - Increased anterior-posterior thoracic diameter (barrel chest)
  - Increased respiratory rate
  - Dyspnea on exertion
  - Prolonged exhalation with pursed-lip breathing
  - Hypertrophy (overdevelopment) of respiratory muscles
  - Dyspnea on exertion
  - Sometimes referred to as a "pink puffer"

- Emergency care
  - Inadequate breathing, oxygen 10 to 15 lpm by non-rebreather mask
  - Adequate breathing—Oxygen by nasal cannula to match rate of patient's home oxygen supply
  - Ongoing assessment every 5 minutes
  - As protocols allow, assist patient with prescribed inhaler or give nebulized bronchodilators
  - Call for ALS if needed

Pneumonia

- Infection of lungs, causing accumulation of fluid (pus) in alveoli and interfering with gas exchange
- Caused by bacterial, viral, or fungus infections
- Signs and symptoms
  - Fever and chills
  - Increased respiratory rate (tachypnea)
  - Increased heart rate (tachycardia)
  - Cough
  - Possible pleuritic chest pain
  - Wheezing and crackles in affected areas of lung
- Emergency care
  - Position of comfort
  - Oxygen 10 to 15 lpm by non-rebreather mask
  - Ongoing assessment every 5 minutes
  - Call for ALS if needed

Acute Pulmonary Edema

- Fluid accumulation in and around alveoli increasing work of breathing and interfering with gas exchange
- Cardiogenic pulmonary edema caused by failure of left ventricle resulting in backup of fluid into lungs
- Noncardiogenic pulmonary edema caused by near-drowning, trauma, overdoses, or inhalation injury
- Signs and symptoms
  - Dyspnea on exertion
  - Increased respiratory rate (tachypnea)
  - Increased heart rate (tachycardia)
  - Restlessness, anxiety
  - Inability to breathe while lying down (orthopnea)
  - Cool, moist skin
  - Accessory muscle use
  - Wheezes and crackles, particularly in lung bases
  - Frothy, blood-tinged sputum
- Emergency care
  - Have patient sit upright, dangle legs over edge of stretcher
  - Oxygen at 15 lpm by non-rebreather mask
  - Ongoing assessment every 5 minutes
  - Call ALS

Spontaneous Pneumothorax

- Lung surface ruptures allowing air to leak into pleural space
- Most common in tall, thin, young males
- May be caused by coughing, exertion, and air travel
- Signs and symptoms
  - Shortness of breath
  - Decreased breath sounds on affected side
  - Sharp chest pain worsened by inhaling on affected side
- Emergency care
  - Position of comfort
  - Oxygen at 10 to 15 lpm by non-rebreather mask
  - Ongoing assessment every 5 minutes
  - Monitor for signs and symptoms of tension pneumothorax
  - Call ALS if patient develops signs and symptoms of tension pneumothorax

Pulmonary Embolism

- Caused by a blood clot that lodges in the pulmonary circulation causing partial or complete obstruction of blood flow
- Part of lung is ventilated but not perfused
- Blood returns from affected part of lung to heart without being oxygenated
- Causes
  - Prolonged bed rest
  - Prolonged immobility (long motor vehicle or airplane trips)
  - Recent surgery, especially of legs, pelvis, or abdomen
  - Leg or pelvic fractures
  - Birth control pills, particularly in patients who also smoke
  - Pregnancy
  - Chronic atrial fibrillation
- Signs and symptoms
  - Sudden onset of dyspnea
  - Possible cough
  - Sharp, stabbing chest pain associated with breathing (pleuritic pain)
  - Tachypnea
  - Tachycardia
  - Possible low blood pressure
  - Possible blood-tinged sputum
- Emergency care
  - Position of comfort
  - Oxygen at 10 to 15 lpm by non-rebreather mask
  - Ongoing assessment every 5 minutes
  - Call for ALS

REVIEW QUESTIONS
Scenario One

It is a Tuesday morning in mid-January. The temperature is 45° F. At 10:30 AM you are dispatched to a report of "difficulty breathing" at a middle school. The patient is a 13-y.o. female who developed shortness of breath while running outside during a physical education class. According to the school nurse, the patient does not have any significant past medical history. Vital signs are blood pressure (BP)—120/78; pulse (P)—108, strong, regular; and respiration (R)—32, regular, labored with expiratory wheezing in both lung fields.

Your Plan of Action

Fill in the blank lines with your treatment plan for this patient. Then compare your plan with the questions, answers, and rationale.

1. _____
2. _____
3. _____
4. _____
5. _____
6. _____
7. _____
8. _____
9. _____

Multiple Choice

15.1. What causes wheezing?
   a. Partially obstructed airway passages
   b. Infection of the alveoli
   c. Narrowing of the cricoid cartilage
   d. A partially blocked trachea

15.2. All of the following statements about asthma are correct *except:*
   a. asthma presents with bronchospasm, increased mucus production, and bronchial edema.
   b. an asthma attack usually is self-correcting.
   c. an asthma attack may result from exposure to an allergen, a respiratory infection, emotional stress, or exercise.
   d. asthma can be serious enough to produce respiratory arrest.

True/False

15.3. Tachypnea and tachycardia are common findings with pediatric asthma.
   a. True
   b. False

Multiple Choice

15.4. Wheezing is characterized by:
   a. rattling sounds caused by fluid in the larger airways.
   b. sounds like those produced by rubbing strands of hair through your fingers.
   c. a crowing sound heard on inspiration.
   d. high-pitched sounds caused by narrowing of the small airways.

15.5. Your treatment for this patient would include:
    a. giving oxygen by nasal cannula at 6 lpm.
    b. assisting ventilations with a bag-valve mask (BVM).
    c. giving oxygen at 10 to 15 lpm by non-rebreather mask.
    d. keeping the patient calm.

Scenario Two

The patient is a 68-y.o. male with respiratory distress that has worsened progressively during the past 2 days. The patient is conscious, restless, and anxious. He is oriented to person, place, time, and events. Cyanosis of the lips and nail beds is present. Rhonchi and crackles can be auscultated in the lower portion of right lung field. The patient says he caught a "cold" approximately 1 week ago and has been coughing up yellow-green sputum for 3 or 4 days. He is receiving home oxygen therapy with a nasal cannula at 2 lpm. He tells you he has a history of emphysema, angina pectoris, and osteoarthritis. His medications include Theobid Duracaps, Nitrostat, and ibuprofen as needed. Vital signs are BP—138/70; P—116, weak, regular; R—26, regular, labored; SaO_2— 82%; and temperature (T)—100.6° F.

Your Plan of Action

Fill in the blank lines with your treatment plan for this patient. Then compare your plan with the questions, answers, and rationale.

1. _____
2. _____
3. _____
4. _____
5. _____
6. _____
7. _____
8. _____
9. _____

Labelling

15.6. Label the components of the respiratory system on the diagram at the top of p. 293.

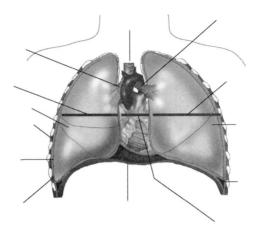

Multiple Choice

15.7. Chronic obstructive pulmonary disease (COPD) includes:
    a. chronic bronchitis.
    b. constant reoccurring episodes of asthma.
    c. emphysema.
    d. either chronic bronchitis or emphysema.

15.8. All of the following statements about COPD are correct *except:*
    a. COPD is a progressive, irreversible respiratory disease that causes decreased inspiratory and expiratory capacity of the lungs.
    b. most patients with COPD have a combination of chronic bronchitis and emphysema.
    c. COPD develops more rapidly than other respiratory diseases and produces bronchospasms.
    d. COPD patients will c/o shortness of breath gradually increasing over several days.

15.9. Treatment of your patient would include:
    a. giving oxygen at 2 to 4 lpm by nasal cannula and calling for ALS.
    b. preparing for intubation and calling for ALS.
    c. giving oxygen at 10 to 15 lpm by non-rebreather mask and calling for ALS.
    d. giving oxygen at 15 lpm via non-rebreather mask, keeping the patient supine, keeping the patient warm, and calling for ALS.

15.10. COPD is characterized by:
    a. patients found sitting in the "tripod" position.
    b. filling of the lungs with fluid so patients feel as if they are drowning.
    c. an underlying bacterial, viral, or fungal infection.
    d. pedal edema, shortness of breath, and abdominal tenderness.

15.11. Your approach to caring for this patient would include:
    a. calling for ALS, preparing for immediate transport, and allowing the paramedic to do the patient examination.
    b. applying oxygen and doing a history of present illness (HPI), SAMPLE, and focused physical examination.
    c. BSI, applying oxygen, and doing a rapid physical examination and ongoing assessment on the way to the hospital.
    d. BSI, performing an initial assessment, applying oxygen, and obtaining baseline vital signs.

Scenario Three

The patient is a 45-y.o. female who is complaining of difficulty breathing. She is speaking in full sentences but tells you she has had a "cough and congestion" for the past 2 weeks. Earlier today she began to experience sharp, left-sided chest pain when she coughed. Her skin is flushed, moist, and warm. Fine crackles are present in the lower half of the left lung field. She has no significant past medical history and does not take any medications on a regular basis. Vital signs are BP—110/72; P—112, strong, regular; R—20, regular, slightly labored because of the coughing; SaO_2—96%; and T—102.8° F.

Your Plan of Action

Fill in the blank lines with your treatment plan for this patient. Then compare your plan with the questions, answers, and rationale.

1. _____
2. _____
3. _____
4. _____
5. _____
6. _____
7. _____
8. _____
9. _____

Multiple Choice

15.12. This patient *most likely* has:
    a. asthma.
    b. COPD.
    c. pulmonary edema.
    d. pneumonia.

True/False

15.13. Pneumonia is an inflammatory condition of the lungs caused by either a bacterial or a viral infection that has a slow onset.
    a. True
    b. False

Multiple Choice

15.14. Which of the following descriptions of a patient with pneumonia is *most* correct?
    a. Fever and chills, cough productive of rust-colored or green sputum, and crackles in one lung field
    b. Acute onset of shortness of breath, cough productive of pink sputum, orthopnea, and crackles heard in both lung fields
    c. A "silent" chest on auscultation, anxiety, and shortness of breath
    d. Pedal edema, crackles in the lung bases

15.15. Your treatment of this patient would include:
   a. calling for an ALS unit so she may be evaluated for a possible myocardial infarction.
   b. applying oxygen and doing an HPI, SAMPLE, and focused physical examination.
   c. BSI, applying oxygen, and performing a rapid physical examination and ongoing assessment on the way to the hospital.
   d. BSI, performing an initial assessment, applying oxygen, and obtaining baseline vital signs.

Scenario Four

A 68-y.o. female is sitting on the edge of her bed in severe respiratory distress. She is unable to speak in complete sentences and is using her accessory muscles to breathe. Her husband tells you she was fine when she went to bed but awoke with difficulty breathing approximately 15 minutes ago. He says she also has been having a problem with her ankles swelling for the past 3 to 4 weeks. The patient's lips and nail beds are cyanotic. Crackles can be heard in the lower halves of both lung fields. Pitting edema of both feet and ankles is present. The patient has a past history of angina pectoris and hypertension. She has smoked one pack of cigarettes per day for the past 30 years. Medications include Cardizem, nitroglycerin as needed, 1 baby aspirin a day, furosemide, and an Atrovent inhaler as needed. Vital signs are BP—186/100; P—124, weak, regular; R—34, regular, labored; and SaO_2—88%.

Your Plan of Action

Fill in the blank lines with your treatment plan for this patient. Then compare your plan with the questions, answers, and rationale.

1. _____
2. _____
3. _____
4. _____
5. _____
6. _____
7. _____
8. _____
9. _____

Multiple Choice

15.16. What problem is this patient *most likely* suffering from?
   a. Asthma
   b. COPD
   c. Pulmonary edema
   d. Pneumonia

15.17. Which of the following descriptions of a patient with pulmonary edema is *most* correct?

    a. Fever and chills, cough productive of rust-colored or green sputum, and crackles in one lung field

    b. Acute onset of shortness of breath, cough productive of pink sputum, orthopnea, and crackles heard in both lung fields

    c. A "silent" chest on auscultation, anxiety, and shortness of breath

    d. Pedal edema, crackles in the lung bases

15.18. Which of the following *best* describes a patient with a severe asthma attack?

    a. Fever and chills, cough productive of rust-colored or green sputum, and crackles in one lung field

    b. Acute onset of shortness of breath, cough productive of pink sputum, orthopnea, and crackles heard in both lung fields

    c. A "silent" chest on auscultation, anxiety, and shortness of breath

    d. Pedal edema, crackles in the lung bases

15.19. Treatment of this patient would include:

    a. applying oxygen 2 to 4 lpm and calling for an ALS unit so she may be evaluated for a possible myocardial infarction.

    b. performing an initial assessment, applying oxygen at 15 lpm, and calling for an ALS unit.

    c. not applying oxygen because she is breathing on the hypoxic drive, performing an initial assessment, and calling for an ALS unit.

    d. BSI, performing an initial assessment, applying oxygen at 15 lpm by non-rebreather mask, and obtaining baseline vital signs.

Scenario Five

A 14-y.o. female is in severe respiratory distress with audible wheezing. According to her mother, the patient has been having an asthma attack for the past 3 hours. She has used her inhalers several times, but the medications are not working. The patient is using her accessory muscles to breathe, and you can hear expiratory wheezes over both lung fields. She is very anxious. Her skin is pale, cool, and diaphoretic. Cyanosis of the lips and nail beds is present. Vital signs are BP—112/60, P—120, strong, regular; R—32, regular, labored; and SaO_2—90%.

Your Plan of Action

Fill in the blank lines with your treatment plan for this patient. Then compare your plan with the questions, answers, and rationale.

1. _____

2. _____

3. _____

4. _____

5. _____

6. _____

7. _____

8. _____

9. _____

Multiple Choice

15.20. Your *greatest* concern for this patient should be that:
  a. she may have overused her inhalers, which may make her condition worse.
  b. she is overmedicated, so you should reduce the flow of oxygen.
  c. she is in danger of going into respiratory arrest.
  d. she may have some problem in addition to asthma.

15.21. This patient probably:
  a. has asthma complicated by pneumonia.
  b. is having a chronic attack.
  c. is breathing on a "hypoxic drive."
  d. has status asthmaticus.

15.22. A patient in this age group has a normal respiratory rate of:
  a. 8 to 16 breaths/min.
  b. 20 to 30 breaths/min.
  c. 12 to 30 breaths/min.
  d. 12 to 20 breaths/min.

15.23. Asthma may be caused by all of the following *except:*
  a. dry, warm weather.
  b. cigarette smoke, air pollution, and dust.
  c. exercising in cold weather.
  d. emotional stress.

True/False

15.24. Certain chemicals such as red and yellow food dye may cause an asthma attack.
  a. True
  b. False

Multiple Choice

15.25. All of the following statements about status asthmaticus are correct *except:*
  a. status asthmaticus usually does not respond to nebulized bronchodilators.
  b. status asthmaticus can only be caused by exposure to allergens.
  c. status asthmaticus frequently is precipitated by a respiratory infection.
  d. the patient may require endotracheal intubation.

15.26. Your treatment of this patient would include:
  a. giving oxygen at 2 lpm to override the hypoxic drive.
  b. monitoring the respiratory rate closely to ensure it does not go over 12 breaths/min.
  c. skipping the initial assessment and transporting immediately because the patient is critically ill.
  d. doing an initial assessment, giving oxygen at 15 lpm, calling for an ALS unit, preparing for intubation, and transporting.

Scenario Six

You respond to a "possible heart attack." The patient is a 39-y.o. male c/o sharp right-sided chest pain. He says the pain began approximately 1 hour ago and is becoming worse, especially when he takes a deep breath. He has coughed up some pink-tinged sputum. The patient is conscious and oriented to person, place, time, and events. His skin is pink, cool, and moist. Wheezing can be heard in the middle portion of the right lung field. He has no significant past medical history except for a fracture of the right tibia from a motor vehicle crash 4 weeks ago that was surgically repaired. He takes no medications and has no known allergies. Vital signs are BP—104/50; P—116, weak, regular; R—24, regular, labored; and SaO$_2$—92%.

Your Plan of Action

Fill in the blank lines with your treatment plan for this patient. Then compare your plan with the questions, answers, and rationale.

1. _____
2. _____
3. _____
4. _____
5. _____
6. _____
7. _____
8. _____
9. _____

Multiple Choice

15.27. What problem is this patient *most likely* suffering from?
  a. Acute myocardial infarction
  b. Severe pneumonia
  c. Pulmonary embolism
  d. Early onset COPD

15.28. Your treatment of this patient would include:
  a. assisting the patient in taking a nitroglycerin tablet.
  b. keeping the patient warm, applying oxygen, and transporting the patient for antibiotic therapy.
  c. performing an initial assessment, applying oxygen at 15 lpm, and calling for an ALS unit.
  d. performing an initial assessment, applying oxygen at 2 to 4 lpm so it does not override the hypoxic drive, and transporting.

True/False

15.29. Obstructive airway diseases include asthma, chronic bronchitis, and emphysema.
  a. True
  b. False

Multiple Choice

15.30. All of the following may cause a pulmonary embolism *except:*
  a. recent surgery.
  b. extreme exercise.
  c. long air or auto trips.
  d. a recent long bone fracture.

Scenario Seven

A 26-y.o. male experienced a sudden onset of "stabbing" left-sided chest pain accompanied by shortness of breath. He is conscious and oriented to person, place, and time. However, he is very anxious. Breath sounds are diminished over the left lung field. The patient's only past medical history is a "cold" with a nonproductive cough approximately 1 week ago. He has no chronic medical problems and runs on a daily basis because he is training for a marathon. He takes no medications except vitamins and has no allergies. Vital signs are BP—100 /62; P—110, weak, regular; R—26, regular, labored; and SaO$_2$—97%.

Your Plan of Action

Fill in the blank lines with your treatment plan for this patient. Then compare your plan with the questions, answers, and rationale.

1. _____
2. _____
3. _____
4. _____
5. _____
6. _____
7. _____
8. _____
9. _____

Multiple Choice

15.31. What problem is this patient *most likely* suffering from?
   a. Acute myocardial infarction
   b. Severe pneumonia
   c. Spontaneous pneumothorax
   d. Pulmonary embolism

15.32. Your treatment for this patient would include all of the following *except:*
   a. giving high-concentration oxygen at 15 lpm and performing a focused examination of the chest.
   b. performing an initial assessment and giving oxygen 2 to 4 lpm by nasal cannula.
   c. assisting the patient in a position of comfort.
   d. obtaining baseline vital signs and noting breath sounds during the ongoing assessment.

15.33. Signs and symptoms of a spontaneous pneumothorax may include:
   a. increased blood pressure, decreased pulse rate, and increased respiratory rate.
   b. respiratory distress, decreased breath sounds, anxiety, weak pulse, distended neck veins, tracheal deviation, and subcutaneous emphysema.
   c. chest pain, crackles on the affected side, and hypotension.
   d. respiratory distress, flat neck veins, hypotension, and subcutaneous emphysema.

True/False

15.34. A spontaneous pneumothorax may be caused by a congenital defect or by COPD.

    a. True

    b. False

Scenario Eight

You are dispatched to a report of a "child not breathing." The patient is a 3-y.o. female who is lying on the floor. Your initial assessment reveals the patient is not breathing but has a carotid pulse of 128. Cyanosis of the face and oral mucous membranes is present. According to her mother, the patient had been playing with her brother's marbles when she began "acting funny" and then lost consciousness.

Your Plan of Action

Fill in the blank lines with your treatment plan for this patient. Then compare your plan with the questions, answers, and rationale.

1. _____

2. _____

3. _____

4. _____

5. _____

6. _____

7. _____

8. _____

9. _____

Multiple Choice

15.35. When you attempt to ventilate with a BVM, the chest does not rise. You should:

    a. immediately call for a paramedic to intubate the patient.

    b. continue to ventilate the patient at a rate of 20 breaths/min.

    c. prepare for spinal immobilization because trauma might be involved.

    d. reposition the head and attempt to ventilate again.

True/False

15.36. You should perform a blind finger sweep to relieve a foreign body airway obstruction.

    a. True

    b. False

Multiple Choice

15.37. Which of the following sequences for managing a foreign body airway obstruction in a child is *correct*?

    a. Attempt to ventilate; if no relief, reposition and attempt again; perform abdominal thrusts until the object is removed; repeat the ventilation-abdominal thrust sequence.

    b. Attempt to ventilate; if no success, reposition the head and attempt again; do a blind finger sweep followed by five back blows and five abdominal thrusts.

    c. Attempt to ventilate; if no success, reposition the head and attempt again; open the airway and attempt to visualize the object; and perform five back blows and five abdominal thrusts.

    d. Attempt to ventilate; if no success, reposition the head and attempt again; if no success, perform CPR; open mouth; if object is seen, remove it; repeat sequence of attempt to ventilate—perform CPR—check mouth until object is removed or patient is ventilated.

Scenario Nine

You are dispatched to "assist the police—unknown illness." When you arrive a police officer takes you to a 30-y.o. male who she found lying unconscious in an alley. The patient smells of alcohol, urine, and feces. His clothes are disheveled and torn. An empty whiskey bottle is lying nearby. The patient responds to painful stimuli by moaning but does not open his eyes or speak. There are no bystanders around to tell you what happened, and there is no evidence of trauma. Vital signs are BP—108/70; P—82, weak, regular; R—8, shallow, regular, and unlabored; and SaO$_2$—90%.

Your Plan of Action

Fill in the blank lines with your treatment plan for this patient. Then compare your plan with the questions, answers, and rationale.

1. _____
2. _____
3. _____
4. _____
5. _____
6. _____
7. _____
8. _____
9. _____

Multiple Choice

15.38. Which of the following actions should you be prepared to take?

    a. Treat the patient for impending shock.

    b. Treat the patient for altered mental status.

    c. Begin ventilating the patient to increase the respiratory rate.

    d. Treat the patient for alcohol intoxication.

15.39. Another term for a slow respiratory rate is:
    a. tachypnea.
    b. bradypnea.
    c. apnea.
    d. dyspnea.

15.40. The patient no longer responds to painful stimuli. What should you do now?
    a. Increase the amount of oxygen being given.
    b. Intubate the patient.
    c. Insert an oropharyngeal airway.
    d. Obtain another set of vital signs.

15.41. The patient begins to vomit. What should you do?
    a. Suction the patient with a tonsil-tip suction catheter.
    b. Suction the patient with a flexible catheter.
    c. Turn the head to the side to prevent aspiration.
    d. Sit the patient up to ensure an open airway.

Scenario Ten

You are dispatched to an "explosion" at a grocery store. When you arrive, you see staff and customers frantically running from the store. Their eyes are tearing, and they are complaining of dim or blurred vision. They all have pinpoint pupils and excessive secretions from their airways, noses, and eyes. Two are nauseated and beginning to vomit. One patient says she feels like she cannot breathe. The owner says someone threw a canister about the size of a hairspray can through the window. It exploded, releasing a vapor with a fruity odor. He also tells you there is one person still inside in the store whom he does not think is breathing.

Your Plan of Action

Fill in the blank lines with your treatment plan for these patients. Then compare your plan with the questions, answers, and rationale.

1. _____
2. _____
3. _____
4. _____
5. _____
6. _____
7. _____
8. _____
9. _____

Multiple Choice

15.42. These patients probably have been exposed to a:
    a. nerve agent, such as sarin.
    b. choking agent, such as phosgene or chlorine.
    c. blood agent, such as cyanide.
    d. blister agent, such as mustard gas or phosgene oxime.

15.43. Nerve agents are:
    a. chemical asphyxiants that interfere with oxygen use by cells.
    b. toxins that can produce increased secretions and paralysis.
    c. respiratory irritants that can cause pulmonary edema.
    d. skin irritants that can cause blistering or intense itching.

15.44. Sarin's odor is best described as being like that of:
    a. almonds.
    b. fruit.
    c. a swimming pool.
    d. freshly cut hay or grass.

15.45. All of the following statements about sarin are true *except:*
    a. factors that affect sarin are temperature, humidity, wind speed, and the nature of the terrain.
    b. skin exposure to a nerve agent may cause respiratory arrest and death.
    c. a small amount of sarin will cause increased saliva, mucus in the nose and mouth, pinpoint pupils, tightness in the chest, and shortness of breath.
    d. the effects of a small amount of nerve agents will begin within seconds to 1 minute and will include choking, gagging, and uncontrollable coughing.

15.46. Which of these statements *best* describes the action you should take?
    a. Enter the building to ensure there are no patients to be rescued.
    b. Call for the hazard materials (Hazmat) team.
    c. Begin triage and transport the critical patients to meet an ALS unit.
    d. Ensure no one else goes into the building; clear everyone back at least 1500 feet; call for the Hazmat team; and notify the police.

SCENARIO ONE

Plan of Action

1. Body Substance Isolation (BSI)
2. Is the scene safe? Yes. Assess nature of illness, number of patients, and need for additional resources.
3. Assess mental status. Ensure an open airway, assess breathing, apply oxygen at 10-15 lpm by non-rebreather mask, and assess circulatory status.
4. Determine priority, consider ALS.
5. HPI, SAMPLE
6. Focused physical examination
7. Baseline vital signs
8. Assist patient to use metered-dose inhaler or give bronchodilators by small volume nebulizer if authorized by local protocol.
9. Transport, perform ongoing assessment, and meet ALS unit.

Rationale

This patient is having an asthma attack. She should be given high-concentration oxygen by non-rebreather mask. If local protocols allow, a small volume nebulizer should used to give her a bronchodilator treatment. A response by an ALS unit should be requested because endotracheal intubation may be required if the patient's condition continues to worsen.

15.1. **A,** Wheezing during an asthma attack is caused by bronchospasm, swelling of the bronchial walls, and increased mucus secretion into the lower airway that partially obstructs airflow. As air moves through the partially obstructed passages, it produces the high-pitched, whistling sound called wheezing.

15.2. **B,** Asthma usually is *not* self-correcting. Asthma can be serious enough to cause respiratory arrest. When the wheezing is no longer present and the chest becomes "quiet," anticipate a possible respiratory arrest.

15.3. **A,** Tachycardia (rapid pulse rate) and tachypnea (rapid respiratory rate) are common in cases of pediatric asthma.

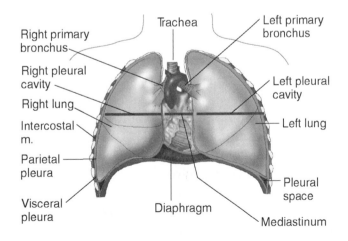

15.4. D, Wheezing is characterized by high-pitched breath sounds caused by narrowing of the small airways. Rattling sounds caused by fluid in the larger airways are called rhonchi. A crowing sound heard on inspiration is called stridor. Sounds like those produced by rubbing strands of hair through your fingers are crackles, which indicate presence of fluid in the alveoli and small airways.

15.5. C, This patient should receive oxygen at 10 to 15 lpm by non-rebreather mask. Restlessness and anxiety during an asthma attack are associated with hypoxia and can be relieved by adequately oxygenating the patient.

SCENARIO TWO

Plan of Action

1. BSI
2. Is the scene safe? Yes. Assess nature of illness, number of patients, and need for additional resources.
3. Assess mental status. Ensure an open airway, assess breathing, apply oxygen 10-15 lpm by non-rebreather mask, and assess circulatory status.
4. Determine priority, consider ALS.
5. HPI, SAMPLE
6. Focused physical examination
7. Baseline vital signs
8. Transport, perform ongoing assessment, and meet ALS unit.

Rationale

This patient appears to have COPD complicated by pneumonia. He should receive high-concentration oxygen by non-rebreather mask, and a meeting with an ALS unit should be coordinated.

15.6

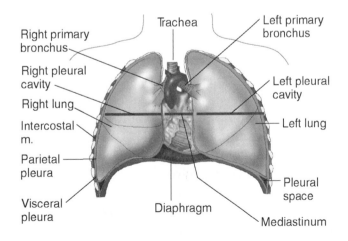

15.7. D, COPD includes either chronic bronchitis or emphysema. Most COPD patients have signs and symptoms characteristic of both diseases.

15.8. C, COPD has a gradual onset. However, the patient may have acute episodes resulting in increased difficulty breathing. These acute episodes may last for days and may require treatment with bronchodilators and antibiotics.

15.9. C, The patient should receive oxygen at 10 to 15 lpm by non-rebreather mask, and an ALS unit should be requested. Patients with difficulty breathing usually are most comfortable when they can sit upright.

15.10. A, A COPD patient often is found sitting upright and leaning forward in the "tripod" position. Filling of the lungs with fluid (pulmonary edema) characterizes congestive heart failure. Although pulmonary infections can worsen COPD, the disease is not caused by an underlying infection. Abdominal tenderness does not occur in COPD.

15.11. B, After performing an initial assessment, you should apply oxygen, perform an HPI, SAMPLE, and focused physical examination.

Scenario Three

Plan of Action
1. BSI
2. Is the scene safe? Yes. Assess nature of illness, number of patients, and need for additional resources.
3. Assess mental status. Ensure an open airway, assess breathing, apply oxygen 10-15 lpm by non-rebreather mask, and assess circulatory status.
4. Determine priority, consider ALS.
5. HPI, SAMPLE
6. Focused physical examination
7. Baseline vital signs
8. Transport, perform ongoing assessment.

Rationale
Difficulty breathing, fever, cough, sharp chest pain, and crackles in the lower left lung field suggest pneumonia. The patient should be given high-concentration oxygen and transported to the hospital for antibiotic therapy.

15.12. D, Sharp chest pain, a cough, a fever, and the presence of crackles in part of one lung indicate the presence of pneumonia. Asthma would be characterized by wheezing throughout both lung fields. A patient with COPD would have a past history of increasing difficulty breathing with diminished breath sounds and rhonchi in both lung fields. A patient with pulmonary edema would have crackles in both lungs. Asthma, COPD, and pulmonary edema do not cause chest pain.

15.13. A, Pneumonia is an inflammatory disease of the lungs. It is caused by either a bacterial or vital infection and has an onset over several days.

15.14. A, Pneumonia typically presents with a cough productive of green or rust-colored sputum, fever and chills, possible pain worsened by coughing or deep breathing, and crackles over the infected area of the lung. Pink, frothy sputum and crackles over both lung fields indicate pulmonary edema. Pulmonary edema caused by heart failure can present with pedal edema and crackles in the lung bases. A silent chest, anxiety, and shortness of breath characterize a severe asthma attack.

15.15. B, Because this patient is responsive and has a medical problem, you would apply oxygen, then do an HPI, SAMPLE, and a focused physical examination.

SCENARIO FOUR

Plan of Action

1. BSI

2. Is the scene safe? Yes. Assess nature of illness, number of patients, and need for additional resources.

3. Assess mental status. Ensure an open airway, assess breathing, apply oxygen 10-15 lpm by non-rebreather mask, and assess circulatory status.

4. Determine priority, consider ALS.

5. HPI, SAMPLE

6. Focused physical examination

7. Baseline vital signs

8. Transport, perform ongoing assessment, and meet ALS unit.

Rationale

Shortness of breath that begins suddenly at night (paroxysmal nocturnal dyspnea), crackles in both lung bases, peripheral edema, and a history of hypertension and angina pectoris indicate this patient has congestive heart failure with pulmonary edema. The patient should receive high-concentration oxygen by non-rebreather mask. Placing her in a sitting position with her legs dangling off the side of the stretcher will decrease blood return to her heart and decrease the amount of fluid entering her lungs. If she shows signs of tiring, her breathing should be assisted with a BVM. An ALS unit should be requested to begin drug therapy with nitroglycerin, furosemide, and morphine to reduce the amount of fluid reaching her lungs.

15.16. C, Severe difficulty breathing with sudden onset + peripheral edema + history of angina + coarse crackles = pulmonary edema. Asthma has a sudden onset, but it produces wheezes and is not associated with peripheral edema. COPD does not usually have a sudden onset. Pneumonia does not have a sudden onset and is associated with fever and a cough that produces infected sputum.

15.17. B, Pulmonary edema produces a rapid onset of shortness of breath; a cough productive of pink, frothy sputum; orthopnea; and crackles in both lung fields.

15.18. C, Severe asthma can present with a "silent" chest, anxiety secondary to hypoxia, and shortness of breath.

15.19. B, After performing an initial assessment, you should apply high-concentration oxygen and call for an ALS unit, so the paramedics can begin drug therapy for congestive heart failure and pulmonary edema. Oxygen at 2 to 4 lpm would be inadequate for this patient. This patient does not have COPD and therefore is unlikely to be breathing on the hypoxic drive.

SCENARIO FIVE

Plan of Action

1. BSI

2. Is the scene safe? Yes. Assess nature of illness, number of patients, and need for additional resources.

3. Assess mental status. Ensure an open airway, assess breathing, apply oxygen 10-15 lpm by non-rebreather mask, consider assisting ventilations with BVM if patient shows signs of tiring, and assess circulatory status.

4. Determine priority, consider ALS.

5. HPI, SAMPLE

6. Focused physical examination

7. Baseline vital signs

8. Assist patient to use metered-dose inhaler or give nebulized bronchodilators using a small volume nebulizer if permitted by local protocol.

9. Transport, perform ongoing assessment, and meet ALS unit.

Rationale

This patient has status asthmaticus—a severe asthma attack that is not responding to nebulized bronchodilators. Give high-concentration oxygen by non-rebreather mask, request an ALS unit, and if protocols allow, give the patient another bronchodilator treatment with a small volume nebulizer. If the patient shows signs of tiring, assist her ventilations with a BVM and oxygen.

15.20. C, This patient is in danger of going into respiratory arrest. Patients who experience prolonged asthma attacks become exhausted by the increased work of moving air through their narrowed airways. If they become tired enough, they may be unable to continue breathing.

15.21. D, A prolonged asthma attack that will not respond to the bronchodilators commonly supplied in metered-dose inhalers is called status asthmaticus.

15.22. D, The normal adult respiratory rate is 12 to 20 breaths/min.

15.23. A, Irritants such as cigarette smoke, air pollutants, and dust; exercise; cold air; and emotional stress can act as triggers for asthma attacks. Dry, warm weather tends to decrease the frequency of attacks.

15.24. A, Certain chemicals in red and yellow food dyes may initiate an asthma attack.

15.25. B, Status asthmaticus can be caused exposure to cold air, heavy exercise, respiratory infections, and allergens.

15.26. D, Treatment of this patient would include performing the initial assessment, giving oxygen at 15 lpm, calling for an ALS unit, preparing to intubate the patient if she stops breathing, and transporting.

SCENARIO SIX

Plan of Action

1. BSI

2. Is the scene safe? Yes. Assess nature of illness, number of patients, and need for additional resources.

3. Assess mental status. Ensure an open airway, assess breathing, apply oxygen 10-15 lpm by non-rebreather mask, and assess circulatory status.

4. Determine priority, consider ALS.

5. HPI, SAMPLE

6. Focused physical examination

7. Baseline vital signs

8. Transport, perform ongoing assessment, and meet ALS unit.

Rationale

This patient has a pulmonary embolism caused by a blood clot that formed in his leg after surgical repair of his tibia fracture. Pulmonary embolism should be suspected whenever a patient develops a sudden onset of shortness of breath without a readily identifiable cause. Presence of factors that promote blood clot formation, such as prolonged immobility, injury to the lower extremities, inflammation of lower extremity veins (phlebitis), or use of birth control pills, should raise suspicion that a pulmonary embolism has occurred.

15.27. C, This patient probably has a pulmonary embolism caused by a blood clot that formed in his leg after surgical repair of his tibia fracture. Pulmonary embolism is characterized by a rapid onset of shortness of breath, often accompanied by sharp chest pain in one side of the chest. An acute myocardial infarction (heart attack) causes pain in the center of the chest that usually is described as being "squeezing," "heavy," or "tight." Pneumonia would be associated with a fever and a cough productive of infected sputum. COPD is a chronic disease that produces a gradual onset of increasing shortness of breath.

15.28. C, After performing an initial assessment, you should give the patient high-concentration oxygen and call for an ALS unit. Nitroglycerin is indicated for chest pain caused by inadequate blood flow to the myocardium (myocardial ischemia). Antibiotic therapy would be indicated for pneumonia, not a pulmonary embolism.

15.29. A, Asthma, chronic bronchitis, and emphysema are all obstructive airway diseases that result in widespread reduction of airflow in the lower airways.

15.30. B, A pulmonary embolism is not caused by extreme exercise. Recent surgery, long air or auto trips, and long bone fractures, particularly in the lower extremities, all predispose patients to clot formation that can lead to pulmonary embolism.

SCENARIO SEVEN

Plan of Action

1. BSI

2. Is the scene safe? Yes. Assess nature of illness, number of patients, and need for additional resources.

3. Assess mental status. Ensure an open airway, assess breathing, apply oxygen 10-15 lpm by non-rebreather mask, and assess circulatory status.

4. Determine priority, consider ALS.

5. HPI, SAMPLE

6. Focused physical examination

7. Baseline vital signs

8. Transport, perform ongoing assessment, monitor closely for signs of tension pneumothorax, and meet ALS unit.

Rationale

Sudden onset of one-sided chest pain accompanied by difficulty breathing and decreased breath sounds indicates spontaneous pneumothorax. Spontaneous pneumothorax tends to occur in tall, thin, young males who cough or strain, rupturing a weak place on the lung's surface. Patients with COPD also develop spontaneous pneumothorax when air-filled spaces on the lung's surface (blebs) rupture into the pleural space. Spontaneous pneumothorax can progress to tension pneumothorax, a life-threatening problem. The patient should be given high-concentration oxygen, monitored carefully for signs of tension pneumothorax, and transported to the hospital for chest tube placement. If the patient shows signs of a tension pneumothorax or of worsening respiratory distress, a meeting with an ALS unit should be arranged.

15.31. C, A sudden onset of stabbing pain on one side of the chest, shortness of breath, and diminished breath sounds suggest the presence of a spontaneous pneumothorax.

15.32. B, Oxygen at 2 to 4 lpm by nasal cannula would not be sufficient to meet this patient's needs.

15.33. B, Signs and symptoms of a spontaneous pneumothorax may include respiratory distress, decreased breath sounds, anxiety, weak pulse, distended neck veins, tracheal deviation, and subcutaneous emphysema. Spontaneous pneumothorax can progress to tension pneumothorax, which is life threatening.

15.34. A, Spontaneous pneumothorax can be caused by rupture of a congenitally weak area of the lung surface or by rupture of one of the large, air-filled spaces (blebs) that form on the lungs of COPD patients.

SCENARIO EIGHT

Plan of Action

1. BSI
2. Is the scene safe? Yes. Assess nature of illness, number of patients, and need for additional resources.
3. Assess mental status. Ensure an open airway, assess breathing, and attempt to ventilate.
4. Reposition head, reattempt to ventilate.
5. Give up to five abdominal thrusts.
6. Open mouth, look for foreign body, and remove if seen (no blind finger sweeps).
7. Continue to attempt to ventilate, perform abdominal thrusts, and look for foreign body until object is removed or chest rises with ventilations.
8. After airway is cleared, assess breathing. Ventilate with BVM and oxygen or give high-concentration oxygen by non-rebreather mask. Assess circulation.
9. Transport, perform ongoing assessment.

Rationale

This patient has a foreign body airway obstruction. Foreign body airway obstruction should be suspected whenever a previously healthy child develops a sudden onset of respiratory distress or rapidly loses consciousness. You will not progress beyond "A" in the initial ABCD assessment until the object is dislodged and the airway is opened. Once the airway is cleared, ensure the patient is oxygenating and ventilating adequately, then evaluate for adequate circulation.

15.35. D, If the chest does not rise when you attempt to ventilate a patient, your first action should be to reposition the head and try to ventilate again. The most common cause of airway obstruction in an unconscious person is the tongue. Repositioning the head may lift the tongue from the airway and allow the patient to be ventilated.

15.36. B, Blind finger sweeps should *not* be attempted to relieve a foreign body airway obstruction. Blind finger sweeps may force the object deeper, worsening the obstruction.

15.37. D, Attempt to ventilate; if chest does not rise, reposition head and chin, and try to ventilate again; if ventilation is unsuccessful, perform CPR; open the airway; if you see the object, remove it (no blind finger sweeps); repeat attempt to ventilate—CPR—check for object sequence until successful.

Scenario Nine

Plan of Action

1. BSI
2. Is the scene safe? Probably. The police are present but use caution because of the situation in which the patient was found. Assess nature of illness, number of patients, and need for additional resources.
3. Assess mental status. Ensure an open airway, use a jaw-thrust to open the airway, assess breathing, ventilate with a BVM and oxygen, and assess circulatory status.
4. Determine priority, consider ALS.
5. Rapid physical examination
6. Baseline vital signs
7. HPI, SAMPLE
8. Transport, perform ongoing assessment.

Rationale

Although you may be tempted to think of this patient as being "just another drunk," you should consider the possibility of other problems being present. Although there are no obvious signs of injury, the patient could have fallen or been assaulted. Depending on the weather conditions, he could be hypothermic. The patient's airway should be opened using a jaw-thrust maneuver until a cervical spine fracture can be ruled out. Because his breathing is slow and shallow, he should be ventilated using a BVM and oxygen. A rapid head-to-toe physical examination should be performed in an attempt to identify the cause of unconsciousness, and a response by an ALS unit should be requested.

15.38. **C,** Because the patient has slow, shallow breathing and a decreased level of consciousness, you should ventilate the patient with a BVM and oxygen to increase the respiratory rate.

15.39. **B,** Bradypnea is a slow respiratory rate.

15.40. **C,** Because the patient is unresponsive, an oral airway should be inserted to help keep the tongue from obstructing the pharynx.

15.41. **A,** A tonsil-tip or rigid suction catheter should be used to suction vomitus from the patient's airway. Flexible catheters tend to obstruct or kink too easily to make them useful to clear vomitus from the airway. Attempting to sit the patient up would increase his risk of aspiration. Until a better history can be obtained, rolling the patient on his side to prevent aspiration would be safer than just turning his head because a neck injury may be present.

SCENARIO TEN

Plan of Action

1. BSI
2. Is the scene safe? No. Avoid entering contaminated areas. Initiate steps to isolate the scene and avoid spread of contaminants. Be aware of the possible presence of secondary devices.
3. Establish command.
4. Request a response by the fire department, including the Hazmat team, the police, and several ALS units.
5. Work with fire department to decontaminate patients.
6. Triage patients using the START method after they have been decontaminated.
7. Ensure patients with significant exposure are adequately oxygenated and ventilated.
8. Ensure response by advanced personnel who can begin management of nerve agent poisoning with atropine.
9. Ensure that patients with significant exposure are transported to facilities that can provide definitive treatment with the antidote for organophosphate poisoning (2-PAM).

Rationale

The combination of pinpoint pupils, increased secretions, and difficulty breathing suggests the patients have been exposed to a nerve agent. Chemical terrorism incidents are a combination of a hazardous materials release, a mass casualty incident, and a major crime scene. First responders should be aware of the possible presence of secondary devices designed to kill or injure them. Steps should be taken to prevent spread of contamination from the scene. Patients should be decontaminated appropriately and triaged for care using the START system. The principal danger with nerve agent poisoning is paralysis of the chest wall muscles and diaphragm, leading to respiratory failure or arrest. ALS personnel can give atropine to reverse the production of excess secretions. Patients should be transported to facilities that can give 2-PAM, the definitive antidote for nerve agent poisoning.

15.42. **A,** Pinpoint pupils, tearing, and increased airway secretions are characteristic of a nerve agent such as sarin gas.
15.43. **B,** Nerve agents are toxins that cause increased production of secretions and paralysis of the skeletal muscles and diaphragm.
15.44. **B,** Sarin has a fruity odor. Cyanide's odor has been described as being like that of bitter almonds. Chlorine has an odor like a swimming pool. Phosgene smells like freshly cut grass or hay.
15.45. **D,** Sarin does not cause choking, gagging, or uncontrollable coughing. Sarin is affected by temperature, humidity, wind speed, and also the nature of the terrain. A small amount of sarin will cause increased saliva and mucus production, pinpoint pupils, chest tightness, and shortness of breath. Skin exposure to nerve agents can cause respiratory arrest from paralysis of the chest wall and diaphragm.
15.46. **D,** Make sure no one else goes into the building unless they are wearing appropriate personal protective equipment; move everyone back at least 1500 feet; call the Hazmat team; and also notify the police.

16

Cardiovascular Emergencies

ANATOMY

- Heart
  - Lies in thoracic cavity between lungs and behind sternum
  - Top of heart is the base; bottom is the apex.
  - Four chambers—Two atria, two ventricles
  - Right atrium and ventricle are a low-pressure pump, receiving blood from the superior and inferior venae cavae and pumping it to the lungs through the pulmonary artery
  - Left atrium and ventricle are a high-pressure pump, receiving blood from the lungs through pulmonary veins and pumping it to the body via the aorta.
- Arteries
  - Thick-walled, high-pressure vessels
  - Carry blood away from heart
  - Smaller arteries (arterioles) control peripheral resistance to blood flow, help regulate blood pressure (BP).
  - Major arteries—Aorta, carotids, femorals, brachials, radials, posterior tibials, and dorsal pedals
- Veins
  - Thin-walled, low-pressure vessels
  - Carry blood toward the heart
  - Contain valves that prevent backflow of blood
  - Major veins—Superior and inferior venae cavae, jugulars, and femorals
- Capillaries
  - Vessels connecting arterial and venous circulation
  - Only one-cell-layer thick
  - Allow for diffusion of materials between bloodstream and body tissues

PHYSIOLOGY

- Definitions
  - *Systole*—Contraction of heart; causes blood to be pumped out
  - *Diastole*—Relaxation of heart; allows heart chambers to fill
  - *Stroke volume*—Amount of blood pumped out of heart during each contraction
  - *Cardiac output*—Amount of blood pumped out of heart each minute; equal to heart rate × stroke volume
- Pathway of blood through heart
  - Inferior and superior venae cavae
  - Right atrium
  - Tricuspid atrioventricular valve
  - Right ventricle
  - Pulmonic semilunar valve
  - Pulmonary artery (only artery carrying unoxygenated blood)
  - Pulmonary capillary bed
  - Pulmonary veins (only veins carrying oxygenated blood)
  - Left atrium
  - Mitral (bicuspid) atrioventricular valve
  - Left ventricle
  - Aortic semilunar valve
  - Aorta

CARDIOVASCULAR DISEASE

- Coronary arteries supply blood to heart muscle
- Atherosclerosis—Accumulation of fat deposits on arterial walls; can narrow vessels resulting in ischemia
- Ischemia—Deficiency in blood supply and oxygen delivery to tissues caused by blood vessel obstruction
- Risk factors for atherosclerosis
  - Age
  - Male gender
  - Race
  - Family history
  - Hypertension
  - Cigarette smoking
  - Diet
  - High blood cholesterol
  - Sedentary lifestyle
  - Stress
  - Type A personality
  - Obesity

Stable Angina Pectoris

- Literally, "a choking in the chest"
- Chest pain that occurs when narrowed coronary arteries are unable to deliver enough blood to meet the heart muscle's need for oxygen during periods of increased work
- Episodes of angina are triggered by exercise, eating, or emotional stress and relieved by rest, nitroglycerin, and oxygen.
- Episodes typically last no longer than 10 to 15 minutes, are brought on by predictable amounts of stress, and are relieved by predictable amounts of rest, nitroglycerin, and oxygen.
- Other signs and symptoms such as weakness, shortness of breath, sweating, or nausea may accompany chest pain.

Unstable Angina Pectoris

- Caused by worsening of narrowing of coronary arteries caused by atherosclerosis
- Episodes of angina occur at rest, are triggered by less stress, or require longer periods of rest and more nitroglycerin to relieve them.
- Signs and symptoms such as weakness, shortness of breath, sweating, or nausea may appear if not previously associated with angina attacks.
- Frequently precedes an acute myocardial infarction (MI)

Acute Myocardial Infarction

- "Heart attack"
- Caused by obstruction of a diseased coronary artery leading to infarction (death) of heart muscle (myocardium) from inadequate oxygen supply
- Most commonly caused by clot formation (thrombosis) in coronary arteries narrowed by atherosclerosis
- May occur in younger persons who abuse stimulants as a result of spasms of coronary arteries
- Signs and symptoms

- ○ Squeezing substernal chest pain that may radiate to the neck and jaw, upper back, upper abdomen, shoulder, or arm
  - ○ May also experience weakness, anxiety, shortness of breath, heavy sweating (diaphoresis), nausea, vomiting, palpitations, or sense of impending doom
  - ○ Elderly patients and diabetic patients may have "silent MIs" with absence of chest pain.
- Management
  - ○ Position of comfort, keep patient calm
  - ○ High-concentration oxygen by non-rebreather mask at 15 lpm
  - ○ Aspirin to reduce tendency of blood to clot
  - ○ Nitroglycerin if BP is >100 mm Hg systolic to reduce heart's workload and improve blood flow through coronary arteries
  - ○ Do not allow patient to walk
  - ○ Transport without lights and siren to avoid increasing patient's anxiety
  - ○ Call for advanced life support (ALS) unit
  - ○ Ensure transport to a facility that can open the blocked coronary arteries with thrombolytic agents ("clot busters") or angioplasty

Congestive Heart Failure

- Left ventricular failure—Blood backs up into lungs, causing pulmonary edema and respiratory distress.
- Signs and symptoms include dyspnea, difficulty breathing while lying flat (orthopnea), tachycardia, diaphoresis, crackles and wheezing in the lung fields, coughing frothy pink or white sputum, and cyanosis.
- Right ventricular failure—Blood backs up into peripheral circulatory system, causing peripheral edema.
- Signs and symptoms include tachycardia, pedal or sacral edema, abdominal distension, and jugular vein distension.
- Management of congestive heart failure (CHF) with pulmonary edema
  - ○ If BP is within normal limits or elevated, sit patient up and dangle legs off of stretcher
  - ○ High-concentration oxygen by non-rebreather mask at 15 lpm
  - ○ Nitroglycerin if BP is >100 mm Hg systolic to reduce blood return to heart and decrease amount of blood being pumped into lungs
  - ○ Aspirin if patient is experiencing chest pain to reduce tendency to form clots in coronary arteries
  - ○ Call for ALS unit

Sudden Cardiac Death

- Rapid, unexpected cessation of heartbeat and breathing
- Frequently results from acute MI, typically during first 2 hours after onset of symptoms
- Most common cause of sudden cardiac death is ventricular arrhythmias (ventricular fibrillation or pulseless ventricular tachycardia) that do not produce blood flow in cardiovascular system.
- Chain of survival
  - ○ Early access
  - ○ Early cardiopulmonary resuscitation (CPR)
  - ○ Early defibrillation of ventricular fibrillation or pulseless ventricular tachycardia
  - ○ Early ALS
- Management

○ Scene survey
○ Initial assessment
○ Have partner and/or first responders begin CPR; consider providing 5cycles (2 minutes) of CPR if response time was >4 to 5 minutes.
○ Turn on automated external defibrillator (AED)
○ Apply AED pads to patient
○ Stop CPR, if necessary push "Analyze" button on AED
○ If AED advises shock, direct other rescuers to stand back, and ensure no one is touching patient
○ Deliver shock if advised by AED
○ Resume CPR immediately after shock delivered
○ Repeat sequence after 2 minutes or as indicated by AED
○ If AED advised "no shock," always check for a pulse. A patient can be in cardiac arrest with a nonshockable rhythm. The nonshockable arrest rhythms are:
  ■ Asystole, which appears as a flat line on the electrocardiographic (ECG) monitor
  ■ Pulseless electrical activity, which can look like any cardiac rhythm other than ventricular fibrillation, pulseless ventricular tachycardia, or asystole but does not produce a pulse

COMMON RHYTHMS

• Normal sinus rhythm—The heart's typical rhythm (Figure 16-1)
  ○ Normal sinus rhythm results from the SA node in the right atrium regularly pacing the heart at 60 to 100 beats/min.

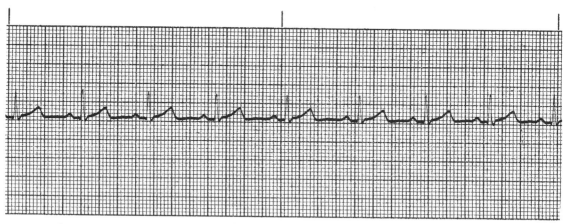

Figure 16-1 Normal sinus rhythm. (From Nagell K, Nagell R: *A case-based approach to ECG interpretation*, St Louis, 2003, Mosby.)

• Ventricular fibrillation—The most common rhythm of cardiac arrest
  ○ Ventricular fibrillation occurs when the ventricles quiver chaotically rather than contracting in an organized fashion.
  ○ A defibrillator shock interrupts the chaotic quivering of ventricular fibrillation and allows the SA node to begin pacing the heart again.
  ○ Ventricular fibrillation sometimes is described as being "fine" (Figure 16-2) or "coarse" (Figure 16-3).

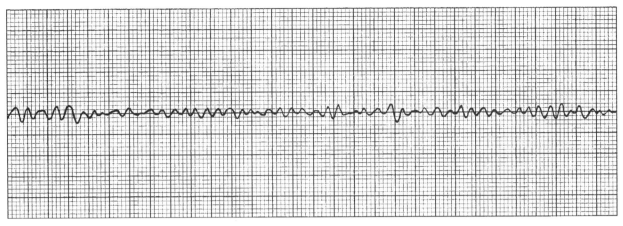

Figure 16-2   Fine ventricular fibrillation. (From Nagell K, Nagell R: *A case-based approach to ECG interpretation,* St Louis, 2003, Mosby.)

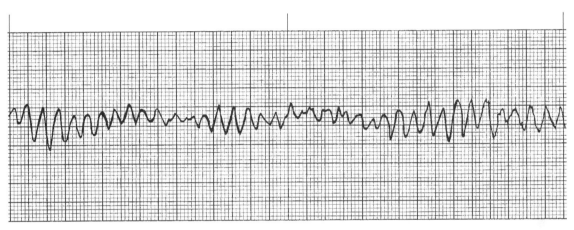

Figure 16-3   Coarse ventricular fibrillation. (From Nagell K, Nagell R: *A case-based approach to ECG interpretation,* St Louis, 2003, Mosby.)

- Asystole—A complete lack of electrical activity in the heart
  - Appears on the ECG as a flat or nearly flat line (Figure 16-4)
  - Asystole should *not* be shocked.
  - AEDs are programmed to identify asystole as a nonshockable rhythm.

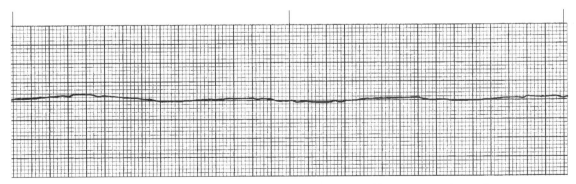

Figure 16-4   Asystole. (From Nagell K, Nagell R: *A case-based approach to ECG-interpretation,* St Louis, 2003, Mosby.)

REVIEW QUESTIONS
Scenario One

At 3:00 AM you respond to a residence for a report of "chest pain." The patient is an 83-y.o. male who is sitting in the living room. He complains of "crushing" substernal chest pain that began at approximately 10:00 PM. He rates the pain as a 5 on the 1 to 10 scale and says his left arm feels "numb." He denies nausea, lightheadedness, or syncope, but he says he felt weak when the symptoms began. He has a past medical history of type II diabetes mellitus, hypertension, and arthritis. He also had a duodenal ulcer approximately 30 years ago. His medications include Glucovance, HCTZ, and ibuprofen as needed. He has no known drug allergies. Vital signs are BP—168/106; pulse (P)—78, strong, regular; respiration (R)—24, regular, nonlabored; and SaO$_2$—95%.

Your Plan of Action

Fill in the blank lines with your treatment plan for this patient. Then compare your plan with the questions, answers, and rationale.

1. _____
2. _____
3. _____
4. _____
5. _____
6. _____
7. _____
8. _____
9. _____

Multiple Choice

16.1. All of the following are risk factors for cardiovascular disease *except:*
   a. cigarette smoking.
   b. high cholesterol.
   c. lack of exercise.
   d. female gender.

16.2. All of the following are signs and symptoms of a possible heart attack *except:*
   a. sweating, nausea, and lightheadedness.
   b. substernal chest pain.
   c. left arm numbness or tingling.
   d. left-sided facial weakness or drooping.

16.3. All of the following statements about the anatomy of the heart are correct *except:*
   a. the heart contains four chambers; the top two chambers are the right and left atria, and the bottom two chambers are the right and left ventricles.
   b. the heart is located just above the diaphragm, posterior to and just slightly to the right of the sternum.
   c. the heart contains four valves: the tricuspid, pulmonic, bicuspid, and aortic valves.
   d. the heart is surrounded by a fibrous sac called the pericardium.

16.4. A heart attack is often referred to as a/an:
   a. acute MI.
   b. transient ischemic attack if arm numbness is present.
   c. coronary vascular accident.
   d. anginal attack.
16.5. What is ischemia?
   a. Blood clots traveling through the bloodstream
   b. A decreased supply of oxygenated blood to tissue
   c. Lack of oxygen leading to a pulmonary embolism
   d. An air embolism blocking blood flow through the heart
16.6. The AV node is located superior to the:
   a. ventricles.
   b. atrium.
   c. SA node.
   d. tricuspid valve.
16.7. The heart's primary pacemaker is the:
   a. bundle of His.
   b. AV node.
   c. left bundle branch.
   d. SA node.
16.8. What is cardiac output?
   a. The amount of blood pumped into a ventricle with each contraction
   b. The amount of blood pumped into the right and left ventricles with each contraction
   c. The amount of blood that is pumped out of either ventricle, measured in lpm
   d. Blood pressure × systemic vascular resistance
16.9. Cardiac output is equal to:
   a. heart rate × BP.
   b. heart rate × stroke volume.
   c. stroke volume × BP.
   d. stroke volume × peripheral resistance.
16.10. Nitroglycerin should *not* be given unless the:
   a. BP is >100 mm Hg systolic.
   b. pulse is <100 beats/min.
   c. BP is <140/90 mm Hg.
   d. pulse rate is >60 beats/min.
16.11. Which of the following statements about giving nitroglycerin is *correct?*
   a. It should be taken with a full glass of water to ensure proper absorption.
   b. It is placed under the patient's tongue.
   c. Three tablets should be taken at a time to ensure full effect.
   d. The patient should chew the tablet well and then swallow it.
16.12. Nitroglycerin relieves chest pain by:
   a. increasing BP, which improves blood flow to the heart muscle.
   b. constricting peripheral blood vessels, which decreases the heart's workload.
   c. dilating the coronary arteries and decreasing the cardiac workload.
   d. constricting blood vessels and decreasing the cardiac workload.

16.13. The *first* action to take when you are caring for a patient with cardiac problems is to:
    a. give oxygen.
    b. give nitroglycerin.
    c. call for ALS.
    d. prepare for intubation because cardiac arrest may be imminent.

16.14. The patient denies any nausea, lightheadedness, or syncope. These symptoms would be:
    a. positive findings.
    b. a part of his past medical history.
    c. not relevant to a chest pain patient.
    d. pertinent negative findings.

Scenario Two

At 10:30 AM you are dispatched to a residence for a report of "difficulty breathing." The patient is an 83-y.o. female who is experiencing shortness of breath accompanied by mild chest pain. She is unable to speak in complete sentences. The patient says she has been having trouble breathing for the past 3 to 4 days, but this morning it suddenly became worse. Her husband tells you his wife has a problem with high BP, her heart "fluttering," and her gallbladder if she eats a fatty meal. She also takes a "water pill" and has to watch her diet so she does not eat too much sugar. The patient's medications include diltiazem, furosemide, K-Dur, and nitroglycerin SL as needed. Vital signs are BP—168/114; P—142, weak, irregularly irregular; R—28, regular, labored; and SaO_2—90%.

Your Plan of Action

Fill in the blank lines with your treatment plan for this patient. Then compare your plan with the questions, answers, and rationale.

1. _____
2. _____
3. _____
4. _____
5. _____
6. _____
7. _____
8. _____
9. _____

Multiple Choice

16.15. Which of the following is the normal pathway of an impulse through the heart's electrical conduction system?
    a. SA node, AV node, bundle of His, right and left bundle branches, and Purkinje fibers
    b. AV node, SA node, right and left bundle branches, bundle of His, and Purkinje fibers
    c. Pericardium, myocardium, endocardium, and ventricles
    d. SA node, internodal atrial pathways, bundle branches, AV node, and Purkinje fibers

16.16. Right ventricular failure in a cardiac patient is indicated by which of the following signs and symptoms:
   a. flat neck veins.
   b. a harsh cough with wheezing or crackles.
   c. ankle edema and abdominal distension.
   d. extremity pain.

16.17. CHF is best described as:
   a. an MI that leads to fluid accumulations in the lungs and extremities.
   b. a blockage of coronary arteries causing a buildup of fluid in the tissues.
   c. an accumulation of fluid in the pericardium.
   d. a condition in which the heart does not pump adequately, causing the blood to back up into the lungs and/or extremities.

16.18. The heart chambers that pump blood into the arteries are the:
   a. right and left atrium.
   b. right and left bundle branches.
   c. right and left ventricles.
   d. pulmonary artery and aorta.

16.19. When blood enters the capillary bed it is:
   a. high in oxygen and high in carbon dioxide.
   b. low in oxygen and low in carbon dioxide.
   c. high in oxygen and low in carbon dioxide.
   d. low in oxygen and high in carbon dioxide.

16.20. The major artery that originates directly from the heart and supplies the peripheral circulatory system is the:
   a. pulmonary artery.
   b. aorta.
   c. carotid artery.
   d. subclavian artery.

16.21. Unoxygenated blood travels from the heart to the lungs via the:
   a. pulmonary artery.
   b. pulmonary vein.
   c. coronary arteries.
   d. bronchial artery.

16.22. All of the following are part of the focused history and physical examination for a patient with chest pain *except:*
   a. a past history of diabetes and hypertension.
   b. medications the patient is currently taking.
   c. the quality, location, and duration of any chest pain.
   d. checking for presence of facial droop, slurred speech, or extremity weakness.

16.23. The left ventricle pumps blood to the:
   a. lungs by way of the pulmonary vein.
   b. lungs by way of the pulmonary artery.
   c. peripheral circulation through the aorta.
   d. peripheral circulation through the carotid artery.

16.24. Which of the following describes the flow of blood from the time it enters the heart until it enters the peripheral circulation?
   a. Right atrium, tricuspid valve, right ventricle, pulmonary artery, lungs, pulmonary vein, left atrium, mitral valve, left ventricle, and aorta
   b. Right atrium, mitral valve, right ventricle, pulmonary artery, lungs, pulmonary vein, left atrium, tricuspid valve, left ventricle, and aorta
   c. Right atrium, tricuspid valve, right ventricle, pulmonary vein, lungs, pulmonary artery, left atrium, mitral valve, left ventricle, and aorta
   d. Right atrium, mitral valve, right ventricle, pulmonary vein, lungs, pulmonary artery, left ventricle, tricuspid valve, left ventricle, and aorta

16.25. All of the following can be detected by auscultation *except:*
   a. lung sounds.
   b. heart sounds.
   c. presence of normal arterial blood flow.
   d. carotid bruits.

True/False

16.26. Atherosclerosis results from buildup of fatty deposits on the inner walls of the arteries.
   a. True
   b. False

Multiple Choice

16.27. The *most common* cause of right ventricular failure is:
   a. chronic obstructive pulmonary disease (COPD).
   b. acute MI.
   c. left ventricular failure.
   d. chronic hypertension.

16.28. Abdominal distension, ankle swelling, shortness of breath, and jugular venous distension indicate:
   a. COPD.
   b. CHF.
   c. congestive pulmonary embolism.
   d. obstructive heart failure.

16.29. Pedal edema is:
   a. swelling of the feet and ankles.
   b. abdominal distension caused by failure of the right ventricle.
   c. accumulation of fluid in the sacral area.
   d. bluish discoloration of the lips and nail beds.

16.30. Which of the following statements about the onset of CHF is *most* correct?
   a. Signs and symptoms always appear suddenly.
   b. Signs and symptoms usually develop over time with a buildup of fluid.
   c. The onset of signs and symptoms indicates that an MI has occurred.
   d. The onset is slow, and the symptoms will gradually resolve.

Scenario Three

An 81-y.o. female is sitting on the edge of her bed in severe respiratory distress. Her family tells you she was fine when she went to bed 4 hours ago and she awakened short of breath 15 minutes ago. The patient's skin is cold, pale, and diaphoretic. Jugular venous distension is present. Capillary refill is >3 seconds. She has a history of CHF, angina, hypertension, and type II diabetes mellitus. Her medications include Glucovance, nitroglycerin as needed, furosemide, K-Dur, and Cardizem. She has no known allergies. Vital signs are BP—198/140; P—160, weak, irregularly irregular; R—40, regular, gasping; and SaO_2—79%.

Your Plan of Action

Fill in the blank lines with your treatment plan for this patient. Then compare your plan with the questions, answers, and rationale.

1. _____
2. _____
3. _____
4. _____
5. _____
6. _____
7. _____
8. _____
9. _____

Multiple Choice

16.31. This patient's problem is *most* likely:
   a. pulmonary embolism.
   b. pulmonary artery occlusion.
   c. pulmonary edema.
   d. unstable pulmonary congestion.

16.32. Pulmonary edema is characterized by a:
   a. sudden onset with mild difficulty breathing.
   b. slow onset with mild difficulty breathing.
   c. slow onset with severe difficulty breathing.
   d. sudden onset with severe difficulty breathing.

16.33. Findings in a patient with pulmonary edema would *most* likely include:
   a. crackles, flat jugular veins, and a rapid respiratory rate.
   b. crackles, distended jugular veins, and a slow respiratory rate.
   c. crackles, flat jugular veins, a rapid pulse, and rapid respiratory rate.
   d. crackles, distended jugular veins, rapid pulse, and rapid respiratory rate.

16.34. Treatment of this patient would include:
  a. keeping the patient sitting and giving oxygen at 4 to 6 lpm.
  b. keeping the patient supine and giving oxygen at 10 to 15 lpm.
  c. keeping the patient sitting and giving oxygen at 10 to 15 lpm.
  d. having the patient sit on the edge of the stretcher and breathe into a paper bag.

16.35. Pulmonary edema is caused by:
  a. a backup of blood into the peripheral venous system.
  b. failure of the left ventricle, resulting in a backup of blood into the lungs.
  c. failure of the right ventricle, resulting in a backup of blood into the abdomen.
  d. failure of the right ventricle, resulting in a backup of blood into the lungs.

16.36. An average adult's stroke volume is:
  a. 50 mL.
  b. 70 mL.
  c. 100 mL.
  d. 150 mL.

16.37. Which valve prevents backflow of blood into the right atrium?
  a. Tricuspid valve
  b. Pulmonic valve
  c. Aortic valve
  d. Mitral valve

16.38. The amount of blood ejected during a ventricular contraction is:
  a. preload.
  b. stroke volume.
  c. stroke output.
  d. cardiac output.

16.39. Which chamber of the heart generates the greatest pressure?
  a. Right atrium
  b. Left atrium
  c. Right ventricle
  d. Left ventricle

Scenario Four

A 61-y.o. female complains of "squeezing" substernal chest pain that began 20 minutes ago when she was mowing the lawn. The pain does not radiate. After the pain began, the patient went inside and lay down. During the next 5 minutes, the pain decreased in severity from 8 to 3 on the 1 to 10 scale. The patient denies nausea, dizziness, and syncope but says she experienced some sweating when the pain started. She has past medical history of asthma. She takes no medications and has no known drug allergies. Vital signs are BP—148/98; P—78, strong, regular; R—20, regular, unlabored; and SaO_2—98%.

Your Plan of Action

Fill in the blank lines with your treatment plan for this patient. Then compare your plan with the questions, answers, and rationale.

1. _____
2. _____
3. _____
4. _____
5. _____
6. _____
7. _____
8. _____
9. _____

Multiple Choice

16.40. Which of the following statements about the chest pain of an MI is *correct?*
   a. The pain is typically relieved with rest and/or nitroglycerin.
   b. The pain is worse when the patient coughs.
   c. The pain often radiates to the left arm, shoulder, back, neck, or jaw.
   d. The pain is worse with movement.

16.41. The "S" in OPQRST stands for:
   a. signs and symptoms.
   b. syncope.
   c. skin color.
   d. severity.

16.42. The "P" in OPQRST of refers to:
   a. prescription medications the patient is taking.
   b. pulse rate.
   c. what factors, if any, caused the pain to develop.
   d. the position in which the patient was found.

16.43. The rapid physical examination of an unresponsive patient is done:
   a. during the initial assessment.
   b. after the initial assessment and before the vital signs.
   c. after the vital signs.
   d. en route to the hospital.

16.44. The vital signs of a conscious patient with chest pain are done:
   a. after the initial assessment.
   b. at the end of the focused history and physical examination.
   c. before the SAMPLE history as part of the focused history and physical examination.
   d. when first arriving on the scene.

16.45. Vital signs include:
   a. BP, pulse, respirations, and capillary refill.
   b. BP, pulse, respirations, and pupils.
   c. BP, pulse, respirations, skin color and temperature, capillary refill, and pupils.
   d. BP, pulse, and respirations.

Scenario Five

You respond to a report of "difficulty breathing." The patient is a 59-y.o. female who is unable to speak in complete sentences. The patient's family tells you she has had a "cold" for the past week. Two hours ago she began having difficulty breathing and developed a cough productive of pink-tinged sputum. The patient's skin is pale, cool, and diaphoretic. Capillary refill is 2 seconds. Crackles are present over the lower half of both lung fields. The patient has a history of mild emphysema, CHF, angina pectoris, and type II diabetes mellitus. Her medications include a Proventil inhaler, Bumex, one baby aspirin a day, and nitroglycerin as needed. The vital signs are BP—180/100; P—112, weak, regular; R—28, regular, labored; and SaO_2—94%.

> **Your Plan of Action**
> *Fill in the blank lines with your treatment plan for this patient. Then compare your plan with the questions, answers, and rationale.*
> 1. _____
> 2. _____
> 3. _____
> 4. _____
> 5. _____
> 6. _____
> 7. _____
> 8. _____
> 9. _____

Multiple Choice

16.46. When a patient has pulmonary edema, the lungs are:
   a. not receiving enough blood from the right ventricle, causing severe dyspnea.
   b. not receiving enough oxygen because of ineffective gas exchange.
   c. filling with fluid because the left ventricle is pumping ineffectively.
   d. collapsed because of an abnormality of the heart.
16.47. A patient in severe distress with pulmonary edema may exhibit:
   a. pink, frothy sputum.
   b. coughing up yellow-green sputum and being unable to talk in full sentences.
   c. a barrel-shaped chest from the respiratory distress.
   d. unequal chest expansion.

16.48. CHF in an elderly patient may present with *only:*
   a. crackles because of narrowed airways.
   b. chest pain because of the heart's increased workload.
   c. confusion because of lack of oxygen.
   d. nausea and vomiting because of decreased blood flow to the stomach and intestine.

True/False

16.49. Patients with pulmonary edema are literally drowning in their own fluid.
   a. True
   b. False

Multiple Choice

16.50. The patient with CHF may present with:
   a. dyspnea, tachycardia, crackles, pedal edema, abdominal distension, prolonged nausea, and vomiting.
   b. dyspnea, tachypnea, crackles, wheezes, pedal edema, abdominal distension, prolonged nausea and vomiting, and abdominal pain worsened by movement.
   c. dyspnea, tachycardia, tachypnea, crackles, wheezes, pedal edema, prolonged nausea and vomiting, and abdominal pain worsened by movement.
   d. dyspnea, tachycardia, tachypnea, crackles, wheezes, pedal edema, and abdominal distension.

True/False

16.51. Abdominal distension (ascites) can be a sign of right heart failure.
   a. True
   b. False

Scenario Six

A 60-y.o. male is experiencing "squeezing" substernal chest pain radiating to his left shoulder and down his left arm that began approximately 1 hour ago while he was sitting quietly watching television. He rates the severity of the pain as a 9 on a 1 to 10 scale. He also experienced weakness, nausea, and an episode of syncope when the pain began. He is alert and oriented to person, place, time, and events. His skin is pale, cool, and diaphoretic. He has a history of angina pectoris and kidney stones. His medications include digoxin and nitroglycerin. He has no known drug allergies. Vital signs are BP—158/98; P—52, strong, regular; R—22, regular, unlabored; and SaO_2—97%.

Your Plan of Action

Fill in the blank lines with your treatment plan for this patient. Then compare your plan with the questions, answers, and rationale.

1. _____
2. _____
3. _____
4. _____
5. _____
6. _____
7. _____
8. _____
9. _____

Multiple Choice

16.52. Oxygen is given to a patient complaining of chest pain because:
   a. it will reduce the patient's anxiety.
   b. the patient usually will have a low BP.
   c. the patient probably has myocardial ischemia.
   d. oxygen will prevent the patient from having an acute heart attack.

16.53. Which of the following statements about arteries is *correct?*
   a. Arteries contain only oxygenated blood.
   b. Arteries travel away from the heart.
   c. Arteries contain only unoxygenated blood.
   d. Arteries travel away from the heart in the systemic circulation and toward the heart in the pulmonary circulation.

16.54. The coronary arteries are responsible for:
   a. providing blood flow to the systemic circulation.
   b. conducting impulses that stimulate the heart to beat.
   c. supplying the myocardium with blood.
   d. controlling the flow of blood through the heart's chambers.

True/False

16.55. A patient can have an acute MI without feeling chest pain.
   a. True
   b. False

Multiple Choice

16.56. A patient with a heart rate of 52 beats/min has:
   a. tachycardia.
   b. bradycardia.
   c. tachypnea.
   d. bradypnea.

Scenario Seven

You respond to a report of an "unresponsive person." The patient is a 59-y.o. male who is lying on the ground beside a lawn mower. There is no evidence of any trauma. Your initial assessment reveals no respirations and no pulse. Your ambulance is equipped with an AED.

Your Plan of Action

Fill in the blank lines with your treatment plan for this patient. Then compare your plan with the questions, answers, and rationale.

1. _____
2. _____
3. _____
4. _____
5. _____
6. _____
7. _____
8. _____
9. _____

Multiple Choice

16.57. Which of the following rhythms can be defibrillated?
  a. Coarse ventricular fibrillation
  b. Fine ventricular fibrillation
  c. Pulseless electrical activity
  d. Both coarse and fine ventricular fibrillation

16.58. The following ECG rhythm is:

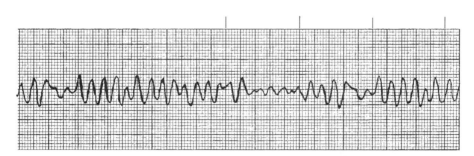

From Nagell K, Nagell R: *A case-based approach to ECG interpretation,* St Louis, 2003, Mosby.

  a. ventricular fibrillation.
  b. asystole.
  c. pulseless electrical activity.
  d. atrial fibrillation.

16.59. The AED pads should be placed on the:
   a. right and left clavicles.
   b. anterior left clavicle and left leg.
   c. right upper anterior chest and left lower chest.
   d. right lower chest and left clavicle.

16.60. All of the following should be done when using the AED *except:*
   a. shocking when advised.
   b. performing CPR for 2 minutes after a shock is delivered.
   c. continuing to ventilate with the bag-valve mask (BVM) while the AED is analyzing the rhythm.
   d. stopping the ambulance while defibrillating.

16.61. The *most important* concern when you use the AED is ensuring:
   a. everyone is clear before defibrillating.
   b. the machine delivers three shocks before resuming CPR
   c. ALS is en route.
   d. the patient is ventilated adequately.

16.62. If the AED advises no shock is indicated, what should you do?
   a. Advise the emergency room the AED is malfunctioning.
   b. Repeat the analysis sequence
   c. Continue with CPR.
   d. Check for a pulse and breathing.

16.63. Complete absence of electrical activity on an ECG monitor is called:
   a. a baseline.
   b. chaotic activity.
   c. asystole.
   d. pulseless electrical activity.

True/False

16.64. Ventricular fibrillation is the only rhythm you would always defibrillate.
   a. True
   b. False

16.65. Ventricular tachycardia may need to be defibrillated even if a pulse is present.
   a. True
   b. False

Multiple Choice

16.66. A chaotic, wavy line on the ECG monitor may be caused by:
   a. ventricular fibrillation.
   b. loose patient leads.
   c. respirations.
   d. either ventricular fibrillation or loose patient leads.

16.67. If a patient has no pulse and respirations, all of the following rhythms should be defibrillated *except:*
   a. ventricular fibrillation.
   b. ventricular tachycardia.
   c. pulseless electrical activity.
   d. ventricular fibrillation and ventricular tachycardia.

16.68. Pulseless electrical activity is:
   a. a cardiac arrest rhythm characterized by uniform, rounded wide T waves.
   b. characterized by a chaotic, wavy rhythm on the ECG monitor.
   c. any organized ECG rhythm that does not generate a pulse.
   d. a cardiac rhythm that presents with hypotension and a slow rate.

16.69. A patient has no pulse and no BP. Your response time was 2 minutes. You should:
   a. perform two-rescuer CPR for 1 minute, apply the AED, and shock if advised.
   b. apply the AED, shock if advised, begin CPR, and call for an ALS unit.
   c. call for an ALS unit, apply the AED, and shock if ventricular fibrillation is present.
   d. apply the AED, shock if advised, call for an ALS unit, and begin CPR.

16.70. Which of the following statements about management of cardiac arrest is *correct?*
   a. An EMT should never transport a cardiac arrest patient before ALS personnel arrive.
   b. An AED will deliver 100 to 200 J of electricity.
   c. When two EMTs are present, one can operate the AED while the other performs CPR.
   d. Two sets of shocks may be delivered without pulse checks or CPR, followed by a pulse check and 2 minutes of CPR before shocking again.

16.71. You are en route to meet the paramedic unit when the patient begins breathing on his own. A pulse and BP are present. You should:
   a. cancel the paramedic unit and continue on to the hospital.
   b. meet the paramedic unit because the patient may need medications.
   c. remove the AED pads because the patient is out of danger.
   d. obtain a history from the patient about what happened before the cardiac arrest.

16.72. The compression-to-ventilation ratio for CPR on an unintubated patient is:
   a. 15 compressions to 1 ventilation.
   b. 30 compressions to 1 ventilation.
   c. 15 compressions to 2 ventilations.
   d. 30 compressions to 2 ventilations.

16.73. After completing 2 minutes of CPR, you should:
   a. check for a pulse.
   b. recheck for signs of circulation.
   c. recheck the status of the ALS unit.
   d. rotate the compressor role.

16.74. When initially ventilating a nonbreathing patient, you should give:
   a. two breaths that produce visible chest rise.
   b. two fast full breaths.
   c. one breath that produces visible chest rise.
   d. one fast breath.

16.75. When supplemental oxygen is used during CPR, the tidal volume should be:
   a. 800 to 1000 mL delivered over 2 seconds.
   b. at least 1000 mL delivered over 1 to 1½ seconds.
   c. 700 to 1000 mL delivered over 2 seconds.
   d. the amount needed to produce chest rise delivered over 1 second.

16.76. When supplemental oxygen is *not* available during CPR, the tidal volume should be:
   a. 500 mL delivered over 2 seconds.
   b. 700 to 1000 mL delivered over 1 to 1½ seconds.
   c. the amount needed to produce chest rise delivered over 1 second.
   d. 500 mL delivered over 1 to 2 seconds.

16.77. When using an AED, you may stop CPR:
  a. for no longer than 30 seconds.
  b. for 1 to 2 minutes between each set of three shocks.
  c. long enough to deliver a set of three shocks.
  d. long enough to analyze and deliver a single shock.

Scenario Eight

An 80-y.o. female is c/o mild, nonradiating substernal chest "tightness." She describes her initial discomfort as a 6 on a 1 to 10 scale but says it now is a 3. She has a past medical history of gastroesophageal reflux disease, an abdominal hernia, gallstones, and leukemia, which has been in remission for 5 years. Her medications include Prilosec and one baby aspirin a day. Vital signs are BP—110/76; P—88, weak, regular; R—22, regular, nonlabored; and SaO_2—95%.

Your Plan of Action

Fill in the blank lines with your treatment plan for this patient. Then compare your plan with the questions, answers, and rationale.

1. _____
2. _____
3. _____
4. _____
5. _____
6. _____
7. _____
8. _____
9. _____

Multiple Choice

16.78. You should suspect this patient has angina pectoris because:
  a. of the past history of leukemia.
  b. the chest pain began as 6 and is now a 3 on the 1 to 10 scale.
  c. the chest pain has subsided with rest.
  d. the patient has no cardiac history.
16.79. Chest pain that is *not* relieved by rest and nitroglycerin should be treated as:
  a. musculoskeletal pain.
  b. stable angina.
  c. unstable angina.
  d. acute MI.

True/False

16.80. Angina may progress to an acute MI if left untreated.
  a. True
  b. False

16.81. Stable angina will usually resolve in 10 to 15 minutes if treated with rest and nitroglycerin.
   a. True
   b. False
16.82. Unstable angina is characterized by a change in the onset, severity, duration, or quality of pain.
   a. True
   b. False

Fill in the Blank

16.83.

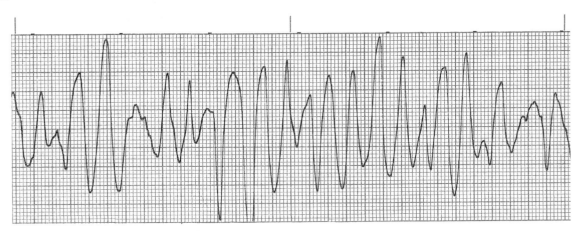

Interpretation: _____

16.84.

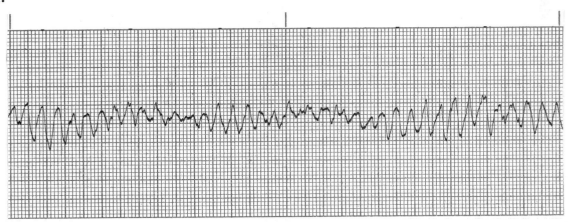

Interpretation: _____

16.85.

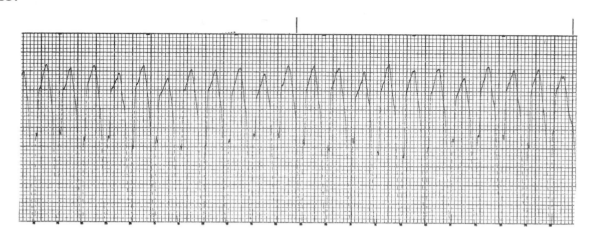

Interpretation: _____

16.86.

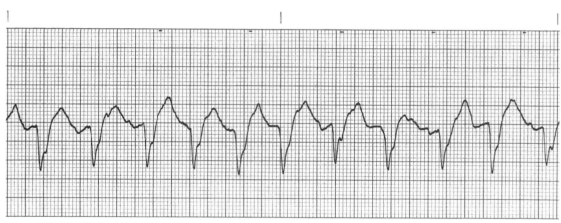

REORDER 40442A/40442B

Interpretation: _____

16.87.

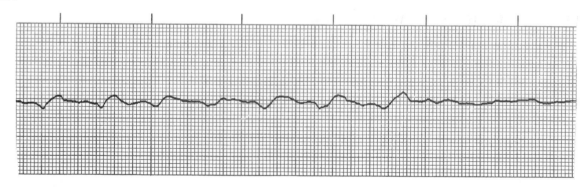

Interpretation: _____

16.88.

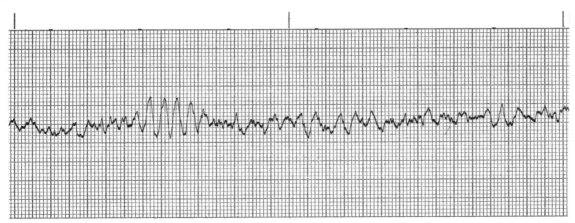

Interpretation: _____

16.89.

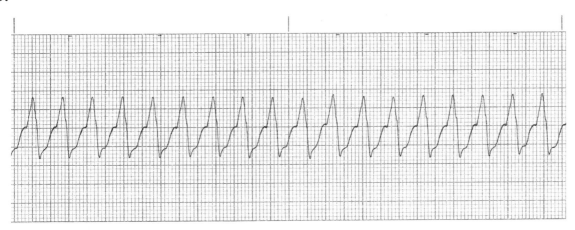

Interpretation: _____

16.90.

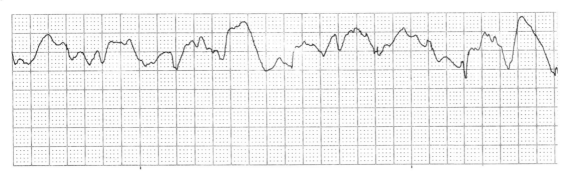

Interpretation: _____

16.91.

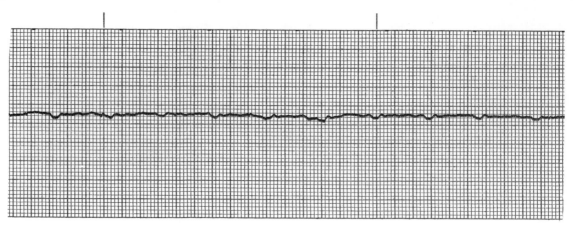

Interpretation: _____

Answer Key—Chapter 16

SCENARIO ONE

Plan of Action

1. Body Substance Isolation (BSI)
2. Is the scene safe? Yes. Assess nature of illness, number of patients, and need for additional resources.
3. Assess mental status. Ensure an open airway, assess breathing, apply oxygen at 10-15 lpm by non-rebreather mask, and assess circulatory status.
4. Determine priority, consider ALS.
5. History of present illness (HPI), SAMPLE
6. Focused physical examination
7. Baseline vital signs
8. Give nitroglycerin and aspirin if permitted by local protocol and not contraindicated.
9. Transport, perform ongoing assessment, and meet ALS unit.

Rationale

A patient who complains of squeezing or crushing substernal chest pain should be treated as if he or she is having an acute MI. The patient should be put at rest physically and psychologically, and high-concentration oxygen should be administered. Based on local protocol the patient should be assisted in taking his or her own nitroglycerin or should be given nitroglycerin and aspirin from the ambulance drug supply. An ALS unit should be called so arrhythmias can be detected by ECG monitoring and treated before they progress to cardiac arrest. The patient should be transported to a hospital that can restore blood flow through the blocked coronary artery. If the patient's vital signs are stable, transport should be without lights and siren to avoid increasing the patient's anxiety, which will increase the heart's workload.

16.1. **D,** All are risk factors except female gender.
16.2. **D,** Left-sided facial weakness or drooping is a sign of a possible stroke.
16.3. **B,** The heart is located in the mediastinum of the thoracic cavity of the pleural cavity. It lies directly behind the sternum with two-thirds of the heart to the *left* of the midline.
16.4. **A,** A heart attack is referred to as an acute MI.
16.5. **B,** "Ischemia" is a decreased supply of oxygenated blood to tissue.
16.6. **A,** The AV node is located superior to the ventricles at the junction of the right atrium and right ventricle.

16.7. D, The heart's primary pacemaker site is the SA node, located in the upper right atrium.

16.8. C, Cardiac output is the volume of blood pumped by the heart in 1 minute. It is measured in lpm and is calculated by multiplying heart rate by stroke volume.

16.9. B, Cardiac output = heart rate × stroke volume

16.10. A, Before giving nitroglycerin you must make sure the BP is >100 mm Hg systolic. Because nitroglycerin dilates blood vessels, it may cause the patient to experience a short episode of hypotension.

16.11. B, Nitroglycerin is given by placing one tablet under the tongue and allowing it to dissolve. The tablet should not be chewed or swallowed. Warn the patient that nitroglycerin tastes bitter and may cause a headache.

16.12. C, Nitroglycerin relieves chest pain by dilating the coronary arteries and decreasing the cardiac workload.

16.13. A, The first step to treat a patient with symptoms of cardiac disease is to give high-concentration oxygen by non-rebreather mask.

16.14. D, Because a patient who is having a heart attack would be expected to experience nausea, lightheadedness, or syncope, the absence of these symptoms makes them pertinent negative findings.

SCENARIO TWO

Plan of Action

1. BSI

2. Is the scene safe? Yes. Assess nature of illness, number of patients, and need for additional resources.

3. Assess mental status. Ensure an open airway, assess breathing, sit patient up and dangle legs and feet off of bed, give oxygen by non-rebreather mask at 10-15 lpm, consider assisting ventilations, and assess circulatory status.

4. Determine priority, consider ALS.

5. HPI, SAMPLE

6. Focused physical examination

7. Baseline vital signs

8. Give nitroglycerin and aspirin if permitted by local protocol and not contraindicated.

9. Transport, perform ongoing assessment, and meet ALS unit.

Rationale

This patient appears to have myocardial ischemia associated with CHF and pulmonary edema. Sitting her up and dangling her feet will help reduce venous return to her heart and relieve the pulmonary edema. She should be given oxygen by non-rebreather mask. If her breathing continues to be labored and she appears to be tiring, her ventilations should be assisted. Because she is experiencing chest pain in association with her shortness of breath, she should be treated as if she is having an acute MI by giving nitroglycerin and aspirin as permitted by local protocol. A response by an ALS unit should be requested so drug therapy for pulmonary edema secondary to CHF can be begun.

16.15. **A,** The pathway of an impulse traveling through the electrical conduction of the heart is SA node, AV node, bundle of His, right and left bundle branches, and Purkinje fibers.

16.16. **C,** Right ventricular failure would cause fluid to back up into the peripheral circulation, producing ankle edema and abdominal distension.

16.17. **D,** CHF is a condition in which the heart does not pump adequately, causing blood to back up into the lungs and/or extremities.

16.18. **C,** The chambers that pump blood into the arteries are the ventricles. The right ventricle pumps blood into the pulmonary artery, and the left ventricle pumps blood into the aorta.

16.19. **C,** When blood enters the capillary bed it is high in oxygen and low in carbon dioxide.

16.20. **B,** The aorta is the major artery that originates directly from the left ventricle and supplies blood to the entire circulatory system.

16.21. **A,** Unoxygenated blood travels through the pulmonary artery to the lungs. A vessel carrying blood away from the heart is an artery, regardless of whether the blood is oxygenated or unoxygenated.

16.22. **D,** Checking for presence of facial droop, slurred speech, or extremity weakness is part of the focused examination of the nervous system, not the cardiovascular system.

16.23. **C,** The left ventricle pumps oxygenated blood to the peripheral circulatory system through the aorta.

16.24. **A,** The pathway of blood from the time it enters the heart until it leaves the heart is right atrium, tricuspid valve, right ventricle, pulmonary artery, lungs, pulmonary vein, left atrium, mitral valve, left ventricle, and aorta.

16.25. **C,** Normal arterial blood flow cannot be heard with a stethoscope.

16.26. **A,** Atherosclerosis is a condition in which there is a buildup of fat deposits on the inner walls of the arteries.

16.27. **C,** The most common cause of right ventricular failure is left ventricular failure, which overworks the right ventricle by increasing the resistance against which it must pump.

16.28. **B,** Abdominal distension, ankle swelling, shortness of breath, and jugular vein distension are signs or symptoms of CHF.

16.29. **A,** Pedal edema refers to swelling of the feet and ankles.

16.30. **B,** Signs and symptoms of CHF usually appear over time as fluid builds up in the circulatory system. Although some patients develop CHF after having an acute MI, most cases of CHF are caused by other problems such as prolonged hypertension, disease of the heart valves, or inflammation of the myocardium. Some patients who have acute MIs will develop an acute onset of CHF with pulmonary edema.

SCENARIO THREE

Plan of Action

1. BSI
2. Is the scene safe? Yes. Assess nature of illness, number of patients, and need for additional resources.
3. Assess mental status. Ensure an open airway, assess breathing, sit patient up, assist ventilations with BVM and oxygen at 12-15 lpm, and assess circulatory status.
4. Determine priority, consider ALS.
5. HPI, SAMPLE
6. Focused physical examination
7. Baseline vital signs
8. Transport, perform ongoing assessment, and meet ALS unit.

Rationale

This patient has severe pulmonary edema caused by CHF. She should be placed in a sitting position with her feet dangling to reduce blood return to her heart. High-concentration oxygen should be administered, and you should consider assisting her breathing with a BVM because she is gasping and having difficulty moving air. A response by an ALS unit should be requested, so the paramedics can give drug therapy to remove the excess fluid from this patient's lungs.

16.31. **C,** This patient has pulmonary edema.
16.32. **D,** Pulmonary edema is characterized by a sudden onset of severe difficulty breathing.
16.33. **D,** A patient with pulmonary edema would be most likely to have crackles, distended neck veins, a rapid pulse, and a rapid respiratory rate.
16.34. **C,** Treatment for pulmonary edema would include keeping the patient sitting upright and giving oxygen by non-rebreather mask at 10 to 15 lpm.
16.35. **B,** Pulmonary edema results from failure of the left ventricle, which causes blood to back up into the lungs.
16.36. **B,** The average adult stroke volume is 70 mL.
16.37. **A,** The tricuspid valve prevents backflow of blood into the right atrium when the right ventricle contracts.
16.38. **B,** The amount of blood ejected from the ventricles during a single contraction of the heart is the stroke volume.
16.39. **D,** The left ventricle generates the greatest pressure because it has to produce flow in the peripheral circulation.

SCENARIO FOUR

Plan of Action

1. BSI

2. Is the scene safe? Yes. Assess nature of illness, number of patients, and need for additional resources.

3. Assess mental status. Ensure an open airway, assess breathing, give oxygen by non-rebreather mask at 10-15 lpm, and assess circulatory status.

4. Determine priority, consider ALS.

5. HPI, SAMPLE

6. Focused physical examination

7. Baseline vital signs

8. Consider administration of nitroglycerin if permitted by local protocol and not contraindicated.

9. Transport, perform ongoing assessment, and meet ALS unit.

Rationale

Because this patient's chest pain began while she was exerting herself mowing the lawn and has rapidly decreased in severity with rest, she probably is having an episode of angina pectoris. She should be placed at rest physically and psychologically. Oxygen should be given by non-rebreather mask. Depending on local protocol, administration of nitroglycerin should be considered. An ALS unit should be requested so the patient's ECG can be monitored en route to the hospital.

16.40. **C,** The pain of an acute MI often radiates to the left arm, left shoulder, back, neck, or jaw. The pain is not relieved by rest or nitroglycerin and does not change when the patient moves or coughs.

16.41. **D,** The "S" in OPQRST stands for severity. The patient is asked to describe how bad the pain is, usually on a 1 to 10 scale.

16.42. **C,** The "P" in OPQRST stands for provokes, what factors caused the pain to develop or worsen.

16.43. **B,** The rapid physical examination of an unresponsive patient is done after the initial assessment and just before vital signs.

16.44. **B,** The vital signs of a conscious patient are taken at the end of the focused history and physical examination.

16.45. **C,** Vital signs include BP, pulse, respirations, pupil responses, skin color, skin temperature, and capillary refill.

SCENARIO FIVE

Plan of Action
1. BSI
2. Is the scene safe? Yes. Assess nature of illness, number of patients, and need for additional resources.
3. Assess mental status. Ensure an open airway, assess breathing, sit patient up, give oxygen by non-rebreather mask at 10-15 lpm, consider assisting ventilations if patient shows signs of tiring, and assess circulatory status.
4. Determine priority, consider ALS.
5. HPI, SAMPLE
6. Focused physical examination
7. Baseline vital signs
8. Transport, performing ongoing assessment.

Rationale
This patient appears to have pulmonary edema secondary to CHF. Because she also has a history of emphysema and a recent "cold," the probable sequence of events is that she became hypoxic from the combination of COPD and a respiratory infection, which depressed the function of her heart enough to worsen her CHF and cause severe pulmonary edema. She should be placed in a sitting position and given high-concentration oxygen. If she shows signs of tiring or continues to have difficulty moving air adequately, her ventilations should be assisted. An ALS unit should be called to begin appropriate drug therapy.

16.46. **C,** When a patient has pulmonary edema, the lungs fill with fluid as a result of the left ventricle pumping ineffectively.

16.47. **A,** Patients in severe distress with pulmonary edema may cough up pink, frothy sputum. The pink, frothy sputum is caused by fluid that has backed up into the lungs from the failing left ventricles, mixing with air in the alveoli.

16.48. **C,** In the elderly population, CHF may present with episodes of confusion from lack of oxygen. These episodes are particularly common at night.

16.49. **A,** In pulmonary edema, the fluid portion of the blood is displaced from the capillaries into the lungs where it interferes with gas exchange, so the patient literally is drowning in his or her own body fluid.

16.50. **D,** A patient with CHF may present with dyspnea, tachycardia, crackles, wheezes, pedal edema, and abdominal distension.

16.51. **A,** Distension from fluid accumulating in the abdominal cavity (ascites) can be a sign of right heart failure.

SCENARIO SIX

Plan of Action

1. BSI

2. Is the scene safe? Yes. Assess nature of illness, number of patients, and need for additional resources.

3. Assess mental status. Ensure an open airway, assess breathing, apply oxygen at 10-15 lpm by non-rebreather mask, and assess circulatory status.

4. Determine priority, consider ALS.

5. HPI, SAMPLE

6. Focused physical examination

7. Baseline vital signs

8. Give nitroglycerin and aspirin if permitted by local protocol and not contraindicated.

9. Transport, perform ongoing assessment, and meet ALS unit.

Rationale

Squeezing substernal chest pain radiating to the left shoulder and arm, nausea, weakness, and syncope suggest this patient is having an acute MI. He should receive high-concentration oxygen by non-rebreather mask, be given nitroglycerin and aspirin as permitted by local protocol, and be transported to a facility where the blocked coronary artery can be unobstructed by angioplasty or thrombolytic agents. Reperfusing the myocardium as quickly as possible will limit the amount of myocardial tissue loss that occurs and preserve heart function.

16.52. C, Oxygen is given to patients with chest pain because they probably have decreased blood flow and oxygen delivery (ischemia) to part of the myocardium.

16.53. B, All arteries travel *away* from the heart.

16.54. C, The coronary arteries supply the myocardium with blood.

16.55. A, A patient may be having an acute MI and have absolutely no chest pain. This condition is called a "silent MI."

16.56. B, A heart rate <60 beats/min is bradycardia.

SCENARIO SEVEN

Plan of Action

1. BSI

2. Is the scene safe? Yes. Assess nature of illness, number of patients, and need for additional resources.

3. Assess mental status. Ensure an open airway, assess breathing, insert oral airway, begin ventilating with BVM and oxygen, and assess circulatory status.

4. Determine priority. Consider ALS.

5. If response time was >4 to 5 minutes provide 5 cycles (about 2 minutes) of CPR before using AED.

6. Attach AED, analyze rhythm, and defibrillate as advised by AED.

7. Following shock by AED, start CPR immediately beginning with chest compressions. Reanalyze with AED after 5 cycles of CPR or 2 minutes.

8. When pulse returns, perform rapid physical assessment and obtain vital signs.

9. HPI, SAMPLE if available. Transport, perform ongoing assessment, and meet ALS unit.

Rationale

In 2 of 3 studies, when the EMS call-to-response interval was 4 to 5 minutes or longer, a period of 1½ to 3 minutes of CPR before defibrillation was associated with improved survival. With witnessed arrests or response times shorter than 4 to 5 minutes, the AED should be used as soon as possible. With most defibrillators, the first shock eliminates VF more than 87% of the time. When the first shock fails, CPR is likely to confer a greater value than another shock. When a shock eliminates VF, a brief period of chest compressions increases the likelihood that the heart will be able to effectively pump blood.

16.57. **D,** Either coarse or fine ventricular fibrillation can be defibrillated. Asystole and pulseless electrical activity are not shockable rhythms.

16.58. **A,** Ventricular fibrillation

16.59. **C,** AED pads are placed on the anterior right chest just under the right clavicle and on the lower left chest in the midaxillary line.

16.60. **C,** While the AED is analyzing the rhythm all contact with the patient must cease, including chest compressions and BVM ventilations. Touching the patient while the AED is analyzing can produce signals that the AED could interpret as a nonshockable rhythm.

16.61. **A,** Your most important concern when you use the AED is to ensure that no one is touching the patient before delivering a shock. After the AED delivers a shock, CPR should be started immediately, beginning with chest compressions. CPR should be performed for 2 minutes (five cycles of 30:2) before the patient is reassessed.

16.62. D, If the AED advises "no shock," you should immediately check for a pulse and breathing. The AED's advising "no shock" does not mean that the patient has a pulse because there are cardiac arrest rhythms that are nonshockable.

16.63. C, Complete absence of electrical activity on an ECG is called asystole.

16.64. B, Ventricular fibrillation and pulseless ventricular tachycardia should be defibrillated.

16.65. B, If a pulse is present, ventricular tachycardia is not defibrillated. Use of an electric shock to terminate a rapid rhythm that is producing a pulse is called cardioversion. AEDs are not designed to cardiovert patients who have a pulse.

16.66. D, A chaotic, wavy line on the ECG monitor may be caused by ventricular fibrillation or by a loose patient lead.

16.67. C, Pulseless electrical activity is not defibrillated. Ventricular fibrillation or pulseless ventricular tachycardia should be shocked.

16.68. C, Pulseless electrical activity is any organized ECG rhythm that does not generate a pulse. In other words, if the patient is pulseless and the monitor shows any rhythm besides ventricular fibrillation, ventricular tachycardia, or asystole, the patient has pulseless electrical activity.

16.69. B, If response time to a cardiac arrest is less than 4 to 5 minutes, apply the AED, shock if advised, begin CPR, and call for ALS.

16.70. C, When only two EMTs are present, one performs CPR while the other operates the defibrillator.

16.71. B, Although the patient is breathing and has a pulse, drug therapy by the paramedics may be needed to completely stabilize the patient. The AED should not be removed in this situation because the patient's heart may fibrillate again before the paramedics arrive.

16.72. D, The compression-to-ventilation ratio for CPR on an unintubated patient is 30 compressions to 2 ventilations. After a patient is intubated, compressions should be continuous with 8 to 10 breaths/minute interposed.

16.73. D, After 2 minutes of CPR the chest compressor role should be rotated. It is difficult to maintain effective compressions at a rate of 100 compressions/minute and a ratio of 30 compressions to 2 ventilations for longer than 2 minutes.

16.74. A, After you determine a patient is not breathing, you should initially give two breaths that produce visible chest rise.

16.75. D, When supplemental oxygen is used with a BVM during CPR, the tidal volume should be the amount needed to produce visible chest rise and should be delivered over 1 second.

16.76. C, When oxygen is not available during CPR, the tidal volume should be the amount needed to produce visible chest rise and should be delivered over 1 second.

16.77. D, When an AED is used, you may stop CPR long enough to analyze and deliver a single shock.

SCENARIO EIGHT

Plan of Action

1. BSI

2. Is the scene safe? Yes. Assess nature of illness, number of patients, and need for additional resources.

3. Assess mental status. Ensure an open airway, assess breathing, give oxygen by non-rebreather mask at 10-15 lpm, and assess circulatory status.

4. Determine priority, consider ALS.

5. HPI, SAMPLE

6. Focused physical examination

7. Baseline vital signs

8. Give nitroglycerin and aspirin if permitted by local protocol and not contraindicated.

9. Transport, perform ongoing assessment, and meet ALS unit.

Rationale

Because this patient has no previous history of heart disease, the most prudent course of action is to treat her as if she is having an acute MI. She should receive high-concentration oxygen, aspirin, and nitroglycerin as indicated by local protocol and should be transported to a facility that can evaluate her for acute MI and perform reperfusion therapy if necessary. A meeting with an ALS unit to ensure continuous monitoring and early treatment of arrhythmias would be appropriate.

16.78. **C,** Angina typically can be relieved with rest, oxygen, and nitroglycerin.

16.79. **D,** Chest pain that is not relieved by rest, oxygen, and nitroglycerin should be treated as an acute MI.

16.80. **A,** Patients who experience chest pain associated with increased cardiac workload and oxygen demand have narrowing of their coronary arteries caused by atherosclerosis. If the patient is not treated appropriately, continued development of the atherosclerotic plaques can cause an MI.

16.81. **A,** Stable angina is relieved by 10 to 15 minutes of rest and nitroglycerin.

16.82. **A,** Unstable angina is present when previously stable angina shows a change in onset, severity, duration, or quality.

16.83. Coarse ventricular fibrillation

16.84. Coarse ventricular fibrillation

16.85. Ventricular tachycardia

16.86. Ventricular tachycardia

16.87. Fine ventricular fibrillation

16.88. Coarse ventricular fibrillation

16.89. Ventricular tachycardia

16.90. Coarse ventricular fibrillation

16.91. Asystole

17

Altered Mental Status

COMMON CAUSES OF ALTERED MENTAL STATUS (AEIOU-TIPS)

- A—Alcohol, acidosis, and apnea
- E—Epilepsy (seizures), environmental, and endocrine
- I—Infection, ischemia
- O—Overdose
- U—Uremia (kidney failure) or other metabolic or endocrine problems
- T—Trauma, temperature regulation
- I—Insulin: hypoglycemia, hyperglycemia
- P—Psychiatric problems, poisonings
- S—Stroke (cerebrovascular accident [CVA]), shock (hypotension)

DIABETES

- Glucose—The "fuel" used by metabolism; necessary for proper functioning of cells
- Blood glucose level—The amount of glucose in the bloodstream; also called "blood sugar"
- Insulin—Hormone secreted by pancreas; insulin must be present for most cells to remove glucose from the bloodstream.
- Diabetes mellitus—A metabolic disease in which insulin production is absent or decreased and cells are unable to remove adequate amounts of sugar from the bloodstream, resulting in increased blood glucose levels
  - ○ Type I diabetes mellitus
    - Usually begins during childhood
    - Pancreas produces no functional insulin.
    - Patients must receive insulin by injection.
  - ○ Type II diabetes mellitus
    - Usually begins in people aged more than 40 years but is becoming more common in severely overweight children
    - Often occurs in persons who are obese
    - Pancreas produces decreased amounts of insulin, and tissues become less responsive to insulin's effects.
  - ○ May be managed with exercise, weight control, diet, and oral medications (Diabinese, Glucotrol, Micronase); some patients may require insulin injections.
  - ○ Complications of diabetes
    - Renal failure
    - Retinal changes leading to blindness
    - Hypertension
    - Increased risk of myocardial infarction (MI; possibly without chest pain)
    - Increased risk of stroke
    - Nerve damage leading to loss of sensation
    - Slow wound healing, increased risk of wound infections
- Diabetic emergencies
  - ○ Hypoglycemia (low blood sugar)
    - Causes
      - Overdose of insulin or other diabetic medications
      - Taking insulin or other diabetic medications but not eating
      - Increased physical activity
    - Signs and symptoms

- Rapid onset
- Hunger
- Headache
- Weakness
- Restlessness, irritability, nervousness, and confusion
- Seizures
- Tachycardia
- Cool, clammy skin
  - Management
    - If alert enough to swallow and protect own airway, give oral glucose
    - If not able to swallow or protect own airway, call for advanced life support (ALS) unit
- Hyperglycemia (high blood sugar)
  - Causes
    - Not taking insulin or other diabetic medications
    - Overeating
    - Infections
    - Emotional stress
  - Signs and symptoms
    - Slow onset
    - Increased urine output (polyuria)
    - Thirst (polydipsia)
    - Hunger (polyphagia)
    - Nausea, vomiting
    - Rapid, deep breathing (Kussmaul's respirations)
    - Acetone or fruity odor on breath
    - Dry skin
    - Tachycardia
    - Hypotension
    - Decreased level of consciousness
  - Management
    - Begin treatment for hypovolemic shock caused by increased urine output
    - Call ALS unit
    - Transport to hospital for insulin injections to decrease blood glucose level
    - If unable to determine whether patient is hypoglycemic or hyperglycemic, give oral glucose unless contraindicated by patient's mental status or ability to swallow

SEIZURES

- Sudden period of altered or abnormal brain activity that causes changes in behavior and/or body function
- Causes
  - Fever
  - Infection
  - Head trauma
  - Brain tumors
  - Hypoxia
  - Hypoglycemia
  - Drug or alcohol withdrawal

- ○ CVA (stroke)
- ○ Pregnancy-induced hypertension (eclampsia)
- ○ Failure to take antiseizure medications
- Types of seizures
  - ○ Grand mal
    - Tonic-clonic, generalized motor seizures
    - Aura—Peculiar sensation that precedes seizure
    - Loss of consciousness
    - Tonic phase—Muscles stiffen for approximately 30 seconds. Patient may be apneic, may bite tongue, and may lose bladder and bowel control.
    - Clonic phase—Muscles alternately stiffen and relax, producing jerking for 1 to 5 minutes.
    - Postictal phase—Drowsiness, confusion, and headache
  - ○ Petit mal
    - Most common in children
    - Loss of consciousness without falling
    - Patient stares blankly into space
    - Typically lasts only a few seconds
  - ○ Status epilepticus
    - Two or more seizures without a period of consciousness
    - Status grand mal seizures may result in death if not treated.
    - Complications include hypoxic brain injury, long bone fractures, dehydration, and hyperthermia.
  - ○ Seizure assessment
    - Scene size-up—Medical or trauma?
    - Initial assessment
    - Physical examination
      - Focused if responsive
      - Rapid head-to-toe if unresponsive
      - Look for medical identification tags or bracelets
    - SAMPLE history
    - Baseline vital signs
  - ○ Management
    - Position on floor
    - Protect from injury, but do *not* restrain
    - Position patient on side to prevent aspiration if vomiting occurs
    - Do *not* insert anything into mouth
    - When seizure ends, give high-concentration oxygen by non-rebreather mask at 15 lpm
    - Examine carefully for trauma caused by or causing the seizure
    - Evaluate for possible hypoglycemia
    - Consider calling ALS unit, particularly if seizures recur or are prolonged

STROKE

- Sudden interruption of blood flow resulting in death of an area of the brain
- Types
  - ○ Ischemic stroke
    - Blood clot travels to brain and obstructs vessel (embolus), or blood clot forms in place within a blood vessel (thrombus), usually on an area of atherosclerotic plaque, causing obstruction of blood flow

- Emboli produce rapid onset of symptoms; onset of symptoms from thrombi is more gradual.
  - ○ Hemorrhagic stroke
    - Blood vessel ruptures, causing hemorrhage into brain.
    - Bleeding into space between brain and arachnoid layer of meninges (subarachnoid hemorrhage), or bleeding from ruptured vessel within brain (intracerebral hemorrhage)
    - Usually produces rapid onset of severe symptoms
- Risk factors
  - ○ High blood pressure (BP)
  - ○ Cardiovascular disease
  - ○ History of acute MI
  - ○ History of diabetes
  - ○ History of transient ischemic attacks (TIAs; "little strokes," strokelike symptoms that resolve in 24 hours or less with no lasting effects)
  - ○ Cigarette smoking
  - ○ Birth control pill use, particularly in combination with smoking
  - ○ History of sickle cell anemia
- Signs and symptoms
  - ○ Weakness (hemiparesis) or paralysis (hemiplegia) of one side of body
  - ○ Loss of sensation on one side of body
  - ○ Visual disturbances
  - ○ Difficulty speaking, slurred speech
  - ○ Confusion
  - ○ Dizziness
  - ○ Headache
  - ○ Altered mental status
  - ○ Inappropriate behavior
- Management
  - ○ Ensure open airway
  - ○ Position patient to reduce risk of aspiration of secretions
  - ○ Give high-concentration oxygen by non-rebreather mask at 15 lpm
  - ○ Protect weak or paralyzed limbs, use caution in lifting by weak or paralyzed extremities
  - ○ Assess patient for possible hypoglycemia
  - ○ Consider calling ALS unit
  - ○ Transport patient to facility where a CT scan can be performed within 25 minutes and read by a radiologist within 45 minutes, with a goal of patients having ischemic strokes being treated with thrombolytic agents within 60 minutes of arrival

REVIEW QUESTIONS
Scenario One

A 78-y.o. male complains of feeling very weak and lightheaded. He also reports being unusually thirsty lately and says he has been urinating more than usual. The patient denies chest pain, nausea, or shortness of breath. His past medical history includes angina pectoris, hypertension, and arthritis. He takes nitroglycerin as needed, captopril, and ibuprofen. He has no known allergies. He is oriented to person and place, but not to time and events. Vital signs are BP—108/62; pulse (P)—96; respiration (R)—22; and SaO$_2$—95%.

Your Plan of Action

Fill in the blank lines with your treatment plan for this patient. Then compare your plan with the questions, answers, and rationale.

1. _____
2. _____
3. _____
4. _____
5. _____
6. _____
7. _____
8. _____
9. _____

Multiple Choice

17.1. As you approach this patient, your scene size-up should include:
  a. talking to the family about his medications, past history, and medical problems.
  b. determining mechanism of injury, past medical history, allergies, and medications the patient takes on a regular basis.
  c. identifying any potential hazards, securing the scene, and determining if any injuries have occurred.
  d. checking his level of responsiveness, skin color, and respiratory effort.

17.2. This patient's problem is *most* likely:
  a. a silent MI.
  b. hyperglycemia.
  c. heat exhaustion.
  d. hypoglycemia.

17.3. Altered mental status in a patient who is hypoglycemic can be confused with all of the following *except*:
  a. alcohol intoxication.
  b. a head injury.
  c. drug overdose.
  d. hypertension.

17.4. A patient who says he has "sugar problems" probably has:
  a. pancreatitis.
  b. gallbladder disease.
  c. kidney failure.
  d. diabetes mellitus.

17.5. The patient's mental status should be determined:
  a. after you have completed your initial assessment.
  b. during a head-to-toe detailed physical examination.
  c. by using the AVPU method.
  d. while obtaining the SAMPLE history.

17.6. Hyperglycemia occurs when:
  a. the pancreas produces too much insulin to use the sugar in the body.
  b. a diabetic patient does not produce enough insulin to use the sugar in body.
  c. a diabetic patient takes insulin but does not eat enough sugar.
  d. the pancreas produces too much glucose.

17.7. Diabetic ketoacidosis (DKA) is a result of:
  a. hypothermia.
  b. hyperglycemia.
  c. hypoglycemia.
  d. hyperthermia.

17.8. DKA is characterized by a:
  a. gradual onset and warm, dry skin.
  b. sudden onset and warm, dry skin.
  c. gradual onset and cool, dry skin.
  d. sudden onset and cool, dry skin.

17.9. All of the following would be part of the history of this patient's *present* illness *except:*
  a. how long he has been sick.
  b. what activities seem to cause or worsen the symptoms.
  c. how rapidly the symptoms developed.
  d. what medications the patient is taking.

Scenario Two

A 35-y.o. female called EMS because she believes she lost consciousness briefly. She has had nausea, vomiting, and diarrhea for 3 days. Her past medical history includes asthma and type I diabetes mellitus. She uses a Proventil inhaler and takes NPH insulin (20 units AM and 10 units PM). The patient appears to be sleepy but is oriented × 4. Vital signs are BP—100/48; P—136, weak, regular; R—24, shallow, regular; SaO_2—96%; and T—101° F.

Your Plan of Action

Fill in the blank lines with your treatment plan for this patient. Then compare your plan with the questions, answers, and rationale.

1. _____
2. _____
3. _____
4. _____
5. _____
6. _____
7. _____
8. _____
9. _____

Multiple Choice

17.10. What kind of drug name is albuterol?

    a. Generic

    b. Trade

    c. Common

    d. Chemical

17.11. Albuterol causes bronchodilation because it is:

    a. an alpha agonist.

    b. an alpha antagonist.

    c. a beta agonist.

    d. a beta antagonist.

17.12. All of the following information would be important during your assessment of this patient *except:*

    a. when she ate and last took her insulin.

    b. any other medications she currently is taking.

    c. a history of yesterday's events.

    d. whether she has any drug allergies.

17.13. Because the patient not able to keep any food down, which of the following conditions would you suspect?

    a. Hypoglycemia

    b. Hyperglycemia

    c. Insulin coma

    d. Hypovolemia

17.14. The focused history and physical examination of a diabetic patient include which of the following:

    a. when the patient last ate, history of present illness (HPI) and SAMPLE, and an assessment of neurologic status.

    b. HPI and SAMPLE, an assessment of neurologic status, and vital signs.

    c. when the patient last ate, HPI and SAMPLE, and vital signs.

    d. when the patient last ate, a neurologic examination, and vital signs.

17.15. In the OPQRST, the "P" stands for:

    a. prescription medications.

    b. pain quality.

    c. physical examination.

    d. what provokes the problem.

17.16. The purpose of the focused history and physical examination is to:

    a. detect changes in the patient's condition en route to the hospital.

    b. discover less obvious signs and symptoms of illness and injury.

    c. identify immediately life-threatening problems.

    d. quickly check mental status.

17.17. The primary organ you are concerned with in hypoglycemia is the:

    a. pancreas.

    b. liver.

    c. stomach.

    d. brain.

17.18. The digestive system breaks down complex sugars food into:
   a. carbohydrates.
   b. insulin.
   c. glucose.
   d. fat.

17.19. If you are unable to determine from the history and physical examination findings whether a patient's blood sugar is too high or too low, you should:
   a. determine the blood glucose level if permitted by local protocol, and give oral glucose if the test indicates the blood sugar is low.
   b. give nothing by mouth because the patient may have a seizure and aspirate.
   c. advise the physician at the emergency room and transport rapidly because you do not want to raise the blood glucose level unnecessarily.
   d. give oral glucose if the patient is awake and alert, and perform a blood glucose check afterwards if permitted by local protocol.

17.20. The *most* common sign of hypoglycemia is:
   a. nausea and vomiting
   b. fruity breath odor.
   c. altered mental status.
   d. warm, dry skin.

17.21. Oral glucose works by:
   a. increasing the blood sugar level.
   b. decreasing the blood sugar level.
   c. increasing the blood insulin level.
   d. decreasing the blood insulin level.

17.22. All of the following characterize DKA *except:*
   a. acetone or fruity breath odor.
   b. rapid, deep respirations.
   c. frequent urination and extreme thirst.
   d. cool, moist skin.

17.23. A diabetic patient who takes a prescribed dose of insulin but does not eat is *most* likely to develop:
   a. hypoglycemia.
   b. hyperglycemia.
   c. DKA.
   d. dehydration.

17.24. After you give oral glucose to a hypoglycemic patient she loses consciousness; you should:
   a. give a second dose of oral glucose.
   b. use a tongue depressor to inspect for glucose that may still be in the mouth.
   c. ensure an open airway.
   d. repeat the initial assessment.

17.25. How would a diabetic patient with low blood sugar be *most* likely to appear?
   a. Energetic and loud
   b. Alert and oriented
   c. Intoxicated
   d. With one-sided weakness and slurred speech

Scenario Three

A 64-y.o. female called EMS because her 68-y.o. husband was "acting strangely." She tells you he will not speak to her and is having trouble walking. The patient appears unable to use his left arm. When you question him, he will not answer. Sensation is present in all four extremities, but the patient does not seem to be able to move his left arm. He has a history of angina pectoris, hypertension, and duodenal ulcer disease. His medications include nitroglycerin as needed, Lotensin, and Zantac. He has no known allergies. Vital signs are BP—192/104; P—88, strong, regular; R—20, regular, unlabored; and SaO_2—96%.

Your Plan of Action

Fill in the blank lines with your treatment plan for this patient. Then compare your plan with the questions, answers, and rationale.

1. _____
2. _____
3. _____
4. _____
5. _____
6. _____
7. _____
8. _____
9. _____

Multiple Choice

17.26. This patient is *most* likely experiencing:
   a. a psychiatric disorder.
   b. an acute MI.
   c. hypoglycemia.
   d. a stroke.

17.27. A stroke is also known as:
   a. a cardiovascular accident.
   b. cerebrovascular angina.
   c. a cerebrovascular accident.
   d. a cerebrovenous accident.

17.28. When a stroke occurs on the brain's right side, which area of the body will be affected?
   a. The right side
   b. The left side
   c. Both sides
   d. Both lower extremities

17.29. Neurologic deficits caused by a stroke would be *least* likely to include:
   a. slurred speech.
   b. inability to speak.
   c. paralysis of the left arm and leg.
   d. numbness in all four extremities.

17.30. After performing the scene survey and initial assessment, the *next* step to assess this patient would be to:
   a. evaluate his mental status.
   b. check for presence and adequacy of breathing.
   c. obtain the vital signs.
   d. do a focused history and physical examination.

17.31. After performing a focused history and physical examination, you would:
   a. check baseline vital signs.
   b. obtain HPI and SAMPLE.
   c. transport.
   d. evaluate the patient's mental status.

17.32. If stroke symptoms suddenly appear but only last a short time and leave no permanent effects, the patient has had a:
   a. transverse ischemic attack.
   b. transient cerebrovascular attack.
   c. transient ischemic attack.
   d. cerebrovascular angina attack.

17.33. En route to the hospital the patient begins talking to you, but he still cannot move his left arm. You should suspect he:
   a. is having psychiatric problems.
   b. was faking when he appeared unable to speak.
   c. had a minor heart attack and is now improving.
   d. had a TIA and now is improving.

Scenario Four

A 48-y.o. female was getting ready to go to work when she developed blurred vision. While she was talking with the EMS dispatcher, she also began experiencing difficulty speaking. By the time you arrive, she can speak in complete sentences, but her vision still is blurred. She tells you she has had an "extremely stressful" month at work and is about to change jobs. She just went through a divorce, and her mother died last month. She has a past medical history of asthma and a duodenal ulcer. She also just finished going through menopause. Her medications include an ipratropium bromide inhaler as needed, cimetidine, and Premarin. Vital signs are BP—178/90; P—96, strong, regular; R—20, regular, unlabored; and SaO_2—98%. Blood glucose is 105 mg/dL.

Your Plan of Action

Fill in the blank lines with your treatment plan for this patient. Then compare your plan with the questions, answers, and rationale.

1. _____
2. _____
3. _____
4. _____
5. _____
6. _____
7. _____
8. _____
9. _____

Multiple Choice

17.34. If the patient is alert and oriented × 4, she is alert and oriented to:
 a. person, place, time, and her normal surroundings.
 b. place, time, event, and her normal surroundings.
 c. person, place, medical history, and allergies.
 d. person, place, time, and events.

17.35. This patient's problem is *most* likely:
 a. hypertension.
 b. a TIA.
 c. related to menopause.
 d. a new onset of diabetes.

17.36. Which of the following would be neurologic deficits?
 a. Weakness in an extremity, an increased pulse rate, facial drooping, and difficulty in speaking
 b. Decreased sensation in area of the body surface, facial drooping, chest pain, and visual disturbances
 c. Weakness in an extremity, decreased sensation in an area of the body surface, facial drooping, and difficulty speaking
 d. Weakness in an extremity, an increased pulse rate, decreased sensation in an area of the body surface, chest pain, and visual disturbances

17.37. The preferred position for transporting this patient would be:
 a. lying supine with her feet elevated.
 b. left lateral recumbent.
 c. Trendelenburg.
 d. lying supine with her head elevated.

17.38. All of the following statements about strokes are correct *except:*
 a. a stroke may be caused by rupturing of an artery in the brain.
 b. an embolism traveling to the brain from elsewhere in the body may cause a stroke.
 c. a stroke that damages the brain's right side will affect the body's left side.
 d. a stroke patient should always be treated for shock.

17.39. Signs and symptoms of a stroke include all of the following *except:*

    a. drooping of the face on one side.

    b. slurred speech.

    c. dilation of the pupil opposite the side of the stroke.

    d. emotional changes, such as alternating between crying and laughing.

Scenario Five

A 5-y.o. male experienced a tonic-clonic seizure that lasted approximately 5 minutes. He currently is sleepy and difficult to arouse, but he will awaken and tell you what his name is and where he is. The patient's mother says he has no past history of seizures. He has had otitis media for approximately 3 days, has been running a low-grade fever, and is taking an antibiotic. He is on no other medications and has no known drug allergies. Vital signs are BP—90/58; P—124, strong, regular; R—22, regular, unlabored; and SaO_2—98%.

> **Your Plan of Action**
>
> *Fill in the blank lines with your treatment plan for this patient. Then compare your plan with the questions, answers, and rationale.*
>
> 1. _____
> 2. _____
> 3. _____
> 4. _____
> 5. _____
> 6. _____
> 7. _____
> 8. _____
> 9. _____

Multiple Choice

17.40. The patient is in which phase of the seizure?

    a. Postictal

    b. Clonic

    c. Tonic

    d. Aura

17.41. The postictal stage of a grand mal seizure:

    a. is characterized by drowsiness.

    b. occurs before the patient begins to convulse.

    c. occurs after the tonic-clonic phase of the seizure.

    d. occurs after the seizure's tonic-clonic phase and is characterized by drowsiness.

17.42. Which type of seizure involves loss of consciousness without any abnormal motor activity?

    a. A grand mal (tonic-clonic) seizure

    b. A Jacksonian seizure

    c. A petit mal (absence) seizure

    d. A hysterical seizure

17.43. A sensation experienced just before the beginning of a seizure is:

    a. the preictal phase of the seizure.

    b. an aura.

    c. a preliminary olfactory sensation.

    d. the hypersensory phase of the seizure.

17.44. The *most* common cause of seizures in children is:

    a. epilepsy.

    b. fever.

    c. head trauma.

    d. hypoxia.

17.45. Petit mal seizures are seizures that:

    a. only involve one part of the body and consist of a tingling sensation and uncontrollable jerking.

    b. last 5 to 10 minutes and involve generalized tonic-clonic convulsions.

    c. occur consecutively without the patient's regaining consciousness.

    d. produce a brief, temporary loss of consciousness without falling or abnormal motor activity.

17.46. Care of a patient who is having a grand mal seizure would include:

    a. protecting the airway, using spinal precautions if needed, removing any objects that may harm the patient, protecting the patient from injury, and using soft restraints if necessary.

    b. protecting the airway, placing the patient on the floor and loosening his or her clothing, protecting the patient from injury, and using soft restraints if necessary.

    c. protecting the airway, placing the patient on the floor and loosening his or her clothing, using spinal precautions if needed, removing objects that may harm the patient, and protecting the patient from injury.

    d. protecting the airway, using spinal precautions if needed, and protecting the patient from injury.

Answer Key—Chapter 17

SCENARIO ONE

Plan of Action

1. Body Substance Isolation (BSI)
2. Is the scene safe? Yes. Assess nature of illness, number of patients, and need for additional resources.
3. Assess mental status. Ensure an open airway, assess breathing, apply oxygen at 10-15 lpm by non-rebreather mask, and assess circulatory status.
4. Determine priority, consider ALS.
5. HPI, SAMPLE
6. Focused physical examination, including blood glucose determination if authorized
7. Baseline vital signs
8. Transport, perform ongoing assessment en route, and meet ALS unit.

Rationale

The combination of polyuria (increased urine output) and polydipsia (extreme thirst with increased fluid intake) suggests this patient may have new-onset diabetes. Patients who have developed diabetes will have elevated blood sugar because they lack the insulin needed to move glucose out to the bloodstream into the cells. The increased urine output these patients experience can lead to hypovolemia and shock. The patient should be treated for volume loss and transported to a hospital where treatment can be started to decrease his blood sugar. If the patient is in shock, requesting a response by an ALS unit would be appropriate so IV fluid replacement can be started.

17.1. C, Your scene size-up should include identifying potential hazards to yourself or your crew, securing the scene, and determining if the patient has been injured.

17.2. B, The history of increasing thirst and urine output suggests the patient may have new-onset diabetes and probably is hyperglycemic.

17.3. D, Altered mental status in a patient who is hypoglycemic can be confused with alcohol intoxication, head injury, or drug overdose. High blood pressure is unlikely to cause alterations of mental status that could be confused with hypoglycemia.

17.4. D, A patient who tells you he or she has a problem with "sugar" probably has diabetes mellitus.

17.5. C, Mental status is determined during the initial assessment by using the AVPU method.

17.6. B, Hyperglycemia occurs when a diabetic patient does not produce enough insulin to use the sugar in the body, resulting in elevated blood glucose levels. As the kidney attempts to clear the excess sugar from the body, a hyperglycemic diabetic patient's urine output will increase, eventually resulting in hypovolemic shock. Patients with type I diabetes, who produce no functional insulin, will begin to use fat as an alternate fuel for metabolism. The byproducts of fat metabolism (ketone bodies) will accumulate in the bloodstream, causing the condition known as DKA. Patients with type II diabetes, who continue to make small amounts of insulin, do not convert to using fat as their primary metabolic fuel when they become hyperglycemic. Therefore, they do not develop ketoacidosis. However, they develop extremely high blood glucose levels that produce increased urine output, leading to life-threatening hypovolemia. This condition is known as hyperglycemic hyperosmolar nonketotic coma (HHNKC).

17.7. **B,** DKA is a result of hyperglycemia. When a diabetic patient is unable to use glucose as fuel for metabolism, he or she begins to burn fat instead. The byproducts of fat metabolism, ketone bodies, accumulate in the bloodstream and cause ketoacidosis.

17.8. **A,** A patient with DKA will experience a gradual onset of symptoms as the blood sugar levels increase. Loss of water caused by increased urine output will lead to the skin being warm and dry.

17.9. **D,** Although medications are an important part of the patient's history, they are not part of the HPI.

SCENARIO TWO

Plan of Action

1. BSI
2. Is the scene safe? Yes. Assess nature of illness, number of patients, and need for additional resources.
3. Assess mental status. Ensure an open airway, assess breathing, apply oxygen at 10-15 lpm by non-rebreather mask, and assess circulatory status.
4. Determine priority, consider ALS.
5. HPI, SAMPLE
6. Focused physical examination, including blood glucose determination if authorized
7. Baseline vital signs
8. Give oral glucose
9. Transport, perform ongoing assessment en route, and meet ALS unit.

Rationale

Because this patient has continued to take her insulin but has been unable to eat, she probably is hypoglycemic. She also may be hypovolemic because of fluid loss from vomiting and diarrhea. Her blood glucose level should be checked. Oral glucose can be used to correct hypoglycemia if it is present. If the patient thinks she may vomit if she swallows the glucose, have her hold it under her tongue or between her gum and cheek. A paramedic unit should be called to give IV glucose if necessary.

17.10. **A,** Albuterol is a generic name for a drug that is sold under the trade names Proventil or Ventolin. The chemical name describes the exact molecular composition of the drug. A generic name usually is an abbreviated form of the chemical name. The name of a drug recognized by the federal government and listed in the *United States Pharmacopeia* or the *National Formulary* is the official name. The letters USP or NF follow official names. The name under which a company chooses to market a particular drug is the trade name. Trade names are capitalized.

17.11. **C,** Albuterol is a beta agonist, a drug that stimulates the beta-2 receptor sites in the lungs, causing relaxation of the smooth muscle in the bronchial walls and bronchodilation.

17.12. **C,** You should ask when the patient ate her last meal, whether she took her insulin today, if she is taking any other medications, and whether she has any drug allergies. You would not need to know yesterday's events to determine the nature of the problem or manage it appropriately.

17.13. **A,** Because the patient has been unable to keep any food down but has been taking her insulin, you would suspect she has hypoglycemia (low blood sugar).

17.14. **C,** The focused history and physical examination should include HPI and SAMPLE, including information about when the patient last ate, and a set of baseline vital signs.

17.15. **D,** The "P" stands for provokes. What caused or worsened the current medical problem?

17.16. **B,** The purpose of the focused history and physical examination is to discover less obvious signs and symptoms of illness and injury that were not detected during the initial assessment for immediately lift-threatening problems.

17.17. **D,** The primary organ you are concerned with in a hypoglycemic patient is the brain. If the brain does not get the proper amount of glucose, permanent brain damage may occur.

17.18. **C,** The digestive system breaks down complex sugars into glucose, which can be absorbed into the cells. However, glucose cannot cross the cell membranes without insulin.

17.19. **A,** If you are authorized to do so by local protocol, determine the patient's blood glucose level. If you cannot do blood glucose determinations, give the patient sugar when you are unable to tell whether the blood sugar is too high or too low. Giving sugar to a patient who is hyperglycemic will not do harm, and giving sugar to a hypoglycemic patient can prevent brain damage.

17.20. **C,** The most common sign of hypoglycemia is altered mental status. Nausea, vomiting, a fruity breath odor, and warm, dry skin are symptoms of hyperglycemia.

17.21. **A,** Oral glucose increases the blood sugar level.

17.22. **D,** DKA is not characterized by cool, moist skin. Cool, moist skin occurs in patients who are hypoglycemic. Signs of DKA include acetone or fruity breath odor; frequent urination; extreme thirst; warm, dry skin; and rapid, deep respirations.

17.23. **A,** A diabetic patient who takes a prescribed dose of insulin but does not eat will become hypoglycemic.

17.24. **D,** Because the patient's condition has changed, you should repeat the initial assessment of mental status, airway, breathing, and circulation to determine if a life-threatening problem has developed.

17.25. **C,** A patient with low blood sugar would be most likely to appear intoxicated. A lack of blood sugar is unlikely to cause a localized neurologic sign like one-sided weakness; however, in some elderly patients hypoglycemia can produce focal deficits.

SCENARIO THREE

Plan of Action

1. BSI

2. Is the scene safe? Yes. Assess nature of illness, number of patients, and need for additional resources.

3. Assess mental status. Ensure an open airway, assess breathing, give oxygen at 10-15 lpm by non-rebreather mask, and assess circulatory status.

4. Determine priority, consider ALS.

5. HPI, SAMPLE

6. Focused physical examination, including blood glucose determination if authorized

7. Baseline vital signs

8. Transport, perform ongoing assessment en route.

Rationale

This patient appears to have had a CVA or stroke. Stroke occurs when a blood vessel in the brain becomes obstructed by a thrombus or embolus or when a vessel ruptures, causing bleeding into the brain. Stroke can cause altered mental status, seizures, or localizing neurologic signs such as difficulty speaking or loss of sensation or movement on the side of the body opposite the area of injury to the brain. The major objective with a patient who is having a stroke is to rapidly transport to a hospital where a CT scan of the brain can be performed within 25 minutes and read by a radiologist within 45 minutes. If the stroke has been caused by vessel obstruction, thrombolytic agents (clot-dissolving drugs) can be given to remove the obstruction and restore blood flow. To be most effective, thrombolytic agents must be given within 3 hours of the onset of stroke symptoms. Blood glucose levels should be checked routinely in all patients with altered mental status, seizures, or localizing neurologic signs.

17.26. **D,** Because the patient's weakness is one-sided and he is unable to speak, you would suspect a possible CVA or stroke.

17.27. **C,** A stroke is a *cerebrovascular accident.*

17.28. **B,** When a CVA occurs on the brain's right side, the body's left side is affected.

17.29. **D,** A stroke would be least likely to cause numbness in all four extremities. To lose sensation in all four extremities, a patient would have to have two CVAs affecting both sides of the brain simultaneously.

17.30. **D,** After completing the scene survey and initial assessment, the next step would be to do a focused history and physical examination.

17.31. **A,** After performing a focused history and physical examination, you would obtain a set of baseline vital signs.

17.32. **C,** Stroke symptoms that appear for a short time and resolve with no permanent effects are called a transient ischemic attack or TIA.

17.33. D, Because the patient has regained the ability to speak, he may only be having a TIA. However, because his arm still is paralyzed, you should continue to treat him as if he is having a stroke. Patients with TIAs are at risk for having strokes that can cause permanent disability.

SCENARIO FOUR

Plan of Action
1. BSI
2. Is the scene safe? Yes. Assess nature of illness, number of patients, and need for additional resources.
3. Assess mental status. Ensure an open airway, assess breathing, give oxygen at 10-15 lpm by non-rebreather mask, and assess circulatory status.
4. Determine priority, consider ALS.
5. HPI, SAMPLE
6. Focused physical examination, including blood glucose determination if authorized
7. Baseline vital signs
8. Transport, perform ongoing assessment en route.

Rationale
Temporary deficits in neurologic function that resolve quickly without permanent effects are called transient ischemic attacks. TIAs frequently precede CVAs (strokes) that can produce permanent disability. A patient who experiences a possible TIA should be transported for evaluation. Early treatment can prevent progression to a stroke. Blood glucose levels should be evaluated routinely in any patient with altered mental status, seizures, or localizing neurologic signs.

17.34. D, Oriented × 4 means oriented to person, place, time, and events.

17.35. B, Because her neurologic symptoms were of short duration, she most likely had a TIA.

17.36. C, Neurologic deficits would include weakness in an extremity, decreased sensation in an area of the body surface, facial drooping, and difficulty speaking.

17.37. D, The position of choice would be supine with the head elevated at a 45-degree angle to help relieve pressure on the brain.

17.38. D, Patients who are having a stroke do not need to be treated for shock. A stroke can be caused by an embolus, a hemorrhage, or a thrombus. Strokes affect the opposite side of the body from the side of the brain in which they occur.

17.39. C, Hemorrhagic strokes will cause dilation of the pupil on the same side as the bleed. As blood accumulates in the cranial cavity, the brain is pushed downward against the nerve that controls the size of the pupils. Because the nerve on the same side as the bleed is compressed first, the pupil on the side of the bleed dilates first. Strokes can cause facial drooping, slurred speech, and altered emotional state. Sudden changes in affect (emotional state) are a common sign of stroke in older persons.

SCENARIO FIVE

Plan of Action

1. BSI
2. Is the scene safe? Yes. Assess nature of illness, number of patients, and need for additional resources.
3. Assess mental status. Ensure an open airway, assess breathing, give oxygen at 10-15 lpm by non-rebreather mask, and assess circulatory status.
4. Determine priority, consider ALS.
5. Rapid head-to-toe physical examination, including blood glucose determination if authorized
6. Baseline vital signs
7. HPI, SAMPLE
8. Transport, perform ongoing assessment en route, and meet ALS unit.

Rationale

This patient appears to be in the postictal phase of a major motor (grand mal) seizure. Although children can have seizures caused by a rapid increase in body temperature (febrile seizures), this patient's seizure probably has some other cause. Febrile seizures usually occur near the beginning of an episode of febrile illness, and this patient has been sick for 3 days. In children, fever plus seizures should equal meningitis until proven otherwise. The patient should receive high-concentration oxygen and be transported immediately. A meeting with an ALS unit is reasonable because the paramedics can give drugs to stop seizures if they recur. Blood glucose levels should be checked routinely in any patient with altered mental status, seizures, or localizing neurologic signs.

17.40. **A,** The patient is in the postictal phase of the seizure.
17.41. **D,** The postictal phase occurs after the tonic-clonic phase and is characterized by drowsiness.
17.42. **C,** Petit mal or absence seizures are caused by a loss of consciousness that lasts only a few seconds. No dramatic motor activity occurs; the patient does not fall; and convulsions do not occur.
17.43. **B,** An aura is an unusual sensation that precedes some types of seizures.
17.44. **B,** The most common cause of seizures in young children is fever.
17.45. **D,** Petit mal seizures cause a brief, temporary loss of consciousness without falling or abnormal motor activity.
17.46. **C,** Caring for a patient having a grand mal seizure would include protecting the airway, placing the patient on the floor, loosening his or her clothing, using spinal precautions if needed, removing objects that may harm the patient, and protecting the patient from injury. Patients who are actively seizing should never be restrained because they may injure themselves as they pull against the restraints.

18

Poisons and Overdoses

POISONING

- Poison—A substance that impairs health or causes death when it comes in contact with the skin or enters the body
- Poisons may enter the body by
  - *Inhalation* through the respiratory tract
  - *Ingestion* through the gastrointestinal (GI) tract
  - *Injection* through a break in the skin, including animal bites and stings
  - *Absorption* through intact skin or mucous membranes
- Assessment
  - Scene size-up
    - Ensure your safety and the safety of your crew *first*
    - Do *not* expose yourself to the poison
    - Use appropriate personal protective equipment or call for appropriately trained and equipped assistance
  - Initial assessment
    - Evaluate airway, breathing, circulation, and mental status *first* with all patients
    - Most victims of poisoning can be treated adequately by supporting the ABCs
  - Focused history and physical examination
    - What was the patient exposed to?
    - By what route? (inhaled, ingested, injected, or absorbed)
    - How much?
    - How long ago?
    - Has anyone attempted to treat the poisoning? How?
    - Does the patient have a psychiatric history? Possible suicide attempt?
    - Does the patient have any underlying medical illnesses, allergies, chronic drug use, or addiction?
    - How much does the patient weigh?
- Ingested poisons
  - Signs and symptoms
    - Nausea
    - Vomiting
    - Diarrhea
    - Altered mental status
    - Abdominal pain
    - Chemical burns around mouth
    - Discoloration of oral mucous membranes
    - Peculiar breath odors
  - Management
    - Maintain airway
    - Provide high-concentration oxygen, assist breathing as needed
    - Give activated charcoal unless contraindicated
    - Bring all containers, bottles, labels, or other clues about poison to receiving facility
- Inhaled poisons
  - Signs and symptoms
    - Difficulty breathing
    - Chest pain
    - Cough

- Hoarseness
- Headache
- Dizziness
- Confusion
- Seizures
- Altered mental status
  ○ Management
    - Remove patient from toxic environment as quickly as possible
    - Maintain airway
    - Give high-concentration oxygen, assist breathing as needed
    - Bring all containers, bottles, labels, or other clues about poison to receiving facility
- Injected poisons
  ○ Signs and symptoms
    - Weakness
    - Dizziness
    - Chills
    - Fever
    - Nausea
    - Vomiting
    - Pain, swelling, and redness at injection site
    - Pupillary changes
    - Difficulty breathing
  ○ Management
    - Maintain airway
    - Give high-concentration oxygen, assist breathing as needed
    - In case of bite or sting, protect yourself and the patient
    - Bring all containers, bottles, labels, or other clues about poison to receiving facility. Do *not* attempt to capture and transport live venomous animals
- Absorbed poisons
  ○ Signs and symptoms
    - Liquid or powder on patient's skin
    - Burns
    - Itching
    - Redness
    - Swelling
  ○ Management
    - Wear appropriate protective clothing
    - Remove patient from source of poison
    - Remove patient's contaminated clothing or jewelry
    - Maintain airway
    - Give high-concentration oxygen, assist breathing as needed
    - Brush any dry chemicals from patient's skin
    - Irrigate all contaminated body surfaces with clean water for at least 20 minutes
- Activated charcoal—Binds with the poisonous substance in the GI tract, prevents movement into body
  ○ Generic name—Activated charcoal
  ○ Trade names—Actidose, LiquiChar, SuperChar, and InstaChar

○ Adult dose—25 to 50 g
○ Pediatric dose—12.5 to 25 g
○ Contraindications
  ▪ Altered mental status
  ▪ Inability to swallow
  ▪ Ingestion of acid or alkali

SUBSTANCE ABUSE

- Drug abuse—Self-administration of a drug or drugs in a manner not consistent with accepted medical and social patterns
- Addiction—Psychological or physiologic dependence on a drug
- Overdose—Poisoning resulting from taking a drug in excessive amounts, may be unintentional or deliberate
- Withdrawal—Physical and/or psychological symptoms resulting from stopping or reducing use of a drug to which a patient is addicted
- Commonly abused drugs
  ○ Stimulants
    ▪ Examples—Amphetamines, caffeine, cocaine, ephedrine, methylphenidate, and nicotine
    ▪ Effects—Agitation, violent behavior, paranoia, increased body temperature, dilated pupils, rapid respirations, hypertension, and seizures
    ▪ Withdrawal—Apathy, depression, and sleepiness
  ○ Central nervous system (CNS) depressants—Narcotics
    ▪ Examples—Codeine, heroin, methadone, morphine, opium, fentanyl, and hydrocodone
    ▪ Effects—Slow breathing, coma, and pinpoint pupils
    ▪ Withdrawal—Restlessness, irritability, rapid pulse, tremors, watery eyes, runny nose, sweating, and chills
  ○ CNS depressants—Sedatives and tranquilizers
    ▪ Examples—Chloral hydrate, barbiturates, and benzodiazepines
    ▪ Effects—Slow breathing, cold and clammy skin, dilated pupils, weak and rapid pulse, and coma
    ▪ Withdrawal—Anxiety, insomnia, tremors, seizures, and delirium
  ○ CNS depressant—Alcohol
    ▪ Effects
      • Low doses—Excitement, decreased inhibitions, increased urine output, and volume depletion
      • High doses—Stupor, coma, hypotension, hypothermia, and respiratory depression or arrest
    ▪ Withdrawal (delirium tremens [DTs])
      • Irritability and anxiety, weakness, tremors, hallucinations, seizures, nausea, vomiting, tachycardia, sweating, and orthostatic hypotension
  ○ Hallucinogens
    ▪ Examples—LSD, PCM, MDA, PCP, DOM, and DMT
    ▪ Effects—Illusions and hallucinations, anxiety, paranoia, delusions of persecution, poor perception of time and distance, and psychosis. PCP may cause violence, rage, status epilepticus, and paralysis.
  ○ Inhalants

- Examples—Aerosol propellants, glues, lighter fluid, typing correction fluid, and lacquer and varnish thinner
        - Effects—Slurred speech, euphoria, delusions, depression, nausea, confusion, hallucinations, unsteady gait, and erratic heartbeat and pulse
        - Withdrawal—Insomnia, decreased appetite, depression, irritability, and headache
    - Cannabis products
        - Examples—Hashish, marijuana, and tetrahydrocannabinol
        - Effects—Euphoria, increased appetite, dry mouth, disorientation, tremors, paranoia, and psychosis
        - Withdrawal—Insomnia, hyperactivity, and decreased appetite
- Management
    - Establish and maintain airway
    - Give high-concentration oxygen, assist breathing as needed
    - Monitor mental status and vital signs frequently
    - Maintain proper body temperature
    - Treat or prevent shock

REVIEW QUESTIONS
Scenario One

A 14-y.o. female tells you she took approximately 50 aspirin because she was angry with her boyfriend. She is conscious and oriented to person, place, time, and events. She has no significant past medical history, takes no medications, and has no known drug allergies. Vital signs are blood pressure (BP)—116 /84; pulse (P)—122, strong, regular; and respiration (R)—24, regular, unlabored.

Your Plan of Action

Fill in the blank lines with your treatment plan for this patient. Then compare your plan with the questions, answers, and rationale.

1. _____
2. _____
3. _____
4. _____
5. _____
6. _____
7. _____
8. _____
9. _____

Multiple Choice

18.1. Which of the following should be your *first* priority?
   a. The patient's airway
   b. Rescuer safety
   c. Assessment of the respiratory and cardiovascular systems
   d. Notification of the hospital as soon as you arrive on the scene

True/False

18.2. If a patient is conscious, ingested poisons should be diluted, and vomiting always should be induced.
   a. True
   b. False

Multiple Choice

18.3. A poisonous substance may have which of the following effects?
   a. An immediate response or a delayed response
   b. An immediate response within 10 to 20 minutes
   c. A delayed response
   d. A delayed response with vomiting

18.4. The usual adult dose for activated charcoal is:
   a. 25 to 50 mg.
   b. 50 to 100 mg.
   c. 25 to 50 g.
   d. 100 to 200 g.

True/False

18.5. You must wait until the parents are contacted to treat this patient.
   a. True
   b. False

Multiple Choice

18.6. Before leaving the scene, you should:
   a. talk with law enforcement officers.
   b. locate any medication bottles and containers and bring them with the patient.
   c. make the patient vomit if you gave activated charcoal.
   d. find out if the patient is taking any other medications.

Scenario Two

You are dispatched to a report of an "unconscious person." You find a 36-y.o. male sitting in his car in the garage with the engine running. The garage door is open only a couple of inches. The patient does not respond to verbal or painful stimuli. No obvious signs of trauma are present. Vital signs are BP—96/58; P—148, bounding, regular; R—28, shallow, regular; and SaO_2—97%.

Your Plan of Action

Fill in the blank lines with your treatment plan for this patient. Then compare your plan with the questions, answers, and rationale.

1. _____
2. _____
3. _____
4. _____
5. _____
6. _____
7. _____
8. _____
9. _____

Multiple Choice

18.7. The *first* step you should take to treat this patient is:
   a. applying high-concentration oxygen.
   b. calling for a paramedic unit.
   c. opening the airway and assessing breathing.
   d. removing the patient from the hazardous environment.

18.8. After removing the patient from the garage, you should:
   a. do an initial assessment.
   b. form a general impression.
   c. determine the patient's priority.
   d. do a rapid focused history and physical examination.

18.9. The patient *most* likely is experiencing:
   a. cyanide poisoning.
   b. an overdose.
   c. carbon monoxide poisoning.
   d. an allergic reaction.

18.10. Early signs and symptoms of carbon monoxide poisoning include:
   a. cherry-red skin.
   b. headache and nausea.
   c. short episodes of syncope.
   d. seizures.

18.11. All of the following statements about carbon monoxide are true *except:*
   a. carbon monoxide is a colorless, odorless, and tasteless gas.
   b. carbon monoxide does not physically harm lung tissue.
   c. carbon monoxide poisoning may cause a low reading on the pulse oximeter.
   d. a hyperbaric chamber may be necessary to adequately manage carbon monoxide poisoning.

Scenario Three

You have been called to a movie theater for a person with "difficulty breathing." When you arrive, you find approximately 20 people standing outside the building. Their eyes are watering, and they are coughing. They tell you approximately 15 to 20 other people are still inside the building. You can smell a sharp "swimming pool odor."

Multiple Choice

18.12. Your *first* concern in this situation should be to:
- **a.** ensure your safety before giving patient care.
- **b.** ensure all patients have adequate airways.
- **c.** transport the patients as quickly as possible because inhaled poisons are absorbed rapidly.
- **d.** contact the hazard materials (Hazmat) team.

Scenario Three—cont'd

You return to the ambulance, don protective clothing, and call for the Hazmat team.

Your Plan of Action

Fill in the blank lines with your treatment plan for this patient. Then compare your plan with the questions, answers, and rationale.

1. _____
2. _____
3. _____
4. _____
5. _____
6. _____
7. _____
8. _____
9. _____

Multiple Choice

18.13. What should you and your partner do *next?*
- **a.** Begin triaging the patients who have come out of the theater
- **b.** Set up an area outside to keep the patients confined in until they can be decontaminated
- **c.** Remove any patients from the theater who cannot walk
- **d.** Begin cardiopulmonary resuscitation (CPR) on the patients who have no pulse or respirations

18.14. During a mass casualty incident, the green triage tag means a patient:
   a. does not need transport.
   b. needs to be transported by ambulance but not immediately.
   c. has low-priority injuries and may be able to be transported on a bus.
   d. is dead.

True/False

18.15. Chlorine gas will *not* affect the skin.
   a. True
   b. False

Multiple Choice

18.16. Signs and symptoms of chlorine gas inhalation could include:
   a. burning of the nose and mouth, respiratory distress, choking, pulmonary edema, skin irritation, inflammation, and possible blisters.
   b. cyanosis, anxiety, dizziness, substernal chest pain, and cardiac arrest.
   c. nausea, vomiting, abdominal pain, and blood in the stools.
   d. both a and b.

True/False

18.17. Chlorine gas may cause easily oxidized organic or combustible materials to ignite or explode.
   a. True
   b. False

18.18. The rescuer must wear a NIOSH/PAPR-approved respirator with a full face piece for >10 ppm of vapor and a protection factor of 50.
   a. True
   b. False

Multiple Choice

18.19. The rescuer dealing with possible chlorine gas should wear:
   a. an approved respirator.
   b. protective gloves and shoes.
   c. impervious clothing and self-contained breathing apparatus.
   d. an approved respirator and protective gloves and shoes.

Scenario Four

A 16-y.o. female was hosting a party at her home while her parents were out of town. She called EMS for a 15-y.o. male who is having a tonic-clonic (grand mal) seizure. The patient has no known history of diabetes or a seizure disorder. There is no evidence of trauma. His skin is pale, moist, and very warm. Several of the other guests at the party seem unusually talkative, excited, and agitated.

Your Plan of Action

Fill in the blank lines with your treatment plan for this patient. Then compare your plan with the questions, answers, and rationale.

1. _____
2. _____
3. _____
4. _____
5. _____
6. _____
7. _____
8. _____
9. _____

Multiple Choice

18.20. You should suspect the patients have taken a:

    a. depressant such as Seconal.

    b. stimulant such as cocaine.

    c. hallucinogen such as LSD.

    d. narcotic such as morphine.

18.21. Your *first* action should be to:

    a. inform the police.

    b. try to find the parents.

    c. protect the seizing patient from injuring himself.

    d. call for a paramedic unit to meet you.

Matching

18.22. _____ Stimulants

18.23. _____ Sedative-hypnotics

18.24. _____ Hallucinogens

18.25. _____ Narcotics

18.26. _____ Volatile chemical

    a. Tachycardia, dilated pupils, flushed face, "hearing things," "seeing things," and not aware of true environment

    b. Excitement, tachycardia, tachypnea, rapid speech, dry mouth, dilated pupils, diaphoresis, apprehensiveness, and possible uncooperativeness

    c. Dazed or showing temporary loss of contact with the environment or reality, linings of mouth and nose may be swollen, numbness, and tingling

    d. Relaxing effect, sluggish actions, poor body coordination, bradycardia, bradypnea, depressant action on the nervous system, drowsiness, staggering gait, hypotension, and respiratory depression

    e. Bradycardia, bradypnea, low skin temperature, constricted pupils, possible pinpoint pupils, muscle relaxation, diaphoresis, and drowsiness

Scenario Five

You respond to a report of an "allergic reaction." The patient is a 21-y.o. male who is in severe respiratory distress. A friend tells you a bee stung the patient, and he is allergic to bee stings. The patient has an epinephrine autoinjector with him, but his friend says she was too scared to help him with it. The patient is diaphoretic, and his speech is slurred. Vital signs are BP—88/48; P—136, weak, regular; R—32, regular, labored, with expiratory wheezing; and SaO_2—92%.

Your Plan of Action

Fill in the blank lines with your treatment plan for this patient. Then compare your plan with the questions, answers, and rationale.

1. _____
2. _____
3. _____
4. _____
5. _____
6. _____
7. _____
8. _____
9. _____

Multiple Choice

18.27. All of the following are signs or symptoms of an allergic reaction *except:*
   a. dyspnea, tightness in the throat.
   b. tachycardia, hypotension.
   c. hives, itching.
   d. muscle cramps, abdominal pain, nausea, and vomiting.

18.28. Allergic reactions may be caused by any of the following *except:*
   a. carbon dioxide gas.
   b. foods such as peanuts or shell fish.
   c. medications such as penicillin.
   d. insects such as bees.

18.29. All of the following are true about allergic reactions *except:*
   a. an allergic reaction can occur in as little as 5 to 10 minutes.
   b. an allergic reaction always involves the respiratory system.
   c. an allergic reaction may occur over several days.
   d. an allergic reaction may or may not have a rash.

18.30. Because the patient has an epinephrine autoinjector, you should *not:*
   a. contact medical control before assisting the patient with the epinephrine autoinjector.
   b. read the label to ensure the medication has not expired.
   c. call for a paramedic unit or transport to the hospital, whichever is closest.
   d. find out if the patient has any allergies before assisting him with the epinephrine autoinjector.

18.31. The epinephrine autoinjector's effects will last approximately:
  a. 2 to 5 minutes.
  b. 10 to 20 minutes.
  c. 30 minutes to 1 hour.
  d. 1 to 2 hours.
18.32. All of the following statements about epinephrine are correct *except:*
  a. epinephrine is contraindicated if the patient is aged <16 years.
  b. the epinephrine autoinjector injects epinephrine intramuscularly.
  c. epinephrine dilates bronchioles and constricts blood vessels.
  d. the usual adult dosage of epinephrine is 0.3 mg.
18.33. An epinephrine autoinjector injection is given in the:
  a. medial portion of the forearm.
  b. abdomen below the navel.
  c. buttocks.
  d. lateral portion of the thigh halfway between the hip and the knee.
18.34. Epinephrine is a:
  a. slow-acting agent that produces bronchoconstriction.
  b. rapid-acting agent that produces bronchoconstriction.
  c. slow-acting agent that produces bronchodilation.
  d. rapid-acting agent that produces bronchodilation.
18.35. Which statement about giving epinephrine during an allergic reaction is *correct?*
  a. Epinephrine is contraindicated if the patient is allergic to penicillin.
  b. Epinephrine is contraindicated if the patient has a history of chronic obstructive pulmonary disease (COPD).
  c. Epinephrine is contraindicated if the patient is aged <8 years.
  d. There are no contraindications to giving epinephrine during an allergic reaction.
18.36. The dose of epinephrine in the pediatric autoinjector is:
  a. 0.015 mg.
  b. 0.03 mg.
  c. 0.15 mg.
  d. 0.3 mg.

Scenario Six

A 6-y.o. female possibly ingested kerosene. Her chief complaint is that her "mouth hurts." She does not appear to be in respiratory distress. The vital signs are BP—94/60; P—116, strong, regular; R—24, regular, unlabored; and SaO_2—99%.

Your Plan of Action

Fill in the blank lines with your treatment plan for this patient. Then compare your plan with the questions, answers, and rationale.

1. _____
2. _____
3. _____
4. _____
5. _____
6. _____
7. _____
8. _____
9. _____

Multiple Choice

18.37. If a child has ingested a petroleum product, you should do all of the following *except:*
  a. notify poison control.
  b. try to induce vomiting before the poison is absorbed into the body.
  c. have the parents keep the child as calm as possible.
  d. do a focused history and physical examination.

18.38. All of the following are ingested poisons *except:*
  a. gasoline.
  b. paint remover.
  c. bleach.
  d. carbon monoxide.

18.39. What type of poison is gasoline?
  a. A hydrocarbon
  b. An acid
  c. A CNS depressant
  d. An alkali

18.40. If this patient begins vomiting, you would be *most* concerned about which of the following?
  a. Suffocation
  b. Aspiration
  c. Hypotension
  d. Damage to the stomach lining

18.41. The system that will *most* likely be affected in this patient is the:
  a. nervous system.
  b. GI system.
  c. immune system.
  d. endocrine system.

Scenario Seven

A 4-y.o. male ingested 25 200-mg ibuprofen tablets approximately 30 minutes ago. He is conscious, alert, and oriented to person, place, time, and events. He has no significant past medical history. Vital signs are BP—108/56; P—112, strong, regular; R—26, regular, unlabored; and SaO_2—97%.

Your Plan of Action

Fill in the blank lines with your treatment plan for this patient. Then compare your plan with the questions, answers, and rationale.

1. _____
2. _____
3. _____
4. _____
5. _____
6. _____
7. _____
8. _____
9. _____

Multiple Choice

18.42. The normal pediatric dose for activated charcoal is:
   a. 12.5 to 25 mg.
   b. 25 to 50 mg.
   c. 12.5 to 25 g.
   d. 25 to 50 g.

18.43. When you give a medication, all of the following are necessary steps *except:*
   a. recording the time and amount given.
   b. ensuring you have the right patient.
   c. asking the patient about any allergies.
   d. determining who the patient's physician is.

18.44. Procedures for giving activated charcoal include:
   a. administering with a full glass of water to prevent vomiting.
   b. *not* giving anything by mouth for at least 1 hour afterward.
   c. shaking well before administering.
   d. ensuring the patient has no allergies.

18.45. All of these patients could be given activated charcoal *except:*
   a. a patient who has had an episode of syncope and is not fully awake.
   b. a patient with a history of cardiac disease.
   c. a patient aged <10 years.
   d. a patient who has just taken an overdose of Ecstasy.

18.46. Treatment for a patient who has ingested a poisonous substance would include all of the following *except:*

    a. applying oxygen by non-rebreather mask.

    b. calling for advanced life support (ALS), if available.

    c. transporting the patient as quickly as possible in a supine position.

    d. recording the time of all your interventions.

18.47. Activated charcoal may cause which of these side effects?

    a. Dizziness

    b. Unusual drowsiness

    c. Black stools

    d. Diarrhea

18.48. All of the following are contraindications to giving activated charcoal *except:*

    a. alkali ingestion.

    b. petroleum product ingestion.

    c. acid ingestion.

    d. aspirin ingestion.

Answer Key—Chapter 18

SCENARIO ONE

Plan of Action

1. Body Substance Isolation (BSI)
2. Is the scene safe? Yes. Assess nature of illness, number of patients, and need for additional resources.
3. Assess mental status. Ensure an open airway, assess breathing, and assess circulatory status.
4. Determine priority, consider ALS.
5. History of present illness (HPI), SAMPLE
6. Focused physical examination
7. Baseline vital signs
8. Give 25 to 50 g of activated charcoal.
9. Transport, perform ongoing assessment.

Rationale

This patient appears to be in no immediate distress. However, untreated aspirin overdose can develop into a life-threatening problem. She should be given activated charcoal to adsorb the aspirin she has ingested and transported for continued care, including a psychiatric evaluation.

18.1. **B,** The number one principle when entering any scene is rescuer safety. You do no one any good if you become a patient yourself.

18.2. **B,** Some poisons are corrosive. If the patient attempts to drink anything or if vomiting is induced, additional damage to the esophagus will occur.

18.3. **A,** Depending on the nature of the substance, the amount taken, the patient's general health, the amount of food in the stomach, and other factors, a poison may have immediate or delayed effects.

18.4. **D,** The usual adult dose of activated charcoal is 25 to 50 g.

18.5. **B,** Because this patient is a minor who is experiencing what reasonably appears to be a life-threatening illness (aspirin overdose), the parents' consent to treat is implied.

18.6. **B,** Locate any medication bottles and containers and bring them with the patient.

SCENARIO TWO

Plan of Action

1. BSI

2. Is the scene safe? No, carbon monoxide probably is present. Open the garage door and move the patient to an uncontaminated area. Assess nature of illness, number of patients, and need for additional resources.

3. Assess mental status. Ensure an open airway, assess breathing, begin assisting ventilations with a bag-valve mask and oxygen at 12-15 lpm, and assess circulatory status.

4. Determine priority, consider ALS.

5. Rapid physical examination

6. Baseline vital signs

7. HPI, SAMPLE

8. Transport, perform ongoing assessment, and meet ALS unit.

Rationale

This patient has been poisoned with carbon monoxide, a toxin that reduces the ability of hemoglobin to bind oxygen for transport to the tissues. He should be removed from the garage as quickly as possible. His ventilations should be assisted with high-concentration oxygen to help displace the carbon monoxide from his red blood cells more rapidly. Hyperbaric (high-pressure) oxygen therapy may be required at the hospital to manage severe cases of carbon monoxide poisoning.

18.7. D, You will want to remove this patient from the hazardous environment as soon as possible.

18.8. A, After removing the patient from the garage, you should perform an initial assessment of mental status, airway, breathing, and circulation.

18.9. C, This patient probably has been poisoned by carbon monoxide—a colorless, odorless, and tasteless gas that is present whenever organic material has been burning incompletely.

18.10. B, The early signs of carbon monoxide poisoning include headache and nausea. Syncope and seizures would be later signs. Cherry-red skin is a *very* late sign of severe carbon monoxide poisoning.

18.11. C, Carbon monoxide binds to the hemoglobin and prevents it from carrying oxygen. Because it produces saturation of hemoglobin, carbon monoxide can cause falsely *high* oximeter readings.

18.12. A, Because a poisonous gas could be present, you should ensure your safety and the safety of your crew before giving patient care.

SCENARIO THREE

Plan of Action

1. BSI and any other appropriate protective equipment
2. Is the scene safe? No. Assess nature of illness/mechanism of injury, number of patients. Request a response by the fire department, including a Hazmat team, the police, and additional ambulances.
3. Establish a command post.
4. Keep patients who have left the theater confined to one location until they can be decontaminated and assessed.
5. Triage patients for treatment and transport using the START method.

Rationale

During a mass casualty incident, the first-arriving EMS crew is responsible for establishing initial EMS command and beginning triage of patients. Because this incident involves a hazardous material (chlorine), patients must be appropriately decontaminated before being treated or transported from the scene. However, prolonged efforts to decontaminate should not be allowed to jeopardize a patient's chance of survival. Only personnel with appropriate protective equipment and training should attempt rescues inside the theater. Because this appears to be a terrorist incident, the possibility of a secondary device designed to injure or kill emergency services personnel should be considered.

18.13. **B,** You should set up an area where patients may be confined until decontamination can be completed. Once this area is established, triage of patients who have come out of the theater can be begun. Until adequate numbers of appropriately equipped rescuers arrive, an attempt should not be made to enter the theater. In a mass casualty incident, CPR is not started on patients in cardiac arrest.

18.14. **C,** A green tag signifies low-priority injuries. These patients can be delayed for transport while other more critical ones are taken to the hospital. If an incident produces a large number of green tag patients, a bus can be used to transport them. A red tag indicates a patient has a treatable, life-threatening problem and should be cared for and transported immediately. Patients who have a yellow tag have problems that are not immediately life threatening but have the potential to become life threatening or produce serious, long-term disability. These patients should be cared for after the red-tagged patients. A black tag indicates a patient who is dead or who is so seriously ill or injured that death will occur despite treatment.

18.15. **B,** Chlorine gas will cause skin burns. It also causes burning and irritation of the eyes, nose, and airway.

18.16. **D,** Chlorine can cause burning of the nose and mouth, respiratory distress, pulmonary edema, skin irritation and blistering, cyanosis, anxiety, dizziness, chest pain, and cardiac arrest.

18.17. **A,** In addition to being toxic and corrosive, chlorine is a potent oxidizer that can cause organic materials to ignite.

18.18. A, The rescuer must wear a NIOSH-approved respirator-type mask for organic vapors. NIOSH has approved an assigned protection factor of 50 for powered air-purifying respirator-type masks with full, tight-fitting face pieces accompanied with an appropriate gas/vapor canister or cartridge.

18.19. C, The rescuer would wear impervious clothing and equipment when dealing with chlorine gas. A respirator worn with protective gloves and shoes would be insufficient because the rescuer's skin surface would not be adequately protected.

SCENARIO FOUR

Plan of Action

1. BSI
2. Is the scene safe? Probably so. However, with a large group of excited teenagers present, calling for police backup would be reasonable. Assess nature of illness, number of patients, and need for additional resources.
3. Assess mental status. Ensure an open airway, assess breathing, and assess circulatory status. While the patient continues to seize, protect him from injury and from aspirating. When the seizure stops, suction the airway (if necessary), and apply oxygen by non-rebreather mask at 10-15 lpm.
4. Determine priority, consider ALS.
5. Rapid physical examination
6. Baseline vital signs
7. HPI, SAMPLE
8. Transport, perform ongoing assessment, and meet ALS unit.

Rationale

This patient probably is seizing because of the effects of a stimulant. While he is actively seizing, he should be protected from injuring himself. He should be placed on his left side to reduce the risk that he will vomit and aspirate. After the seizure stops, the airway should be cleared, and the patient should be given high-concentration oxygen. His vital signs should be monitored, and he should be transported to the hospital or to meet an ALS unit. Patients who are toxic from stimulants are at risk of seizures, high BP, stroke, myocardial infarction, and heat stroke.

18.20. B, Because everyone is excited and very talkative and the patient is seizing, you would suspect a stimulant such as cocaine.

18.21. C, Your first action would be to protect the patient from injuring himself.

18.22. B, Excitement, tachycardia, tachypnea, rapid speech, dry mouth, dilated pupils, diaphoresis, apprehensiveness, and possible uncooperativeness

18.23. D, Relaxing effect, sluggish actions, poor coordination, bradycardia, bradypnea, depressant action on CNS, drowsiness, staggering gait, hypotension, and respiratory depression

18.24. **A,** Tachycardia, dilated pupils, flushed face, "hears things," "sees things," and not aware of true environment

18.25. **E,** Bradycardia, bradypnea, low skin temperature, constricted pupils, possible pinpoint pupils, muscle relaxation, diaphoresis, and drowsiness

18.26. **C,** Dazed or showing temporary loss of contact with the environment or reality, linings of mouth and nose may be swollen, numbness, and tingling

SCENARIO FIVE

Plan of Action

1. BSI

2. Is the scene safe? Yes. Assess nature of illness, number of patients, and need for additional resources.

3. Assess mental status. Ensure an open airway, assess breathing, give oxygen by non-rebreather mask at 10-15 lpm, consider assisting ventilations, and assess circulatory status.

4. Determine priority, consider ALS.

5. Rapid physical examination

6. Baseline vital signs

7. HPI, SAMPLE

8. Give epinephrine using an epinephrine autoinjector.

9. Transport, perform ongoing assessment, and meet ALS unit.

Rationale

This patient has anaphylactic shock. He should receive high-concentration oxygen by non-rebreather mask and should be given epinephrine using an epinephrine autoinjector. Epinephrine will dilate the patient's lower airways, reducing his respiratory difficulty. It also will constrict his peripheral blood vessels, helping to increase his BP. The patient should be transported to the hospital or to a meeting with an ALS unit as quickly as possible.

18.27. **D,** Muscle cramps, abdominal pain, nausea, and vomiting are not typical signs of an allergic reaction.

18.28. **A,** Carbon dioxide is a waste product of metabolism and a normal component of the human body; therefore, it will not cause allergic reactions.

18.29. **B,** An allergic reaction does not always involve the respiratory system. Mild reactions may cause a rash. Some mild allergic reactions develop slowly over several days.

18.30. **D,** Because epinephrine is a normal component of the human body, you do not have to ask about allergies before giving it.

18.31. **B,** The duration of the epinephrine autoinjector's effects is 10 to 20 minutes. If the allergen is still active, signs and symptoms of an allergic reaction may appear again.

18.32. A, You may give epinephrine to any patient of any age if you have a physician's order and the dose is correct for age and weight.

18.33. D, The best site to inject epinephrine is the lateral portion of the thigh halfway between the hip and knee.

18.34. D, Epinephrine is a rapid-acting agent that produces bronchodilation.

18.35. D, There are no contraindications to giving epinephrine during an allergic reaction.

18.36. C, The pediatric dose of epinephrine is 0.15 mg.

SCENARIO SIX

Plan of Action

1. BSI

2. Is the scene safe? Yes. Assess nature of illness, number of patients, and need for additional resources.

3. Assess mental status. Ensure an open airway, assess breathing, give oxygen by non-rebreather mask at 10-15 lpm, and assess circulatory status.

4. Determine priority, consider ALS.

5. HPI, SAMPLE

6. Focused physical examination

7. Baseline vital signs

8. Transport, perform ongoing assessment.

Rationale

The patient appears to be stable at this time. Her ABCs should be monitored, and she should be transported to the hospital.

18.37. B, You would *not* induce vomiting. Hydrocarbons like kerosene are easily aspirated. If the patient vomits, she has an opportunity to get more kerosene into her lungs, where it can cause severe pneumonia.

18.38. D, Carbon monoxide, a gas, is an inhaled poison.

18.39. A, Gasoline is a hydrocarbon.

18.40. B, If the patient vomits, you are most concerned about her aspirating.

18.41. B, The GI system will be most affected. The patient's respiratory system also is at risk if she has aspirated the kerosene.

SCENARIO SEVEN

Plan of Action

1. BSI

2. Is the scene safe? Yes. Assess nature of illness, number of patients, and need for additional resources.

3. Assess mental status. Ensure an open airway, assess breathing, give oxygen 10-15 lpm by non-rebreather mask, and assess circulatory status.

4. Determine priority, consider ALS.

5. HPI, SAMPLE

6. Focused physical examination

7. Baseline vital signs

8. Consider giving 12.5-25 g of activated charcoal.

9. Transport, perform ongoing assessment.

Rationale

This patient appears to be stable. The ABCs should be monitored, and he should be transported to the hospital. Activated charcoal should be considered to slow absorption of the toxin.

18.42. **C,** The pediatric dose of activated charcoal is 12.5 to 25 g.

18.43. **D,** You do *not* need to know the identity of the patient's physician to give a medication. You do need to ask about allergies, ensure you have the right patient, and record the time and amount given.

18.44. **C,** Activated charcoal is a suspension of fine particles of charcoal in water. It should be shaken well before it is administered.

18.45. **A,** A patient who is not fully awake should never be given activated charcoal because of the risk of aspiration.

18.46. **C,** If there is no trauma requiring spinal motion restriction, the patient should be transported in a position that minimizes the risk of aspiration if vomiting occurs.

18.47. **C,** Patients who take activated charcoal will have black stools as the charcoal begins to leave the GI tract.

18.48. **D,** Aspirin ingestion is *not* a contraindication to the use of activated charcoal. Patients who have ingested corrosive substances (acids and alkalis) should not be given activated charcoal because of the risk of damage to the burned esophagus when the patient swallows. Ingestion of petroleum products is a contraindication because of the danger of causing vomiting, which may lead to aspiration of the petroleum product.

19

Environmental Problems

PHYSIOLOGY

- Metabolism runs best at a normal body temperature of 98.6° F.
  - Increased T°—Increased metabolic rates; cell damage
  - Decreased T°—Decreased metabolic rates; cell damage
- Maintaining body temperature requires balancing heat production and loss.
  - Heat production
    - Metabolism
    - Movement of large muscles
    - Shivering
  - Heat loss
    - Radiation—Heat transfer between objects not in direct contact
    - Conduction—Heat transfer between objects in direct contact
    - Convection—Heat transfer by movement of air currents
    - Evaporation—Heat loss by change of water from a liquid to a gas. Results from sweating
    - Respiration—Heat loss by exhaled air, a combination of evaporation and convection
  - Heat production > heat loss = Increased body temperature
  - Heat loss > heat production = Decreased body temperature
- Heat/cold illness results from
  - Effects of increased or decreased body temperature
  - Effects of attempting to compensate for changes in heat production, heat loss

HEAT-RELATED ILLNESS

- Heat cramps
  - Caused by salt loss from sweating
  - Spasms in large muscle groups
  - Patient awake, alert
  - Treatment
    - Stop activity
    - Move to cool environment
    - Oral balanced salt solution (sports drinks)
    - Do *not* give salt or water alone
- Heat exhaustion
  - Sweating causes decreased blood volume.
  - Vasodilation increases size of vascular space.
  - Both decrease perfusion.
  - Signs and symptoms
    - Dizziness
    - Weakness
    - Faintness
    - Headache
    - Nausea, vomiting
    - Pale, cool, and moist skin
  - Treatment
    - Stop activity
    - Move to cool environment
    - Lie down, elevate legs

- ▪ Balanced salt solution (sports drink) orally if not nauseated
- ▪ Transport if symptoms do not improve rapidly
- ● Heat stroke
  - ○ *Most serious* heat-related illness
  - ○ Body temperature increases to >106° F
  - ○ Damage occurs to brain's temperature-regulating center.
  - ○ Sweating mechanism fails
  - ○ Heat stroke types
    - ▪ Classic
    - ▪ Exertional
  - ○ High-risk groups
    - ▪ Classic heat stroke
      - ● Elderly population
      - ● Patients with congestive heart failure
      - ● Obese persons
      - ● Alcoholic patients
    - ▪ Exertional heat stroke
      - ● Small children in closed vehicles
      - ● Athletes, military recruits, or construction workers on hot, humid days
  - ○ Signs and symptoms
    - ▪ Increased body temperature
    - ▪ Hot, flushed, and dry skin (Skin may still be moist in patients with exertional heat stroke.)
    - ▪ Absence of sweating
    - ▪ Altered mental status (confusion, irritability, and coma)
    - ▪ Seizures
    - ▪ Altered mental status + hot environment = heat stroke until proven otherwise
  - ○ Treatment
    - ▪ High-concentration oxygen
    - ▪ Assist ventilations as needed
    - ▪ Rapidly cool to 102° F
    - ▪ Transport

COLD-RELATED INJURIES AND ILLNESS

- ● Frostbite
  - ○ Localized cold injury
  - ○ Tissues exposed to subfreezing temperatures
  - ○ Vasoconstriction occurs
    - ▪ Decreased blood flow to distal circulation (nose, ears, fingers, and toes)
    - ▪ Water in tissues freezes; tissue damage occurs.
  - ○ Signs and symptoms
    - ▪ Mild (frostnip)—Red, burning areas
    - ▪ Superficial—White, waxy, and doughy-feeling
    - ▪ Deep—Dead white, hard, and no sensation
  - ○ Treatment
    - ▪ Remove from cold
    - ▪ Dry areas gently, wrap in sterile dressing

- Transport
- If transport prolonged, rewarm rapidly in 100° to 105° F water
- Do *not* rub frostbite
- Do *not* allow refreezing
- Do *not* allow patient to smoke
- Hypothermia
  - Generalized cooling of body
  - Can occur at temperatures *above* freezing
  - Hypothermia risk groups
    - Homeless persons
    - Alcoholic patients
    - Elderly persons living in poorly heated homes
    - Outdoor sports participants
  - Altered mental status + cool environment = hypothermia until proven otherwise
  - Treatment
    - Remove from cold
    - Support airway, breathing
    - 100% O_2—Warmed, if possible
    - If able to follow instructions, actively rewarm
    - If unable to follow instructions, prevent further heat loss
    - Avoid rough handling
    - Transport
    - Hypothermia can cause apparent absence of vital signs.
    - Resuscitate hypothermic cardiac arrest patients aggressively
    - You are not dead until you are warm and dead.

NEAR DROWNING

Definitions

Drowning—Death by suffocation after immersion in a liquid
Near drowning—An episode in which a person initially survives immersion in a liquid

Near Drowning Types

- Dry lung
  - 15% of cases
  - Aspiration of small amount of H_2O results in laryngospasm
  - Asphyxia occurs
- Wet lung
  - 85% of cases
  - Large amounts of water enter lungs
  - Fluid, electrolyte imbalances occur
  - Freshwater
    - Surfactant lost; alveoli collapse.
    - Water moves from alveoli to bloodstream.
    - Blood is diluted; oxygen-carrying capacity decreases.
    - Red cells swell and rupture.
      - Potassium released, causes arrhythmias
      - Hemoglobin released, causes renal failure

○ Saltwater
  ■ Water moves from bloodstream to alveoli.
  ■ Pulmonary edema occurs.
  ■ Blood volume decreases, causing shock.

Treatment

- Do not attempt swimming rescue without proper training
- Consider possibility of neck injuries with
  ○ Drowning in swimming pools
  ○ Drowning without adequate history
  ○ Diving accidents
- Place patient on spine board in water
- If possible, begin to ventilate patient while removing from water
- Resuscitate all patients who drown in cold water (<70° F)
- Transport all near-drowning patients for observation

SCUBA AND ALTITUDE-RELATED EMERGENCIES

Squeeze

- Inability to equalize pressure in sinuses, middle ear
- Causes severe pain

Ear Drum Rupture

- Caused by inability to equalize pressure in middle ear
- Causes loss of equilibrium

Nitrogen Narcosis

- Caused by breathing compressed air under pressure
- Under pressure, N_2 becomes toxic to central nervous system (CNS).
- Disorientation, confusion result.
- Problem disappears on surfacing.

Air Embolism

- Patient surfaces suddenly holding breath.
- Compressed air in alveoli expands, lung tissue tears, and air enters pulmonary circulation, returns to heart, and is pumped to brain.
- Signs and symptoms
  ○ Sudden extremity weakness or numbness
  ○ Hemiplegia
  ○ Dilated pupil on affected side
  ○ Seizures
  ○ Coma
- Treatment
  ○ High-concentration oxygen
  ○ Assist ventilations as needed
  ○ Transport to recompression chamber

Decompression Sickness (Bends)

- Diver dives deeply or too long.
- Diver does not ascend slowly enough to let dissolved nitrogen leave blood gradually.
- Nitrogen bubbles form and obstruct vessels.
- Decompression sickness can result only if the dive was >33 feet.
- Signs and symptoms may be delayed.
- Types of decompression sickness
  - Pain only (joint) bends—Aching or boring pain in joints
  - CNS bends—Bubbles affect blood flow to brain or spinal cord.
  - "Chokes"—Bubbles affect flow of blood through lungs.
- Treatment
  - High-concentration oxygen
  - Transport to recompression chamber

Acute Mountain Sickness

- Also known as high altitude sickness
- Usually occurs in high altitudes >8000 feet
- Results from decreased atmospheric pressure and hypoxia
- Signs and symptoms
  - Headache
  - Tiredness out of proportion to activity
  - Shortness of breath
  - Swelling of face, hands
- Treatment
  - Rest and do not go any higher
  - Give oxygen for severe cases
  - If symptoms do not improve rapidly, descend.

BURNS
Skin Functions

- Sensation
- Protection
- Temperature regulation
- Fluid retention

Effects of Burns

- Fluid loss
- Inability to maintain body temperature
- Infection

Burn Depth

- First degree (superficial)
  - Involves only epidermis
  - Red
  - Painful
  - Tender
  - Blanches under pressure

- ○ Possible swelling, no blisters
- ○ Heals in approximately 7 days
- Second degree (partial thickness)
  - ○ Extends through epidermis into dermis
  - ○ Salmon pink
  - ○ Moist, shiny
  - ○ Painful
  - ○ Blisters may be present. (Not all second-degree burns blister, but all burns that blister are second degree.)
  - ○ Heals in 7 to 21 days
- Third degree (full thickness)
  - ○ Through epidermis, dermis into subcutaneous tissues
  - ○ Thick, dry
  - ○ Pearly gray or charred black
  - ○ May bleed from vessel damage
  - ○ Painless because nerve endings are destroyed
  - ○ Requires skin grafting to heal

Burn Extent

- Adult rule of nines
  - ○ Head—9%
  - ○ Each upper extremity—9%
  - ○ Anterior chest/abdomen—18%
  - ○ Posterior chest/abdomen—18%
  - ○ Each lower extremity—18%
  - ○ Genitalia—1%
- Pediatric rule of nines
  - ○ For a 1-y.o. child
    - ■ Head—18%
    - ■ Each upper extremity—9%
    - ■ Anterior chest/abdomen—18%
    - ■ Posterior chest/abdomen—18%
    - ■ Each lower extremity—13.5%
    - ■ Genitalia—1%
  - ○ For each year >1 year, subtract 1% from head and add 0.5% to each lower extremity.
- Rule of palm—*Patient's* palm equals 1% of *his or her* body surface area (BSA).

Burn Severity

- Contributing factors
  - ○ Depth
  - ○ Amount of body surface involved
  - ○ Location
  - ○ Cause
  - ○ Patient age
  - ○ Associated injuries or illnesses
- Critical burns
  - ○ Full thickness >10% BSA

- ○ Partial thickness >25% BSA (20% pediatric)
- ○ Face, feet, hands, and genitalia involved
- ○ Airway or respiratory involvement
- ○ Associated trauma (fractures, internal injuries)
- ○ Associated medical disease (diabetes, heart disease, and pulmonary disease)
- ○ Electrical burns
- ○ Deep chemical burns
- Moderate burns
  - ○ Full thickness 2% to 10%
  - ○ Partial thickness 15% to 25% (10% to 20% pediatric)
- Minor burns
  - ○ Third degree <2%
  - ○ Second degree <15% (<10% pediatric)

Thermal Burn Management

- Stop burning process
  - ○ Remove patient from source of injury
  - ○ Remove clothing unless stuck to burn
  - ○ Cut around clothing stuck to burn, leave in place
- Assess airway/breathing
  - ○ Start oxygen if
    - Moderate or critical burn
    - Decreased level of consciousness
    - Signs of respiratory involvement
    - Burn occurred in closed space
    - History of carbon monoxide or smoke exposure
  - ○ Assist ventilations as needed
- Assess circulation
  - ○ Begin treatment of shock, if present
  - ○ Rapid onset of hypovolemic shock in a burn patient suggests presence of other injuries in addition to burn.
- Obtain history
  - ○ How long ago was patient burned?
  - ○ What has been done for the patient?
  - ○ What caused the burn?
  - ○ Was the patient burned in a closed space?
  - ○ Did patient lose consciousness?
  - ○ SAMPLE
- Rapid head-to-toe physical examination
  - ○ Check for other injuries
  - ○ Estimate percent of BSA burned
  - ○ Remove jewelry, other constricting bands
- Treat burn wound
  - ○ Cover with a dry, clean sheet or a sterile burn sheet. (Wet dressings increase speed of heat loss through burn and worsen hypothermia.)
  - ○ Do *not* rupture blisters

    ○ Do *not* apply creams, salves, or ointments
- Transport to appropriate facility

Inhalation Injury

- Carbon monoxide
  - ○ Product of incomplete combustion
  - ○ Colorless, odorless, and tasteless
  - ○ Binds to hemoglobin 200 × stronger than oxygen
  - ○ Headache, nausea, vomiting, and "roaring" in ears
- Upper airway burn
  - ○ Caused by inhalation of heated gases
  - ○ Danger signs
    - ■ Neck, face burns
    - ■ Singeing of nasal hairs, eyebrows
    - ■ Tachypnea, hoarseness, and drooling
    - ■ Red, dry oral/nasal mucosa
- Lower airway burn
  - ○ Caused by chemicals present in inhaled smoke
  - ○ Danger signs
    - ■ Loss of consciousness
    - ■ Burned in a closed space
    - ■ Tachypnea
    - ■ Cough
    - ■ Crackles, wheezes, and rhonchi
    - ■ Carbonaceous (black) sputum

Chemical Burns

- Concerns
  - ○ Damage to skin
  - ○ Absorption of chemical, systemic toxic effects
  - ○ Avoiding EMS personnel exposure
- Management
  - ○ Remove chemical from skin
  - ○ Liquids—Wash away with water
  - ○ Dry chemicals—Brush away as much as possible, wash away what remains with water
- Special concerns
  - ○ Phenol
    - ■ Not water soluble
    - ■ Flush with polyethylene glycol (PEG300 or PEG400), glycerin, or isopropyl alcohol
    - ■ Then wash with large amounts of water, followed by soap and water for at least 15 minutes
  - ○ Sodium/potassium
    - ■ Burn on contact with water
    - ■ Cover with oil
  - ○ Tar
    - ■ Use cold packs to solidify tar
    - ■ Do *not* attempt to remove
    - ■ Tar can be dissolved away later with organic solvents.

○ Chemicals in eyes
  ▪ Wash with water or saline solution
  ▪ Do *not* place any other chemicals into eyes
  ▪ Wash out contact lenses

Electrical Burns

- Considerations
  ○ Intensity of current
  ○ Duration of contact
  ○ Kind of current (AC or DC)
  ○ Width of current path
  ○ Types of tissues exposed (resistance)
  ○ Voltage
- Types of injuries
  ○ Conductive injuries
    ▪ Entrance/exit wounds may be small
    ▪ Massive tissue damage between entrance/exit
  ○ Nonconductive injuries
    ▪ Arc burns
    ▪ Flame burns from ignition of clothing
- Other complications
  ○ Cardiac arrest/arrhythmias
  ○ Respiratory arrest
  ○ Spinal fractures
  ○ Long bone fractures
- Management
  ○ Make sure current is off before you approach the patient!
  ○ Check ABCs
  ○ Assess carefully for other injuries
  ○ Splint, restrict motion of spine as needed
  ○ Patient needs hospital evaluation, observation.

REVIEW QUESTIONS
Scenario One

On a bitterly cold January day, you are called for a "person down." The wind chill factor is 20 degrees below zero, and snow has been falling all morning. The patient is an 89-y.o. female who apparently slipped on the ice and fell when she went outside to get her mail. She is unconscious and unresponsive. Her extremities are extremely cold to the touch, and her skin is very pale. Vital signs are pulse (P)—50, weak, regular at the carotid; respirations (R)—8, shallow, regular; and blood pressure (BP)—unobtainable.

Your Plan of Action

Fill in the blank lines with your treatment plan for this patient. Then compare your plan with the questions, answers, and rationale.

1. _____
2. _____
3. _____
4. _____
5. _____
6. _____
7. _____
8. _____
9. _____

Multiple Choice

19.1. This patient will have lost heat by:
  a. conduction.
  b. convection.
  c. evaporation.
  d. both conduction and convection.

19.2. What is homeostasis?
  a. A medical condition caused by weather-related factors
  b. The normal state of balance between the body's systems
  c. The body's transfer of heat between itself and the environment
  d. The normal body temperature

19.3. Your *first* step to care for this patient would be to:
  a. assist her respirations with high-concentration oxygen.
  b. begin to rewarm her.
  c. move her to the ambulance using spinal precautions.
  d. perform an initial assessment and call for advanced life support (ALS).

19.4. What type of hypothermia would the patient *most* likely have?
  a. Early or mild hypothermia
  b. Localized hypothermia
  c. Transient hypothermia
  d. Late or severe hypothermia

19.5. After moving the patient to the ambulance you would *immediately*:
  a. remove all of her wet clothing.
  b. place warm blankets over her.
  c. examine her from head to toe.
  d. attempt to find a family member so you can obtain a history.

19.6. If this patient goes into cardiac arrest, the *most* likely cause would be:
  a. low core temperature causing increased myocardial irritability.
  b. injuries from the fall causing hypovolemia.
  c. airway obstruction producing hypoxemia.
  d. injury to the myocardium from cold exposure.

19.7. One of the *most important* considerations of this call would be:
  a. starting chest compressions to support the heart rate.
  b. handling the patient carefully.
  c. rapidly rewarming the patient.
  d. calling for an ALS unit so IV therapy can be started.

Scenario Two

Your patient is a 28-y.o. female who was running a 10-kilometer race when she suddenly developed "cramping" leg and abdominal pain. She is very diaphoretic, and her skin is cool and pale. Vital signs are BP—100/66; P—128, weak, regular; and R—26, shallow. The temperature is 96° F, and the humidity is 70%.

Your Plan of Action

Fill in the blank lines with your treatment plan for this patient. Then compare your plan with the questions, answers, and rationale.

1. _____
2. _____
3. _____
4. _____
5. _____
6. _____
7. _____
8. _____
9. _____

Multiple Choice

19.8. This patient probably is experiencing:
  a. an acute myocardial infarction (MI).
  b. bleeding caused by a tubal ectopic pregnancy.
  c. heat stroke.
  d. heat cramps.

True/False

19.9. Heat cramps are caused by failure of the body's temperature-regulation mechanisms.
  a. True
  b. False

Multiple Choice

19.10. Because the patient is conscious, you should:
   a. obtain a complete history.
   b. allow her to drink as long as she is alert and oriented.
   c. tell her she can go home after she rests for 30 minutes.
   d. not give anything by mouth because she has abdominal pain.

19.11. Which of the following patients would be *most* likely to develop heat cramps?
   a. A 19-y.o. female who is 5 months pregnant
   b. A 55-y.o. male who is overstressed at work
   c. A 70-y.o. male who exercises regularly
   d. A 12-y.o. female who has had a respiratory infection for 1 week

Scenario Three

Your patient is a 58-y.o. male who has been running 10 miles a day for several days to prepare for the Senior Olympics. During this period temperatures have been in the upper 90s, and the humidity has been >70%. The patient says he felt very dizzy and weak after his run yesterday. This morning he began experiencing dizziness, nausea, vomiting, and a severe headache. He has no past medical history. Vital signs are BP—94/52; P—138; R—24, shallow; and skin is dry and extremely warm to touch.

Your Plan of Action

Fill in the blank lines with your treatment plan for this patient. Then compare your plan with the questions, answers, and rationale.

1. _____
2. _____
3. _____
4. _____
5. _____
6. _____
7. _____
8. _____
9. _____

Multiple Choice

19.12. This patient is *most* likely experiencing:
   a. heat stroke.
   b. heat exhaustion.
   c. heat cramps.
   d. a cerebrovascular accident (CVA).

19.13. Which of the following statements about this patient is *most* correct?
    a. He will have increased heat loss caused by vasodilatation.
    b. Shivering will help rid the body of additional heat.
    c. He should be cooled as rapidly as possible.
    d. Ice packs may be used but should *not* be placed near the groin, the neck, and the armpits.

19.14. After completing the initial assessment, you should:
    a. apply oxygen at 4 lpm.
    b. call for an ALS unit.
    c. begin cooling the patient rapidly.
    d. have the patient drink water to which salt has been added.

True/False

19.15. This patient could be cooled by immersing him in cold water.
    a. True
    b. False

19.16. Patients with this problem may have body temperatures >106° F.
    a. True
    b. False

Scenario Four

A 16-y.o. male was canoeing down an inlet into a lake with a group of friends. He became separated from them, and approximately 45 minutes later they found him lying face down in the water at the mouth of the inlet. It is a cool September day, and the water temperature is approximately 50° F. He is pulseless and apneic. His friends are trying to perform cardiopulmonary resuscitation (CPR).

Your Plan of Action

Fill in the blank lines with your treatment plan for this patient. Then compare your plan with the questions, answers, and rationale.

1. _____
2. _____
3. _____
4. _____
5. _____
6. _____
7. _____
8. _____
9. _____

Multiple Choice

19.17. What type of drowning has this patient experienced?

    a. Warm, saltwater

    b. Cold, saltwater

    c. Warm, freshwater

    d. Cold, freshwater

19.18. The *most* appropriate action at this point would be to:

    a. attempt to resuscitate the patient.

    b. call for the police and the coroner.

    c. calm the friends and call for the police.

    d. attempt to locate the patient's parents.

19.19. Which statement about near drowning is *most* correct?

    a. Victims of cold water drowning are not dead until they are "warm and dead."

    b. A dry-lung drowning in which the lungs fill with fluid is more likely to occur in saltwater.

    c. In a "wet" drowning, asphyxiation is caused by laryngeal spasms.

    d. Near drowning has occurred if the patient was submerged <3 minutes.

Scenario Five

A 28-y.o. male was scuba diving in a lake with a friend when he disappeared. After 10 minutes, his friend found him floating on top of the water. The patient is experiencing "tightness" in his chest and is complaining of weakness in his right arm and leg. Vital signs are BP—110/78; P—82, strong, regular; and R—22, labored.

Your Plan of Action

Fill in the blank lines with your treatment plan for this patient. Then compare your plan with the questions, answers, and rationale.

1. _____

2. _____

3. _____

4. _____

5. _____

6. _____

7. _____

8. _____

9. _____

Multiple Choice

19.20. The patient is *most* likely experiencing:

    a. acute MI.

    b. nitrogen narcosis.

    c. air embolism.

    d. a near-drowning incident.

True/False
19.21. Patients with nitrogen narcosis experience a euphoric state from the toxic effects of pressurized oxygen.
  a. True
  b. False

Multiple Choice
19.22. All of the following statements about air embolism are correct *except*:
  a. give high-flow oxygen 15 lpm.
  b. position the patient with his head elevated 45 degrees.
  c. air has entered the circulatory system from tearing of the alveolar walls.
  d. air embolism is caused by breath-holding during ascent.

Scenario Six

A 32-y.o. male who was rock climbing in the Rocky Mountains suddenly became dizzy and short of breath. He also is complaining of a headache and appears slightly disoriented. He denies any trauma or significant past medical history and has no known allergies. Vital signs are BP—112/70; P—74, strong, regular; and R—22, deep, regular.

Your Plan of Action
Fill in the blank lines with your treatment plan for this patient. Then compare your plan with the questions, answers, and rationale.

1. _____
2. _____
3. _____
4. _____
5. _____
6. _____
7. _____
8. _____
9. _____

Multiple Choice
19.23. This patient is *most* likely experiencing:
  a. pulmonary embolism.
  b. nitrogen narcosis.
  c. acute mountain sickness (AMS).
  d. decompression sickness.

True/False
19.24. This illness is caused by an unacclimatized climber rapidly ascending to an altitude >8000 feet.
  a. True
  b. False

Multiple Choice

19.25. Which of the following statements about altitude sickness is *most* correct?

    a. It presents with severe chest pain caused by expansion of air trapped in the alveoli.

    b. It is caused by formation of nitrogen bubbles in the blood during a rapid ascent.

    c. It occurs as a result of decreased atmospheric pressure, which causes hypoxia.

    d. It can occur only during a descent from a high altitude.

Scenario Seven

An 18-y.o. hiker became lost overnight in a state park. It is January, and nighttime temperatures have been falling well below freezing. The patient is complaining of pain in his right foot and lower leg and says his left foot feels numb. He denies any trauma. There is no significant past medical history, and the patient takes no medications. Vital signs are BP—104/80; P—68, strong, regular; and R—18, shallow, regular.

Your Plan of Action

Fill in the blank lines with your treatment plan for this patient. Then compare your plan with the questions, answers, and rationale.

1. _____
2. _____
3. _____
4. _____
5. _____
6. _____
7. _____
8. _____
9. _____

Multiple Choice

19.26. As you begin to perform a focused examination of this patient, you should *first:*

    a. remove his shoes and socks.

    b. give him high-concentration oxygen.

    c. place a splint on the right leg.

    d. make sure he does not elevate his feet above the level of his heart.

19.27. The patient is *most* likely to have what problem?

    a. Frostbite of both feet

    b. A right sprained ankle

    c. A blood clot occluding circulation to the left foot

    d. An infection of the right leg and foot

19.28. Treatment of this patient would include:
   a. rubbing the legs and feet to increase circulation.
   b. bandaging both lower extremities tightly to reduce swelling.
   c. opening any blisters to relieve pressure.
   d. removing the socks and shoes and bandaging the extremities.

Scenario Eight

A 91-y.o. female has been working outside in her garden every day for the past 4 days. Each day the temperature has reached the upper 90s. The patient is complaining of nausea, vomiting, dizziness, and fatigue that have been present for approximately 2 days. She denies any pain. Her skin feels dry and very warm. She has a past history of colitis and arthritis and takes ibuprofen as needed. Vital signs are BP—92/60; P—116, strong, regular; and R—22, deep, regular.

> **Your Plan of Action**
>
> *Fill in the blank lines with your treatment plan for this patient. Then compare your plan with the questions, answers, and rationale.*
>
> 1. _____
> 2. _____
> 3. _____
> 4. _____
> 5. _____
> 6. _____
> 7. _____
> 8. _____
> 9. _____

Multiple Choice

19.29. This patient is *most* likely to have what problem?
   a. Influenza
   b. Heat stroke
   c. Heat exhaustion
   d. Acute MI

19.30. All of the following statements about heat stroke are correct *except:*
   a. heat stroke is caused by failure of the body's temperature-regulating mechanisms.
   b. heavy sweating usually is present.
   c. the patient will have altered mental status and increased body temperature.
   d. signs and symptoms of shock may be present.

19.31. Heat stroke also is known as:
   a. hypothermia.
   b. hyperthermia.
   c. hypertensive crisis.
   d. advanced heat exhaustion.

Scenario Nine

A 36-y.o. male removed a radiator cap from an overheated engine and was splashed with hot water. Salmon pink, blistered burns are present on his chest, right arm, and right hand. He is in extreme pain. Vital signs are BP—148/90; P—114, strong, regular; and R—22, shallow, unlabored.

Your Plan of Action

Fill in the blank lines with your treatment plan for this patient. Then compare your plan with the questions, answers, and rationale.

1. _____
2. _____
3. _____
4. _____
5. _____
6. _____
7. _____
8. _____
9. _____

Multiple Choice

19.32. The *first* action to take when caring for a burn patient is to:
    a. apply oxygen at 10 to 15 lpm.
    b. perform an initial assessment.
    c. stop the burning process.
    d. obtain an initial set of vital signs.

19.33. Which statement about a second-degree burn is *correct*?
    a. The burn involves only the epidermis.
    b. The burn extends through all layers of the skin.
    c. Blisters always will be present.
    d. The burn involves the epidermis and part of the dermis.

19.34. Which statement about a third-degree burn is *correct*?
    a. Blisters always will be present.
    b. The burned area usually has a gray, moist appearance.
    c. The skin is burned through its full thickness.
    d. The burned area is painful.

19.35. The *most* significant concern in the emergency care of burns is:
    a. preventing infection by applying moist, sterile dressings.
    b. preventing shock by managing pain.
    c. preventing contamination of the burn and beginning management of fluid loss.
    d. initiating care to prevent scar formation.

19.36. A burn of the right leg, right arm, face, and head involves what percentage of the BSA?
    a. 18%
    b. 27%
    c. 36%
    d. 45%

19.37. A patient's palm is equal to what percentage of his or her total BSA?

    a. 1%

    b. 3%

    c. 5%

    d. 6%

Scenario Ten

A 1-y.o. female pulled a hot cup of coffee off the table, splashing herself. She has burned her left arm and hand. Vital signs are BP—98/60; P—124, strong, regular; and R—26, regular.

Your Plan of Action

Fill in the blank lines with your treatment plan for this patient. Then compare your plan with the questions, answers, and rationale.

1. _____

2. _____

3. _____

4. _____

5. _____

6. _____

7. _____

8. _____

9. _____

Multiple Choice

19.38. Approximately what percentage of this patient's total BSA has been burned?

    a. 4.5%

    b. 9%

    c. 14%

    d. 18%

19.39. Which of the following would be considered a *critical* burn?

    a. A second-degree burn of the anterior chest

    b. A second-degree burn of 9% or more

    c. Burns involving the hands or feet

    d. A sunburn of 20% of total BSA

19.40. All of the following pieces of information about a burn are important to obtain *except:*

    a. if the patient has been burned before.

    b. what caused the burn.

    c. what time the burn occurred.

    d. if the patient has any allergies.

Answer Key—*Chapter 19*

SCENARIO ONE

Plan of Action

1. Body Substance Isolation (BSI)

2. Is the scene safe? No. The extreme cold is a hazard to you and to the patient. Rapidly remove the patient from the cold to the protection of the ambulance patient compartment while maintaining spinal precautions. Assess nature of illness, number of patients, and need for additional resources.

3. Assess mental status. Ensure open airway, assist oxygen with a bag-valve mask (BVM) and oxygen at 12-15 lpm, and assess circulatory status.

4. Determine priority, consider ALS.

5. Remove wet clothing, perform rapid head-to-toe examination, and wrap patient in warm, dry blankets.

6. Baseline vital signs

7. SAMPLE

8. During transport perform detailed physical examination if time permits, perform ongoing assessment.

Rationale

This scene is not safe. You and your patient are in immediate danger because of the low temperatures and extreme wind chill. Using appropriate spinal precautions, the patient should be moved to the ambulance as quickly as possible. Because her breathing is slow, it should be assisted with a BVM and oxygen. The patient's wet clothing should be removed to prevent further cooling and to allow a head-to-toe examination for any injuries to be performed. After the examination is completed, the patient should be covered with warm blankets. The patient should be transported to the hospital so she can be rewarmed from the body's core outward. She should be handled gently at all times because rough handling can cause cardiac arrest in hypothermic patients.

19.1. D, This patient will have lost heat by conduction to the cold air and ground and by convection to the cold wind.

19.2. B, Homeostasis is the normal state of balance between the body's systems that maintains a stable internal environment.

19.3. C, Because the extreme cold is a hazard to you and your patient, you should move her to the ambulance as quickly as possible while taking appropriate spinal precautions.

19.4. D, The patient probably has late or severe hypothermia.

19.5. A, You should immediately remove all of the patient's wet clothing to reduce further heat loss. After you have removed her wet clothing, you can then cover her with warm blankets.

19.6. A, This patient would be most likely to go into cardiac arrest from her low core body temperature, which would cause increased myocardial irritability and arrhythmias.

19.7. B, Hypothermic patients should be handled with extreme care. The heart becomes increasingly irritable as body temperature decreases. Rough handling can produce cardiac arrest. Severely hypothermic patients must be rewarmed gradually from the core outward to avoid causing shock. Chest compressions should not be started on an adult unless a pulse is absent.

SCENARIO TWO

Plan of Action

1. BSI

2. Is the scene safe? Yes. Assess nature of illness, number of patients, and need for additional resources.

3. Assess mental status. Ensure an open airway, assess breathing, apply oxygen at 10-15 lpm by non-rebreather mask, and assess circulatory status.

4. Determine priority, consider ALS.

5. History of present illness (HPI), SAMPLE

6. Focused physical examination

7. Baseline vital signs

8. Provide patient with balanced electrolyte solution to drink.

9. Transport, perform ongoing assessment.

Rationale

The patient appears to have heat cramps. Heat cramps are painful spasms in the large skeletal muscles caused by excess loss of salt and water from heavy sweating. Heat cramps are not associated with the alterations in mental status that accompany heat exhaustion and heat stroke. The patient should be moved to a cool environment to stop her sweating and should drink a balanced electrolyte solution (sports drink).

19.8. D, This patient probably has heat cramps.

19.9. B, Heat cramps are caused by excessive lost of salt and water from sweating. Failure of the body's temperature-regulating mechanisms causes heat stroke.

19.10. B, Because the patient's mental status is unaltered and she has an open airway, she can drink a balanced electrolyte solution such as any of the commercially available sports drinks. Drinking large amounts of water without salt may worsen the patient's cramps.

19.11. D, A child who has already lost body water and salt because of an infection would have an increased risk of heat cramps.

SCENARIO THREE

Plan of Action

1. BSI
2. Is the scene safe? Yes. Assess nature of illness, number of patients, and need for additional resources.
3. Assess mental status. Ensure an open airway, assess breathing, apply oxygen at 10-15 lpm by non-rebreather mask, and assess circulatory status.
4. Determine priority, consider ALS.
5. HPI, SAMPLE
6. Focused physical examination
7. Baseline vital signs
8. Begin rapid cooling.
9. Transport, perform ongoing assessment.

Rationale

This patient is having a heat stroke. Heat stroke occurs when an increase in the body's core temperature overwhelms the mechanisms that regulate body temperature. Sweating ceases, and the core temperature rapidly increases to >106° F. Heat stroke victims have altered mental status and warm, dry skin. They complain of nausea and severe headache. Patients with heat stroke must be cooled rapidly to prevent permanent brain damage or death.

19.12. A, This patient has heat stroke. Heat stroke is characterized by a core temperature >106° F, warm skin, and altered mental status. Although most heat stroke patients are not sweating and have dry skin, young people who develop heat stroke rapidly as a result of intense exertion in hot, humid environments may still be sweating.

19.13. C, The patient should be cooled as rapidly as possible. Steps to produce cooling can include placing cold packs on the groin, neck, and armpits. Shivering should be avoided because it generates heat and can increase body temperature.

19.14. C, After completing the initial assessment, you should begin cooling the patient rapidly. Oxygen should be given by non-rebreather mask at 10 to 15 lpm. Because heat stroke alters mental status, fluids should not be given by mouth.

19.15. A, Medical control may ask you to cool the patient by immersing him in cold water, especially if transport times are likely to be long.

19.16. A, A patient with heat stroke will have a body temperature of >106° F.

SCENARIO FOUR

Plan of Action

1. BSI

2. Is the scene safe? Yes. Assess nature of illness, number of patients, and need for additional resources.

3. Assess mental status. Ensure open airway using spinal precautions, ventilate with BVM and oxygen at 12-15 lpm, assess circulatory status, and continue CPR.

4. Apply semi-automated external defibrillator (SAED), and deliver shocks as indicated.

5. Determine priority, consider ALS.

6. Rapid trauma examination

7. SAMPLE

8. Secure to long spine board with cervical collar and cervical immobilization device.

9. During transport do a detailed physical examination if time permits, perform ongoing assessment, and meet ALS unit.

Rationale

After determining the patient is in cardiac arrest, continue CPR. Because the patient appears to have drowned in cold water, resuscitation may be possible even after an extended period of submersion. Apply the SAED, and deliver shocks as indicated. If the patient does not respond, perform a rapid examination for any injuries, immobilize the patient's spine, and transport. Arrange a meeting with an ALS unit if one is available. Restricting motion of the spine is indicated because the history of the events leading to the cardiac arrest is incomplete.

19.17. **D,** This patient has experienced a cold, freshwater drowning. Freshwater drowning leads to loss of surfactant, a chemical needed to keep the alveoli from collapsing. It also causes dilution of the blood and rupturing of red cells as the freshwater shifts from the alveoli into the bloodstream. Exposure to cold water decreases core temperature, slows metabolism, and increases the body's tolerance of hypoxia.

19.18. **A,** You should attempt to resuscitate the patient. Cold-water exposure slows the metabolic rate, increasing the body's ability to tolerate hypoxia. Victims of cold-water drowning have been successfully resuscitated after being submerged for >1 hour.

19.19. **A,** Cold-water drowning victims are not considered dead until they are "warm and dead" because of the tendency of hypothermia to protect the body tissues from the effects of hypoxia. Dry-lung drowning results from spasms of the vocal cords caused by water entering the upper airway. Wet-lung drowning occurs when the patient aspirates water into the lower airway. A near drowning has occurred when the patient initially survives being submerged in water or some other liquid.

SCENARIO FIVE

Plan of Action

1. BSI

2. Is the scene safe? Yes. Assess nature of illness, number of patients, and need for additional resources.

3. Assess mental status. Ensure an open airway, assess breathing, apply oxygen at 10-15 lpm by non-rebreather mask, assist ventilations as needed, and assess circulatory status.

4. Determine priority, consider ALS.

5. HPI, SAMPLE

6. Focused physical examination

7. Baseline vital signs

8. Transport to a recompression chamber, perform ongoing assessment during transport.

Rationale

Arterial air embolism occurs when a scuba diver holds his or her breath while ascending. Air in the alveoli expands and tears the alveolar walls, entering the pulmonary circulation. The air then returns to the heart and is pumped into the systemic circulation, causing emboli that can obstruct blood flow in the brain, coronary arteries, and other structures. The patient should receive oxygen and be transported to a facility that has a recompression chamber. At one time, the recommended transport position for patients with arterial air embolism was 30 degrees head down (Trendelenburg position). However, most diving medicine specialists now suggest that these patients be transported in a supine position.

19.20. C, The patient probably has an arterial air embolism. Scuba divers develop arterial air embolism when they surface rapidly while holding their breath. Air trapped in the alveoli expands, tears the alveolar walls, enters the pulmonary circulation, returns to the heart, and is pumped into the systemic circulation. Air bubbles that reach the brain can obstruct vessels, causing stroke symptoms. Arterial air emboli also can enter the coronary arteries, causing an acute MI.

19.21. B, Nitrogen narcosis is a euphoric effect caused by toxic effect of pressurized nitrogen on the CNS.

19.22. B, The patient should *not* be placed in a semi-sitting position. Air rises! Position the patient supine or with his head lower than his feet to keep air from traveling to the brain.

SCENARIO SIX

Plan of Action
1. BSI
2. Is the scene safe? Yes. Assess nature of illness, number of patients, and need for additional resources.
3. Assess mental status. Ensure an open airway, assess breathing, apply oxygen at 10-15 lpm by non-rebreather mask, and assess circulatory status.
4. Determine priority, consider ALS.
5. HPI, SAMPLE
6. Focused physical examination
7. Baseline vital signs
8. Transport, perform ongoing assessment.

Rationale
AMS occurs after a rapid ascent to an altitude >8000 feet by a person who is not used to the effects of high altitude. Symptoms include dizziness, headache, agitation, irritability, shortness of breath, and euphoria. The patient should be given high-concentration oxygen and observed carefully. If symptoms do not resolve rapidly with rest and oxygen, the patient should be taken to a lower altitude.

19.23. **C,** This patient has AMS. AMS occurs when an unacclimatized person rapidly ascends to an altitude >8000 feet. AMS may take up to 6 hours to develop and can last up to 3 to 4 days. Signs and symptoms include dizziness, headache, malaise, vomiting, impaired memory, shortness of breath, euphoria, and irritability.

19.24. **A,** AMS is caused by a rapid ascent to an altitude >8000 feet.

19.25. **C,** AMS is caused by decreased atmospheric pressures at higher altitudes that cause hypoxia.

SCENARIO SEVEN

Plan of Action
1. BSI
2. Is the scene safe? Yes. Assess nature of illness, number of patients, and need for additional resources.
3. Assess mental status. Ensure open airway, assess breathing, apply oxygen at 10-15 lpm by non-rebreather mask, and assess circulatory status.
4. Determine priority, consider ALS.

Continued

SCENARIO SEVEN—cont'd

5. Remove wet shoes and socks, perform focused trauma assessment, and bandage frozen areas loosely.

6. Baseline vital signs

7. SAMPLE

8. Transport, perform ongoing assessment en route.

Rationale

The patient has frostbite of both feet and the right leg. Remove any wet clothing and loosely bandage the frostbitten areas. Unless transport times are very long, frostbitten tissue should be rewarmed in the hospital, not in the field. If rewarming is attempted in the field, ensure that injured areas do not refreeze. Do not rub a frozen extremity in an attempt to improve circulation. This will cause further damage by moving ice crystals that have formed in the tissues.

19.26. **A,** To perform the focused examination, you should remove the patient's shoes and socks and examine his feet for signs of frostbite.

19.27. **A,** This patient probably has frostbite of both feet and the right lower leg.

19.28. **D,** After the patient's shoes and socks are removed, his frostbitten feet should be loosely bandaged to protect the frozen tissues. Rubbing frostbitten areas can worsen damage by moving ice crystals that have formed in the tissues. Tight bandages can increase damage because injured tissues swell. Blisters help protect underlying tissue and should not be opened in the field.

SCENARIO EIGHT

Plan of Action

1. BSI

2. Is the scene safe? Yes. Assess nature of illness, number of patients, and need for additional resources.

3. Assess mental status. Ensure an open airway, assess breathing, apply oxygen at 10-15 lpm by non-rebreather mask, and assess circulatory status.

4. Determine priority, consider ALS.

5. HPI, SAMPLE

Continued

SCENARIO EIGHT—cont'd

6. Focused physical examination

7. Baseline vital signs

8. Begin rapid cooling.

9. Transport, perform ongoing assessment en route.

Rationale

Heat stroke is common in elderly patients after exposure to several days of high temperatures. Any patient with warm skin and altered mental status after being in a hot environment should be suspected of having had a heat stroke and should have his or her temperature taken. Heat stroke victims should be cooled rapidly to prevent permanent brain damage or death.

19.29. **B,** This patient probably has heat stroke. Heat stroke is common in the elderly population and typically occurs after exposure to several days of high temperatures. Patients with heat stroke have altered mental status, headache, and warm, dry skin.

19.30. **B,** Heat stroke patients usually do *not* sweat because the body's temperature-regulating mechanisms have failed. However, it is possible to still see sweating in young, healthy victims of heat stroke who have been exerting themselves in hot, humid environments. Heat stroke should be suspected in any person who develops altered mental status after exposure to a hot environment. The only completely reliable way to identify heat stroke is to take the patient's temperature.

19.31. **B,** Heat stroke also is known as hyperthermia.

SCENARIO NINE

Plan of Action

1. BSI

2. Is the scene safe? Yes. Assess mechanism of injury, number of patients, and need for additional resources.

3. Ensure burning process has stopped.

Continued

SCENARIO NINE—cont'd

4. Assess mental status. Ensure open airway, assess breathing, apply oxygen at 10-15 lpm by non-rebreather mask, and assess circulatory status.

5. Determine priority, consider ALS.

6. Focused trauma assessment

7. Baseline vital signs

8. SAMPLE

9. Cover burned areas with dry, clean dressing; transport; perform ongoing assessment; and meet ALS unit.

Rationale

The patient has partial thickness burns. After ensuring the burning process has stopped and the ABCs are not compromised, you should cover the burned areas with a dry, clean dressing. When a patient has a large burn, an ALS unit should be called so fluid replacement can be begun as quickly as possible.

19.32. C, The first action to take to care for a burn patient is to stop the burning process.

19.33. D, Second-degree (partial-thickness) burns involve the epidermis and part of the dermis. Although the presence of blisters indicates a burn is second degree, not all second-degree burns blister.

19.34. C, Third-degree burns involve the full thickness of the skin and extend through the epidermis and dermis into the subcutaneous tissues. Full-thickness burns have a gray, dry appearance. Blisters are not present. Third-degree burns are not painful because the burning process destroys nerve endings.

19.35. C, The most significant concerns in emergency care of burns are limiting contamination of the injury and replacing the fluid lost through burned areas. The patient should be covered with a dry, clean sheet or a sterile burn sheet to reduce further contamination. An ALS unit should be called so IV fluid replacement can be begun. Moist dressings should *not* be applied to large burns because they increase heat loss and can cause hypothermia.

19.36. C, One leg is 18% of the body surface. One arm is 9% of the body surface. The head and face are 9% of the body surface.

19.37. A, The patient's palm equals approximately 1% of his or her BSA.

SCENARIO TEN

Plan of Action

1. BSI

2. Is the scene safe? Yes. Consider mechanism of injury, number of patients, and need for additional resources.

3. Ensure burning process has stopped.

4. Assess mental status. Ensure open airway, assess breathing, apply oxygen at 10-15 lpm by non-rebreather mask, and assess circulatory status.

5. Determine priority, consider ALS.

6. Focused trauma assessment

7. Baseline vital signs

8. SAMPLE

9. Cover burned areas with dry, clean dressing; transport; perform ongoing assessment; and meet ALS unit.

Rationale

The principles of burn management are the same for pediatric patients as for adults. The burning process should be stopped. The ABCs should be evaluated, and any immediately life-threatening problems should be corrected. The burn should be covered with a clean, dry dressing. A response by an ALS unit should be requested so fluid therapy can be started. Because children have a much larger surface area in proportion to their body mass than adults, they tend to suffer more severe effects than adults when an equivalent area of body surface is burned.

19.38. **B,** A 1-y.o.'s arm and hand are 9% of the BSA.

19.39. **C,** Burns of the hands and feet are critical because of the potential for lasting disability.

19.40. **A,** Knowing whether the patient has been burned before is not important. The cause of the burn is important because it helps determine the appropriate treatment and identify the possible presence of associated injuries. The time the burn occurred will be important to guide fluid therapy. The patient's allergies are important to determine what medications can be given safely.

20

Behavioral Emergencies

DEFINITIONS

Behavior—The manner in which a person acts or performs

Behavioral emergency—Abnormal behavior within a given situation that is unacceptable or intolerable to the patient, the family, or the community

CAUSES OF BEHAVIORAL EMERGENCIES

- Physical causes (Never assume a patient has a psychiatric disorder until all possible physical causes are ruled out.)
  - Low blood sugar
  - Hypoxia
  - Inadequate cerebral blood flow
  - Head trauma
  - Drugs, alcohol abuse, or withdrawal
  - Excessive heat, cold
  - Central nervous system (CNS) infections
  - Alzheimer's disease and other organic brain syndromes
- Psychiatric disorders
  - Anxiety
    - Most common psychiatric illness (10% of adults)
    - Painful uneasiness about impending problems, situations
    - Characterized by agitation, restlessness
    - Frequently misdiagnosed as other disorders
  - Panic attack
    - Intense fear, tension, and restlessness
    - Patient overwhelmed, cannot concentrate
    - Signs and symptoms may include sweating, shortness of breath, palpitations, numbness, and tingling in extremities.
    - May also cause anxiety, agitation among family, bystanders
  - Phobias
    - Closely related to anxiety
    - Stimulated by specific things, places, and situations
    - Signs, symptoms resemble panic attack.
    - Most common is agoraphobia (fear of open places)
  - Depression
    - Deep feelings of sadness, worthlessness, and discouragement
    - May be triggered by significant losses (death of loved one, job loss, and divorce)
    - Characterized by crying, irritability, loss of appetite, inability to sleep, weight loss, and lack of interest in personal appearance
    - Factor in 50% of suicides
    - Ask all depressed patients about suicidal thoughts
  - Bipolar disorder
    - "Manic-depressive" disorder
    - Swings from one end of mood spectrum to other
    - *Manic* phase—Inflated self-image, elation, and feelings of being very powerful
    - *Depressed* phase—Loss of interest, feelings of worthlessness, and suicidal thoughts
    - Delusions, hallucinations occur in either phase.

- ○ Paranoia
  - ■ Exaggerated, unwarranted mistrust
  - ■ Often elaborate delusions of persecution
  - ■ Tend to carry grudges
  - ■ Cold, aloof, hypersensitive, defensive, and argumentative
  - ■ Cannot accept fault
  - ■ Excitable, unpredictable
- ○ Schizophrenia
  - ■ Debilitating distortions of speech, thought
  - ■ Bizarre hallucinations
  - ■ Social withdrawal
  - ■ Lack of emotional expressiveness
  - ■ *Not* the same as multiple personality disorder

VIOLENCE AND BEHAVIORAL EMERGENCIES

- • Suicide
  - ○ Statistics
    - ■ 10th leading cause of death in the United States
    - ■ Second among college students
    - ■ Women *attempt* more often; men *succeed* more often
    - ■ 50% who succeed attempted previously
    - ■ 75% gave clear warning of intent
  - ○ Risk factors
    - ■ Age—15 to 25 years or >40
    - ■ Male gender
    - ■ Single, widowed, or divorced
    - ■ Severe depression
    - ■ Previous attempts, gestures
    - ■ Highly specific plans
    - ■ Obtaining means of suicide (e.g., gun, pills)
    - ■ Previous self-destructive behavior
    - ■ Current diagnosis of serious illness
    - ■ Recent loss of loved one
    - ■ Arrest, imprisonment, or loss of job
    - ■ Violence to others
  - ○ 60% to 70% of behavioral emergency patients become assaultive or violent
  - ○ Causes include
    - ■ Real, perceived mismanagement
    - ■ Psychosis
    - ■ Alcohol, drugs
    - ■ Fear
    - ■ Panic
    - ■ Head injury
  - ○ Warning signs
    - ■ Nervous pacing
    - ■ Shouting
    - ■ Threatening

- Cursing
- Throwing objects
- Clenched teeth or fists

BASIC PRINCIPLES FOR DEALING WITH BEHAVIORAL EMERGENCIES

- We all have limitations.
- We all have a right to our feelings.
- We have more coping ability than we think.
- We all feel some disturbance when injured or involved in an extraordinary event.
- Emotional injury is as real as physical injury.
- People who have been through a crisis do not just "get better."
- Cultural differences have special meaning in behavioral emergencies.

BASIC TECHNIQUES FOR DEALING WITH BEHAVIORAL EMERGENCIES

- Speak calmly, reassuringly, and directly
- Maintain comfortable distance
- Seek patient's cooperation
- Maintain eye contact
- No quick movements
- Respond honestly
- *Never* threaten, challenge, belittle, or argue
- Always tell the truth
- Do *not* "play along" with hallucinations
- Involve *trusted* family, friends
- Be prepared to spend time
- *Never* leave patient alone
- Avoid using restraints if possible
- Do *not* force patient to make decisions
- Encourage patient to perform simple, noncompetitive tasks
- Disperse crowds that have gathered

BEHAVIORAL EMERGENCIES ASSESSMENT

- Scene size-up
  - Pay careful attention to dispatch information for indications of potential violence
  - Never enter potentially violent situations without police support
  - If personal safety uncertain, stand by for police
  - In suicide cases, be alert for hazards
    - Automobile running in closed garage
    - Gas stove pilot lights blown out
    - Electrical devices in water
    - Toxins on or around patient
  - Quickly locate patient
  - Stay between patient and door
  - Scan quickly for dangerous articles
  - If patient has weapon, back out and wait for police

- ○ Look for
  - ■ Signs of possible underlying medical problems
  - ■ Methods, means of committing suicide
  - ■ Multiple patients
- Initial assessment
  - ○ Identification of life-threatening injuries or medical problems has priority over behavioral problem.
- Focused history, physical examination
  - ○ Be polite, respectful
  - ○ Preserve patient's dignity
  - ○ Use open-ended questions
  - ○ Encourage patient to talk; show you are listening
  - ○ Acknowledge patient's feelings

Assessment: Suicidal Patients

- Injuries, medical conditions related to attempt are primary concern.
- Listen carefully
- Accept patient's complaints, feelings
- Do *not* show disgust, horror
- Do *not* trust "rapid recoveries"
- Do something tangible for the patient
- Do *not* try to deny that the attempt occurred
- *Never* challenge patient to go ahead, do it

Assessment: Violent Patients

- Find out if patient has threatened or has history of violence, aggression, or combativeness
- Assess body language for clues to potential violence
- Listen to clues to violence in patient's speech
- Monitor movements, physical activity
- Be firm, clear
- Be prepared to restrain, but *only* if necessary

MANAGEMENT

- Your safety comes first.
- Trauma, medical problems have priority.
- Calm the patient, *never* leave him or her alone
- Use restraints as needed to protect yourself, the patient, and others
- Transport to facility with appropriate resources

USE OF FORCE

- Force may be used against a patient if it is reasonably necessary to protect
  - ○ Yourself or your partner
  - ○ The patient
  - ○ Other people
- Use the minimum amount of force needed to keep patient from injuring self, others
- Force must *never* be punitive in nature.

USE OF RESTRAINTS

- Understand state and local laws related to use of restraints by EMS personnel
- Generally, restraint and involuntary transport must be authorized by a law enforcement officer or a court of law.
- Have sufficient manpower
- Have a plan, know who will do what
- Use only as much force as needed
- When the time comes, act quickly, take the patient by surprise
- At least four rescuers, one for each extremity
- Use humane restraints (soft leather, cloth) on limbs, do not use handcuffs or disposable plastic criminal restraints
- Secure patient to stretcher with straps at chest, waist, and thighs
- Do *not* "hog-tie" patients; patients restrained in a prone position should be monitored closely to avoid positional asphyxia.
- If patient spits, cover his or her face with surgical mask or apply an oxygen mask
- Monitor extremity circulation and neurologic status carefully
- Do *not* remove restraints until the patient has reached a health care facility and has been evaluated by a physician
- Carefully document the behavior that led to the patient being restrained, the personnel who participated, and the techniques used

REVIEW QUESTIONS

Scenario One

You are dispatched to an "unknown illness." On arrival you find a 22-y.o. female sitting on the porch. She looks very anxious. She tells you her three children—ages 1, 2, and 4—have been overactive all day. She recently lost her job, and last month her husband decided he needed some time to himself, so he left for awhile. The patient is c/o of dizziness and nausea, and she keeps saying, "I cannot do this any longer." She has no past medical history and no known allergies. Vital signs are blood pressure (BP)—132/90; pulse (P)—114, strong, regular; and respiration (R)—20, regular, unlabored.

Your Plan of Action

Fill in the blank lines with your treatment plan for this patient. Then compare your plan with the questions, answers, and rationale.

1. _____
2. _____
3. _____
4. _____
5. _____
6. _____
7. _____
8. _____
9. _____

Multiple Choice

20.1. What is the *most likely* cause of this patient's problem?
  a. Bipolar disorder
  b. An anxiety attack
  c. Depression
  d. A phobia

20.2. Which of the following statements about bipolar disorder is *correct?*
  a. The patient alternates between depression and mania.
  b. The patient experiences depression, no episodes of relief or improvement.
  c. The patient almost always commits suicide.
  d. The patient experiences anxiety, hyperventilation, trembling, and chest discomfort.

20.3. The *best* approach to communicate with this patient would be to:
  a. speak in a firm, commanding tone.
  b. tell her to "snap out of it" because everything is going to be okay.
  c. play along with the situation to avoid aggravating her.
  d. act in a calm, reassuring manner and always be honest.

20.4. During your assessment and treatment of this patient, what should be your *greatest* concern?
  a. Whether additional help is needed
  b. Ensuring the safety of yourself and your crew
  c. Preparing to call the police if needed
  d. Gathering evidence of any drugs the patient may taken

20.5. A behavioral emergency occurs only when the patient:
  a. is declared mentally incompetent by a court of law.
  b. displays behavior unacceptable to the community, the patient's family, or the patient.
  c. has experienced the loss of a friend or family member.
  d. is acting strangely.

Scenario Two

You have been dispatched to an "unknown medical emergency." The patient is a 36-y.o. male who is pacing around his living room. He keeps repeating, "My neighbor is out to get me" and "He hates me, I know he hates me." He appears very angry and is uncooperative and belligerent toward you. He does not live with any other family members, has no significant past medical history, and no known allergies. Vitals signs are BP—130/86; P—76, strong, regular; and R—22, regular, unlabored.

Your Plan of Action

Fill in the blank lines with your treatment plan for this patient. Then compare your plan with the questions, answers, and rationale.

1. _____
2. _____
3. _____
4. _____
5. _____
6. _____
7. _____
8. _____
9. _____

Multiple Choice

20.6. This patient is *most likely* experiencing:
   a. paranoia.
   b. substance abuse.
   c. bipolar disorder.
   d. a panic attack.

20.7. All of the following statements about paranoia are correct *except:*
   a. the patient just wants to be left alone.
   b. the patient is experiencing a major interruption in his life and is delusional.
   c. the patient may think other people are saying things about him or conspiring against him.
   d. the patient may experience hostile feelings and pose a danger to himself and those around him.

20.8. To help calm this patient, you should:
   a. avoid slow, deliberate movements.
   b. insist the patient do exactly what you say at all times.
   c. maintain direct eye contact.
   d. give the patient time alone to get control of himself.

20.9. Suddenly the patient becomes violent and tries to hit you. You should:
   a. repeat the initial assessment and recheck the patient's vital signs.
   b. immediately restrain the patient.
   c. continue to talk to the patient quietly.
   d. call for the police and back off until they have arrived.

20.10. Restraints are used only for patients who:
   a. are out of control.
   b. pose a danger to themselves, their families, or the EMS crew.
   c. already have an established history of a psychological problem.
   d. exhibit delusional thinking.

20.11. As a general rule, the *minimum* number of people needed to restrain a patient is:
 a. two.
 b. four.
 c. five.
 d. six.

20.12. After the patient has been restrained, he becomes calm again and begins to complain about the restraints hurting him. What would be your *best* response?
 a. Contact on-line medical control for permission to remove the restraints.
 b. Remove the restraints if the patient will agree to cooperate and stay calm.
 c. Leave the restraints in place but continue to assess extremity circulation, sensation, and movement.
 d. Remove the restraints if a police officer can accompany the patient to the hospital.

20.13. All of the following statements about restraining a patient are correct *except:*
 a. patients may be restrained in either the supine or prone position.
 b. in most areas, use of restraints must be authorized by law enforcement officers.
 c. EMS personnel may use handcuffs or plastic criminal restraints to restrain patients.
 d. a surgical mask may be placed on a patient who is spitting or biting.

20.14. Documentation of restraint application should include all of the following *except:*
 a. the behavior that led to the decision to restrain the patient.
 b. the type of restraints used and the time they were applied.
 c. the number of persons who helped to restrain the patient.
 d. any bystander descriptions of patient behavior before EMS arrived.

Scenario Three

You are dispatched to a residence for an "unknown medical emergency." When you arrive, a 17-y.o. male tells you his friend, who is inside the house, is threatening suicide. When you enter, you find a 16-y.o. male sitting on the edge of a chair. He looks very sad and will not make eye contact with you. He is holding a shotgun.

Your Plan of Action
Fill in the blank lines with your treatment plan for this patient. Then compare your plan with the questions, answers, and rationale.

1. _____
2. _____
3. _____
4. _____
5. _____
6. _____
7. _____
8. _____
9. _____

Multiple Choice

20.15. Your *best* response to this situation would be to:

   a. request a response by the police, then began to talk with the patient in a calm, quiet manner.

   b. back out of the house, request a response by the police, and wait for them to secure the scene before reentering.

   c. tell the patient to put the gun down immediately.

   d. approach the patient, ask him to give you the gun, and then try to talk to him about what is wrong.

20.16. The *most* effective way to treat a suicidal person is to:

   a. allow any family members who are present to talk with the patient first.

   b. encourage the patient to talk, think about alternative solutions, and consider the effects the suicide would have on others.

   c. tell the patient in a calm, quiet manner that suicide is not what he or she wants to do.

   d. talk to the patient only after applying restraints.

20.17. All of the following statements about assessing suicide risk are correct *except:*

   a. suicide is most common in persons who are aged 15 to 25 years or >40.

   b. detailed suicide plans or selection of very lethal methods indicates a higher risk.

   c. EMS personnel should not ask patients whether they have thought about killing themselves.

   d. sudden improvement from depression can indicate an increased suicide risk.

20.18. One of the best ways to determine if a patient has the potential to be violent is:

   a. what his family or friends tell the EMT.

   b. the patient's past medical history.

   c. the patient's body language and actions.

   d. if the patient is making eye contact.

Scenario Four

You have been dispatched to a report of a "behavioral problem." The patient is a 38-y.o. male who keeps shouting he is "the king." He is talking very rapidly, wringing his hands, and quickly pacing.

> **Your Plan of Action**
>
> *Fill in the blank lines with your treatment plan for this patient. Then compare your plan with the questions, answers, and rationale.*
>
> 1. _____
> 2. _____
> 3. _____
> 4. _____
> 5. _____
> 6. _____
> 7. _____
> 8. _____
> 9. _____

Multiple Choice

20.19. What problem is the patient *most* likely experiencing?
    a. A phobia
    b. Bipolar disorder
    c. Paranoia
    d. An anxiety disorder

20.20. The patient begins to scream obscenities and moves between you and the door. You should:
    a. shout for help from your partner.
    b. politely ask the patient to move away from the door.
    c. threaten the patient with arrest if he does not move.
    d. talk to the patient calmly while trying to move toward the door.

20.21. After the patient has been restrained on the stretcher he continues to scream and begins to spit at you. Your *best* response would be to:
    a. isolate the patient in the patient compartment and ride up front with your partner.
    b. cover the patient's mouth with roller gauze while maintaining the airway.
    c. request a response by an advanced life support (ALS) unit so the patient can be sedated.
    d. place a surgical mask or oxygen mask over the patient's face.

True/False

20.22. The patient will probably be able to talk to you more easily if his or her family members are present.
    a. True
    b. False

Multiple Choice

20.23. A patient who reports constant feelings of worthlessness, sadness, helplessness, and discouragement probably has:
    a. a phobia.
    b. depression.
    c. an anxiety disorder.
    d. paranoia.

20.24. A patient who experiences extreme, disabling fear when exposed to a particular stimulus or situation has:
    a. paranoia.
    b. a phobia.
    c. bipolar disorder.
    d. delusional thought content.

Answer Key—Chapter 20

SCENARIO ONE

Plan of Action

1. Body Substance Isolation (BSI)
2. Determine if the scene is safe—Any violent or potentially unsafe situations?
3. Assess for potential violence—Posture, speech, physical activity, and history. This patient appears upset and anxious, but she does not appear to be potentially violent.
4. Initial assessment—General impression, mental status, airway, breathing, and circulation
5. Chief complaint, history of present illness (HPI), and SAMPLE
6. Focused physical examination, exclude possible medical causes of problem.
7. Baseline vital signs
8. Transport with ongoing assessment.

Rationale

This patient appears to be having an anxiety attack caused by multiple sources of stress. Approach the patient slowly, and respect her "personal space." Maintain good eye contact, and talk in a calm, reassuring voice. Never promise anything that you cannot deliver. Give the patient time to tell her story, and then explain what you are going to do for her. Never be threatening, challenging, or argumentative with a patient who is experiencing a psychological crisis. Rule out any medical problems that could cause signs and symptoms of anxiety. Hypoxia, shock, or low blood sugar can cause a patient to be restless, anxious, or agitated.

20.1. **B,** This patient is having an anxiety attack, bordering on a panic attack.
20.2. **A,** Patients with bipolar disorder alternate between episodes of depression and episodes of extreme excitement and agitation (mania).
20.3. **D,** Talk in a calm, reassuring voice and always be honest. Do not promise the patient something you cannot deliver. Being overly firm or commanding with your voice tone can upset the patient and possibly trigger a violent response. Patients with emotional or behavioral problems should never be told to "calm down" or "snap out of it." If they were able to handle the problem themselves, they would not need EMS.

20.4. B, Your highest priority should always be your safety and the safety of your crew. Significant numbers of patients with behavioral emergencies become violent or aggressive at some point during their care. Having the police routinely respond with EMS to all behavioral emergency calls is a good strategy.

20.5. B, A behavioral emergency occurs when a patient displays behavior that is unacceptable, disturbing, or dangerous to himself or herself or to the community.

SCENARIO TWO

Plan of Action
1. BSI
2. Determine if the scene is safe—Any violent or potentially unsafe situations?
3. Assess for potential violence—Posture, speech, physical activity, and history. This patient appears to be paranoid. Because they are highly suspicious of the intentions of others, paranoid patients may become violent.
4. Based on assessment of potential for violence, consider police intervention and restraint of patient.
5. Initial assessment—General impression, mental status, airway, breathing, and circulation
6. Chief complaint, HPI, and SAMPLE
7. Focused physical examination, exclude possible medical causes of problem.
8. Baseline vital signs
9. Transport with ongoing assessment.

Rationale
This patient appears to have paranoia. Patients with paranoia think other people are out to get them. They are always suspicious of others and their actions. This situation needs to be handled carefully because the patient is displaying signs of anger, is not cooperating, and is belligerent. If the patient cannot be "talked down" and convinced to come to the hospital voluntarily, intervention by the police and application of restraints may be necessary. If restraints are applied, document the behavior that led to their use, the type of restraints used, the names of those who helped apply them, and the time the restraints were applied. Reassess extremity circulation and neurologic function repeatedly after application of restraints. Once the patient is under control, assess for medical problems that could be causing the abnormal behavior.

20.6. A, This patient appears to have paranoia. Paranoia is a psychiatric disorder characterized by being highly suspicious of others. Patients with paranoia believe others are "out to get them," are jealous and distrustful, display hostile behavior, and are uncooperative. They may show intense rage.

20.7. **A,** The patient does not want to be left alone. He needs help and through his actions is asking for help.

20.8. **C,** When you are managing a behavioral emergency, maintain good eye contact. Respect the patient's "personal space." If you get too close, he or she may feel threatened. Speak in a quiet, calm, and firm manner and never lie or promise things that cannot be delivered. Moving quickly or insisting that the patient do exactly what you say may cause him or her to become agitated or resistant to help. Once you have made contact with a patient with a behavioral emergency, you are responsible for his or her safety. The patient should not be left alone unless he or she becomes an immediate threat to your personal safety.

20.9. **D,** Now the entire situation has changed. The patient has become violent. This is the time to back away and only approach the patient again after the police have arrived and stabilized the situation.

20.10. **B,** Restraints are used as a last resort when patients poses a danger to themselves, their family, those around them, or the EMS crew. Most patients who initially appear to be "out of control" can be treated by talking to them and listening to their concerns or problems. If a patient must be restrained, document the type of restraints used, how many people applied them, the time they were applied, and the condition of the patient after application. The patient's level of consciousness and vital signs should be documented at least every 15 minutes after restraints are applied.

20.11. **B,** As a general rule it takes four people to apply restraints—one person to control each extremity.

20.12. **C,** Once restraints have been applied, they should not be removed until the patient has reached the hospital and has been evaluated by a physician. Extremity circulation and neurologic function should be reassessed regularly to ensure the restraints are not too tight. The level of consciousness and vital signs of a patient in restraints should be assessed and documented at least every 15 minutes.

20.13. **C,** EMS personnel should not use law enforcement restraint devices to restrain patients. These devices potentially can cause significant soft tissue injuries. Patients may be restrained in either the supine or prone position. However, the respirations of patients placed in the prone position should be monitored closely. Patients should never be "hog-tied" because of the risk of positional asphyxia. Although an EMT may temporarily restrain a patient to prevent him or her from injuring himself or herself or someone else, continued restraint and involuntary transportation to a hospital require authorization by the police or a court of law in most areas. Patients may be discouraged from spitting or biting by placing a surgical mask on them.

20.14. **D,** Documentation of restraint application should include an explanation of why restraint became necessary, the type of restraints used, the time they were applied, and the number of persons who helped to restrain the patient. Bystander descriptions of patient behavior before EMS arrived are not relevant to the decision to restrain the patient.

SCENARIO THREE

Plan of Action

1. BSI
2. Determine if the scene is safe—Any violent or potentially unsafe situations? Yes, the patient has a firearm. Back out, call the police, and approach the patient only after the police secure the scene. In the meantime, talk to the patient from a safe location.
3. Assess for potential violence—Posture, speech, physical activity, and history
4. Based on assessment of potential for violence, consider police intervention and restraint of patient.
5. Initial assessment—General impression, mental status, airway, breathing, and circulation
6. Chief complaint, HPI, and SAMPLE
7. Focused physical examination, exclude possible medical causes of problem.
8. Baseline vital signs
9. Transport with ongoing assessment.

Rationale

This is a very dangerous situation. You should slowly back away and leave the house. Attempting to take the gun away from the patient could result in you being shot. Call for law enforcement and a crisis negotiator. While you are waiting for the police, attempt to talk to the patient from a safe location. Try to get him to talk about his feelings and why he is considering suicide. Help him try to identify alternatives for himself. Never dare a suicidal person to "go ahead and do it." Once the police have secured the scene, assess the patient for any underlying medical problems that could have led to the behavioral emergency.

20.15. B, Because this patient has a deadly weapon, you should back out of the house, request a response by the police, and wait for them to secure the scene. Attempting to disarm the patient could result in you being shot.

20.16. B, If you can do so from a safe location, encourage the patient to talk about what may be bothering him and to think about alternatives to suicide. Family members may be part of the problem and allowing them to talk to the patient may worsen the situation. You should help the patient think through the situation and come to the conclusion that suicide is not his or her best option. Restraints should be used only when the patient cannot be controlled by any other means.

20.17. C, To assess the risk of suicide, EMS personnel should ask patients whether they have thought about killing themselves. Contrary to popular belief, asking about suicidal thoughts or plans will *not* "put the idea into the patient's head." Suicide is most common in people aged 15 to 25 years or in persons >40. A detailed plan or selection of highly lethal methods indicates a higher risk. Sudden improvement in depression can indicate that the patient has finally made the decision to kill himself or herself and is relieved that "the end is in sight."

20.18. C, The best way to determine if the patient is violent or going to be violent is by his or her body language. Are the fists clenched? Is the jaw tight? Are movements forceful or relaxed? Are the arms up in front of his or her chest?

SCENARIO FOUR

Plan of Action

1. BSI

2. Determine if the scene is safe—Any violent or potentially unsafe situations?

3. Assess for potential violence—Posture, speech, physical activity, and history. This patient is extremely agitated. Maintain a safe distance while trying to talk to him.

4. Based on assessment of potential for violence, consider police intervention and restraint of patient.

5. Initial assessment—General impression, mental status, airway, breathing, and circulation

6. Chief complaint, HPI, and SAMPLE

7. Focused physical examination, exclude possible medical causes of problem.

8. Baseline vital signs

9. Transport with ongoing assessment.

Rationale

This patient appears to be in the manic phase of bipolar disorder. By talking with him calmly, you may be able to persuade him to come to the hospital. If he becomes increasingly agitated or violent, police intervention and use of restraints may be necessary. When you are talking with agitated or potentially violent patients, always stay between them and the door. Never let a patient get between you and the way out. Although agitated or violent patients can be frustrating to care for, EMS personnel must remain professional and calm at all times. The EMT is responsible for the safety of patients who must be restrained. The status of the ABCs and extremity circulatory and neurologic function should be evaluated frequently. The patient should be assessed carefully for any underlying medical problems that could be responsible for the abnormal behavior.

20.19. B, This patient appears to be in the manic phase of bipolar disorder. Patients with bipolar disorder alternate between depression and mania. During the manic phase, they are talkative and speak loudly and rapidly. Delusions of personal grandeur and strong feelings of elation are present. Their energy level is extremely high, and they display increased motor activity.

20.20. D, You should continue to talk to the patient calmly while moving into a position where your escape route no longer is blocked. Asking the patient to move out of the way, making threats, or calling for help could trigger an assault.

20.21. D, If a patient is spitting, place a surgical mask over his or her mouth and nose. This will discourage spitting or attempts to bite. Once the mask is in place, monitor the patient's airway and breathing closely.

20.22. B, Usually a patient with a behavioral problem will be more open if family members are not present. The family may be the reason for the behavioral crisis.

20.23. B, Feelings of worthlessness, helplessness, sadness, and discouragement are symptoms of depression.

20.24. B, A phobia is a disorder in which extreme fear is triggered by a specific situation or stimulus. The most common phobia is agoraphobia, fear of being in an open space. Some patients with agoraphobia remain inside their homes for years because any attempt to go outside triggers uncontrollable anxiety. Other common phobias include fear of heights (acrophobia) and fear of spiders (arachnophobia).

21

Obstetric and Gynecologic Emergencies

FEMALE REPRODUCTIVE ANATOMY AND PHYSIOLOGY

- Ovaries
  - Located in right and left lower abdominal quadrants within pelvic cavity
  - Produce estrogen and progesterone, store ova (egg cells)
- Fallopian tubes
  - Extend from ovaries to the uterus
  - Most common location of fertilization of ovum by sperm
- Uterus ("womb")
  - Smooth muscle structure in which fetus grows and develops
  - Contracts and expels fetus during childbirth
- Cervix
  - Narrow opening connecting the uterus to the vagina
  - Dilates during labor to allow fetus to pass through
- Vagina ("birth canal")
  - Muscular tube between the cervix and body surface
- Perineum
  - Area of tissue between vagina and anus
  - Commonly tears during delivery of the baby
- Placenta
  - Special structure of pregnancy contained in uterus
  - Attaches to uterine wall and also to baby via umbilical cord
  - Allows transfer of oxygen and nutrients from mother's blood to fetus and carbon dioxide and waste products from fetus to mother's blood
- Umbilical cord
  - "Lifeline" between fetus and mother
  - Attaches to navel (umbilicus) of fetus
  - Contains two arteries and one vein
  - Umbilical arteries carry unoxygenated blood from fetus to the placenta.
  - Umbilical vein carries oxygenated blood from placenta to fetus.
- Amniotic sac ("bag of waters")
  - Membranous bag of fluid
  - Surrounds the baby in the uterus
  - Contains 1 to 2 liters of amniotic fluid at full term
  - Acts as shock absorber to cushion, protect fetus

PREDELIVERY EMERGENCIES

- Spontaneous abortion
  - Termination of pregnancy before fetus can survive (approximately 20 to 24 weeks)
  - Signs and symptoms—Cramping lower abdominal pain, moderate to severe vaginal bleeding, and passage of tissue and blood clots
  - Complete abortion—Uterus completely discharges all products of conception
  - Incomplete abortion—Some products of conception retained in uterus; results in continued bleeding, risk of infection
  - Management—Treat patient for hypovolemic shock, save and transport any tissue she passes, and provide psychological support

- Ectopic pregnancy
  - Pregnancy located outside the uterus, most commonly in fallopian tube
  - Leads to rupture of fallopian tube, life-threatening internal bleeding
  - Signs and symptoms—Missed menstrual period, signs of early pregnancy (morning sickness, breast tenderness/enlargement), mild vaginal bleeding, lower abdominal pain, and signs and symptoms of shock
  - Ectopic pregnancy should be suspected in any female of child-bearing age who complains of abdominal pain.
  - Management—Treat patient for hypovolemic shock, transport to facility with surgical capabilities
- Preeclampsia (pregnancy-induced hypertension)
  - High blood pressure (BP), fluid retention, and edema associated with pregnancy
  - May occur up to 1 week after delivery
  - Signs and symptoms—Elevated BP; swelling of hands, face, and fingers especially when present early in day; rapid weight gain; headache; visual disturbances; decreased urine output; upper abdominal pain; and crackles in lungs
  - Management—Airway, high-concentration oxygen, position patient on left side; place in quiet environment; and transport without lights and siren
- Eclampsia
  - Signs and symptoms of preeclampsia accompanied by seizures
  - Management—Protect patient's airway, prevent injury during seizure activity but do not restrain, give high-concentration oxygen, and request advanced life support (ALS) response or transport to hospital for anticonvulsant drug therapy
- Supine hypotension
  - Uterus compresses inferior vena cava when mother is in supine position.
  - Causes decrease in blood return to heart, hypotension, and decreased blood flow to placenta
  - Management—Position women in last half of pregnancy on left side to keep uterus off of vena cava
- Placenta previa
  - Placenta covers part or all of the cervical opening
  - Signs and symptoms—Heavy, painless, bright red vaginal bleeding during last 3 months of pregnancy
  - Management—Place patient on left side, treat for hypovolemic shock
- Abruptio placentae
  - Partial or complete detachment of placenta from uterine wall before delivery of infant
  - Signs and symptoms—Severe abdominal pain; tender, rigid uterus; possibly mild vaginal bleeding; and signs and symptoms of hypovolemic shock out of proportion to any bleeding observed
  - Management—Place patient on left side, treat for hypovolemic shock
- Uterine rupture
  - Rupture of uterine wall; occurs most commonly during prolonged active labor; and may also rupture as a result of trauma, especially from lap belts or seat belts during a motor vehicle collision (MVC)
  - Signs and symptoms—Continuous, severe abdominal pain; tearing sensation in abdomen; loss of normal shape, continuity of uterus; and signs and symptoms of hypovolemic shock
  - Management—Place patient on left side, treat for hypovolemic shock

STAGES OF LABOR

- First stage—Dilation
  - From time contractions begin until cervix is completely dilated
  - Contractions initially are 10 to 15 minutes apart, last approximately 30 seconds.
  - Near end of first stage, contractions are 3 to 4 minutes apart, lasting 60 seconds.
  - Contractions cause cervix to open (dilate) and thin (efface).
  - Lasts as long as 18 hours for woman having first child
  - May only last 2 or 3 hours after multiple deliveries
- Second stage—Expulsion
  - From complete dilation of cervix until delivery of baby
  - Contractions every 2 to 3 minutes lasting 60 to 90 seconds
  - Amniotic sac ruptures.
  - Mother may experience feeling of needing to move bowels as fetal head pushes on her rectum.
  - Crowning occurs as fetal head is pushed out of vaginal area.
  - Lasts 60 to 90 minutes
- Third stage—Placental delivery
  - From time baby is delivered until delivery of placenta
  - Lasts 5 to 20 minutes

NORMAL DELIVERY

- Allow for adequate privacy and enough space for delivery
- Give high-concentration oxygen
- Position mother on back with knees flexed and thighs apart, provide adequate drapes over legs and under the patient
- Encourage mother to push during the contractions
- Apply gentle pressure on the head as it delivers to prevent a rapid delivery
- If amniotic sac has not broken, use a clamp to puncture it and push it away from infant's head and mouth
- As the head delivers, check to make sure umbilical cord is not around neck
  - If the cord is wrapped around the neck, try to slip it over the head
  - If unable to do so, place fingers between the baby's neck and the cord, clamp cord in two places, and cut between clamps
- After head delivers, suction mouth, then nose using bulb syringe
- Guide head downward to deliver upper shoulder, then guide head upward to deliver lower shoulder
- After baby delivers, position head slightly lower than body and suction mouth, then nose again. Suctioning nose first may stimulate breathing, causing infant to aspirate fluid present in mouth.
- Clamp umbilical cord in two places, cut between clamps
- Record the time of delivery
- Dry the infant, wrap it in a blanket to help keep it warm
- Deliver placenta, transport to hospital with mother and infant
- Control postpartum hemorrhage by
  - Gently massaging mother's uterus
  - Applying a sanitary napkin over the vaginal opening
- Determine, record the infant's Apgar score at 1 and 5 minutes postpartum (Table 21-1)

Table 21-1   Apgar Score

Sign	0	1	2
Appearance	Blue, pale	Body pink, blue extremities	Completely pink
Pulse	Absent	<100 beats/min	>100 beats/min
Grimace (irritability)	No response	Grimace	Cough, sneeze, cry
Activity (muscle tone)	Limp	Some flexion	Active motion
Respirations	Absent	Slow, irregular	Good, crying

Resuscitation of the Newborn

- Follow inverted pyramid approach. Move from less invasive to more invasive therapies
- Dry, warm, position, suction, and stimulate the infant
- If the infant is cyanotic but spontaneous respirations are present and the heart rate is >100 beats/min, give oxygen by blow-by
- If respirations are absent or inadequate, the heart rate is <100 beats/min, or cyanosis continues to be present after oxygen is given, ventilate with a bag-valve mask (BVM) at a rate of 40 to 60 breaths/min
- If the heart rate is <60 beats/min, begin chest compressions to a depth of ⅓ the AP diameter of the chest. The ratio of chest compressions to ventilations should be 3 to 1 with 90 compressions and 30 breaths to achieve 120 events/minute.
- If the infant does not respond to oxygen, ventilation, and chest compressions, ALS (intubation, drug therapy) is needed.

ABNORMAL DELIVERIES AND COMPLICATIONS

- Prolapsed umbilical cord
  - ○ Umbilical cord enters vagina before fetus during delivery.
  - ○ Umbilical cord becomes compressed between baby's head and vaginal wall, cutting off flow of oxygenated blood.
  - ○ Management
    - ▪ Position mother in knee-chest position or Trendelenburg position
    - ▪ Give high-concentration oxygen to mother
    - ▪ Encourage mother *not* to push during contractions
    - ▪ Insert gloved hand into vagina, push up on head to relieve pressure on cord
    - ▪ Cover exposed portions of umbilical cord with moist dressings
    - ▪ Transport while continuing to hold infant's head off cord
- Breech delivery
  - ○ Buttocks or both legs deliver first.
  - ○ Head may become trapped in vagina, compressing umbilical cord and producing suffocation of infant.
  - ○ Management
    - ▪ Proceed as with normal delivery
    - ▪ If head does not deliver within 2 to 3 minutes of body, insert gloved hand into vagina and push vaginal wall away from baby's face to create airway
    - ▪ Do *not* attempt to force delivery by pulling on baby
    - ▪ Transport immediately
- Limb presentation
  - ○ Infant's arm or leg is presenting first
  - ○ Management

- Position mother in knee-chest position or Trendelenburg position
- Give high-concentration oxygen to mother
- Transport immediately
- Do *not* pull on infant's arm or leg
- Multiple births
  - ○ Anticipate complications associated with low birth weight or prematurity
  - ○ Call for assistance, be prepared for more than one resuscitation
  - ○ After the delivery of first infant, clamp and cut umbilical cord
  - ○ Assist with delivery of second infant, clamp and cut umbilical cord
  - ○ There may be a single placenta or two placentas; if two placentas are present, first baby's placenta may deliver either before or after second baby.
- Meconium
  - ○ Meconium—Dark green material that makes up the infant's first bowel movement
  - ○ May be discharged into amniotic fluid and aspirated when an infant is under stress before delivery
  - ○ Routine suctioning of the upper airway during delivery for infants born with meconium in the amniotic fluid is no longer recommended.
- Premature infant
  - ○ Infant born before 38th week of pregnancy or weighs <5.5 pounds
  - ○ Management
    - Avoid heat loss, wrap infant securely, and heat vehicle during transport
    - Prevent bleeding from umbilical cord; premature infants have small blood volumes.
    - Give oxygen by blow-by, do *not* blow oxygen directly into infant's face
    - Prevent contamination; a premature infant's immune system is immature.

REVIEW QUESTIONS

Scenario One

You have been dispatched to a report of a "woman in labor." The patient is a 23-y.o. female who is having contractions every 4 to 5 minutes. This is her second baby, and she is full term. She denies any problems with the pregnancy. Her water has not broken. She has no significant past medical history, takes no medications, and has no known allergies. Vital signs are BP—128/86; pulse (P)—78, strong, regular; and respiration (R)—16, regular, unlabored.

Your Plan of Action

Fill in the blank lines with your treatment plan for this patient. Then compare your plan with the questions, answers, and rationale.

1. _____
2. _____
3. _____
4. _____
5. _____
6. _____
7. _____
8. _____
9. _____

Multiple Choice

21.1. A woman having a second baby is known as a:

   a. primipara.

   b. multipara.

   c. gravida.

   d. nullipara.

21.2. The term gravida refers to:

   a. a woman who is delivering her first child.

   b. the total number of pregnancies a woman has had.

   c. a woman's first pregnancy.

   d. the total number of pregnancies carried to full term.

21.3. The perineum is the:

   a. passageway between the cervix and the outside.

   b. an organ that transfers oxygen and nutrients from mother to baby.

   c. the external female genital region between the vagina and the anus.

   d. the inferior, narrow part of the uterus that opens into the vagina.

21.4. Fetal heart tones may be heard with a stethoscope at approximately ____ months.

   a. 2

   b. 3

   c. 4

   d. 6

21.5. If the contractions are 2 to 3 minutes apart, you should:

   a. call for an ALS unit.

   b. do a rapid physical examination.

   c. transport immediately.

   d. prepare for an imminent delivery.

21.6. To prepare the patient for the delivery, you should:

   a. place her in a sitting position.

   b. place her on her left side.

   c. allow her to use the bathroom one last time before delivery.

   d. place her in a supine position with her knees flexed and her thighs abducted.

21.7. If the patient says she feels like she needs to move her bowels, this is:

   a. a normal sensation caused by the infant's head pressing on the rectum.

   b. a sign something is wrong with the delivery.

   c. an indication to tell the mother to stop pushing so the sterile field does not become contaminated.

   d. a sign the perineum is preparing for delivery.

21.8. After the baby delivers, the *first* thing you should do is:

   a. place extra padding under the mother to absorb blood from delivery.

   b. cut the umbilical cord using sterile scissors.

   c. suction the baby's mouth and nose.

   d. wrap the baby in a clean blanket to preserve warmth.

Scenario Two

You are dispatched to a report of a "pregnant female with heavy bleeding." The patient is a 21-y.o. female who is 7½ months pregnant. She began experiencing moderate, bright red vaginal bleeding approximately 15 minutes ago. The patient denies any pain or recent trauma. Her skin is pale, cool, and moist. Vital signs are BP—108/66; P—122, weak, regular; and R—20, regular, unlabored.

Your Plan of Action

Fill in the blank lines with your treatment plan for this patient. Then compare your plan with the questions, answers, and rationale.

1. _____
2. _____
3. _____
4. _____
5. _____
6. _____
7. _____
8. _____
9. _____

Multiple Choice

21.9. This patient probably has:
   a. placenta previa.
   b. abruptio placentae.
   c. a ruptured uterus.
   d. normal third-trimester bleeding.

True/False

21.10. Placenta previa occurs when all or part of the placenta covers the cervical opening.
   a. True
   b. False

Multiple Choice

21.11. Your care for this patient should include:
   a. having the patient call her doctor just before transport.
   b. placing the patient in a supine position just in case she delivers.
   c. placing the patient on her left side.
   d. preparing for an immediate delivery.
21.12. All of the following are causes of vaginal bleeding in late pregnancy *except:*
   a. placenta previa.
   b. eclampsia.
   c. abruptio placentae.
   d. uterine rupture.

Scenario Three

You are dispatched to a report of "a woman with abdominal pain." The patient is an 18-y.o. female c/o left-sided abdominal pain. She tells you her last menstrual period 6 weeks ago was not as heavy as it normally is and that she has been having intermittent spotting since then. She denies any recent trauma, nausea, vomiting, or diarrhea. The patient's skin is pale and cool. Her left lower abdominal quadrant is tender to palpation. She has no significant past medial history, takes no medications, and has no known drug allergies. Vital signs are BP—110/60; P—106, weak, regular; and R—22, regular, unlabored.

> **Your Plan of Action**
>
> *Fill in the blank lines with your treatment plan for this patient. Then compare your plan with the questions, answers, and rationale.*
>
> 1. _____
> 2. _____
> 3. _____
> 4. _____
> 5. _____
> 6. _____
> 7. _____
> 8. _____
> 9. _____

Multiple Choice

21.13. This patient probably has:
  a. bleeding associated with an early normal pregnancy.
  b. an early abruptio placentae.
  c. a possible ectopic pregnancy.
  d. an unusual heavy period, which could cause hypovolemic shock.

21.14. A patient has had a complete abortion when:
  a. all the products of conception are passed out of the uterus.
  b. hemorrhaging and cramping occur, but the cervix remains closed and the products of conception stay in the uterus.
  c. all of the products of conception are not expelled from the uterus.
  d. the fertilized egg implants itself outside the uterus.

21.15. A patient has had an incomplete abortion when:
  a. all the products of conception are passed out of the uterus.
  b. hemorrhaging and cramping occur, but the cervix remains closed and the products of conception stay in the uterus.
  c. all of the products of conception are not expelled from the uterus.
  d. the fertilized egg implants itself outside the uterus.

21.16. A patient has an ectopic pregnancy when:
- **a.** all the products of conception are passed out of the uterus.
- **b.** hemorrhaging and cramping occur, but the cervix remains closed and the products of conception stay in the uterus.
- **c.** all of the products of conception are not expelled from the uterus.
- **d.** the fertilized egg implants itself outside the uterus.

21.17. Which statement best describes the severity of an ectopic pregnancy?
- **a.** It is a true emergency requiring a rapid transport.
- **b.** It is a nonemergency requiring a normal basic life support transport.
- **c.** It is a nonemergency for which the patient can call her own doctor.
- **d.** It is a true emergency in which the BP becomes extremely high.

Scenario Four

You are dispatched to an "MVC with injuries." It is snowing very hard, so your response time is slowed. On arrival you find a 27-y.o. female, 8-months pregnant, who was a passenger in a head-on collision. The patient was wearing the lap portion of her seat belt but not the shoulder harness. Each vehicle was traveling at approximately 45 mph. The patient is unusually quiet and says her abdomen is very painful and "feels funny." No vaginal bleeding or contractions are present. However, the uterus feels unusually firm and rigid. The firmness is steady, not intermittent like labor pains. The patient has not had any problems with her pregnancy and has no past medical history. Vital signs are BP—88/40; P—136, weak, regular; and R—12, shallow, regular.

Your Plan of Action

Fill in the blank lines with your treatment plan for this patient. Then compare your plan with the questions, answers, and rationale.

1. _____
2. _____
3. _____
4. _____
5. _____
6. _____
7. _____
8. _____
9. _____

Multiple Choice

21.18. This patient probably is experiencing:
- **a.** pregnancy-induced hypotension or traumatic placental abruption.
- **b.** a traumatic placenta previa or a ruptured uterus.
- **c.** a traumatic spontaneous abortion or a traumatic placental abruption.
- **d.** a traumatic placental abruption or a ruptured uterus.

21.19. All of the following statements about placental abruption are correct *except:*
    a. it may be caused by uterine trauma.
    b. it occurs when a part of the placenta covers a part or all of the cervical opening.
    c. it may or may not be associated with external vaginal bleeding.
    d. it usually presents with a rigid or tender abdomen.

21.20. If you cannot hear fetal heart tones, you should:
    a. not be concerned because fetal heart tones are difficult to hear.
    b. prepare for imminent delivery.
    c. apply oxygen and treat the patient for shock.
    d. transport immediately and request a helicopter response.

21.21. This problem most likely resulted from:
    a. compression of the uterus by the lap belt.
    b. a congenital condition in which the uterine wall was too thin.
    c. a malformed placenta.
    d. the patient wearing her shoulder harness incorrectly.

Scenario Five

You are dispatched to a "possible maternity problem." The patient is a 24-y.o. female c/o mild abdominal pain. She is at 38 weeks' gestation. She has no significant past medical history and has had an uncomplicated pregnancy. This is her first baby. Vital signs are BP—108/72; P—110, strong, regular; and R—18, shallow, regular, and unlabored.

Your Plan of Action
Fill in the blank lines with your treatment plan for this patient. Then compare your plan with the questions, answers, and rationale.

  1. _____
  2. _____
  3. _____
  4. _____
  5. _____
  6. _____
  7. _____
  8. _____
  9. _____

Multiple Choice

21.22. Questions you would ask this patient include all of the following *except:*
    a. if the pain comes and goes or is steady.
    b. how many pregnancies she has had.
    c. how far along her pregnancy is.
    d. if the abdominal pain moves or radiates.

21.23. The first stage of labor is from the:
   a. time the EMS service is called until the contractions are 2 minutes apart.
   b. time regular contractions begin until the cervix is completely dilated.
   c. delivery of the baby to the delivery of the placenta.
   d. first contraction to the delivery of the baby.

21.24. The second stage of labor is from the:
   a. time the contractions are 2 minutes apart until the placenta is delivered.
   b. time regular contractions begin until the baby is delivered.
   c. full cervical dilation until the baby is delivered.
   d. delivery of the baby to the delivery of the placenta.

21.25. Outward bulging of the area around the vaginal opening as the baby's head begins to deliver is called:
   a. dilation.
   b. bloody show if bleeding is present.
   c. crowning.
   d. cephalic presentation.

21.26. During delivery, rotation of the baby's head would normally occur:
   a. once the head is delivered.
   b. only if the cord is wrapped around the neck.
   c. only in a shoulder presentation.
   d. while crowning is occurring.

21.27. The third stage of labor is from:
   a. the time contractions are 2 minutes apart until the placenta is delivered.
   b. crowning until the placenta is ready to deliver.
   c. the delivery of the baby until the delivery of the placenta.
   d. full dilation of the cervix until the baby is delivered.

Scenario Six

You are dispatched to a "woman in labor." On arrival you find a 23-y.o. female in the process of delivering on the living room floor. The mother has a normal amount of bleeding after the delivery. Her vital signs are BP—116/76; P—106, strong, regular; and R—18 regular, unlabored. The infant's head and trunk are pink, but the extremities are cyanotic. The heart rate is 118 beats/min. He grimaces and cries intermittently when suctioned. His extremities move with weak flexing motions. He has a respiratory rate of 32 breaths/min with a weak cry.

Your Plan of Action

Fill in the blank lines with your treatment plan for this patient. Then compare your plan with the questions, answers, and rationale.

1. _____
2. _____
3. _____
4. _____
5. _____
6. _____
7. _____
8. _____
9. _____

Multiple Choice

21.28. This infant's Apgar score is:
   a. 4.
   b. 6.
   c. 8.
   d. 9.

21.29. One of the major concerns when caring for a newborn is to:
   a. guard against potential heat loss.
   b. ensure the cord has been cut no more than 2 inches from the navel.
   c. make certain the extremities become pink within 1 minute.
   d. wash the body as soon as possible and then wrap in warm blankets.

21.30. If the infant's heart rate decreases to 90 beats/min, you should:
   a. give oxygen at 10 lpm via non-rebreather mask.
   b. stimulate the child by rubbing its back.
   c. take a new set of vital signs in 5 minutes.
   d. begin artificial respirations.

SCENARIO ONE

Plan of Action

1. Body Substance Isolation (BSI)
2. Is the scene safe? Yes. Evaluate nature of illness, number of patients, and need for additional resources.
3. Assess mental status. Ensure open airway, assess breathing, apply oxygen by non-rebreather mask at 10-15 lpm, and assess circulatory status.
4. Determine priority, consider ALS.
5. History of present illness (HPI), SAMPLE
6. Focused physical examination
7. Baseline vital signs
8. Transport, perform ongoing assessment.

Rationale

This appears to be a normal pregnancy, and the patient probably will deliver without complications. Because this is her second pregnancy, delivery time will most likely shorten. Because contractions are still 4 to 5 minutes apart, begin transport. If necessary, the infant can be delivered during transport to the hospital.

21.1. B, A woman who is having her second baby is a multipara. A woman having her first child is a primipara. A woman who has not had a child is a nullipara. Gravida refers to the total number of pregnancies a woman has had.

21.2. B, Gravida refers to the total number of pregnancies a woman has had.

21.3. C, The perineum is the region between the vagina and the anus. The perineum frequently tears during childbirth.

21.4. C, Fetal heart tones can be heard at approximately 4 months.

21.5. D, If the contractions are 2 minutes apart, prepare for an immediate delivery.

21.6. D, To prepare for delivery, the patient should be placed supine (on her back) with her knees flexed and her thighs abducted (spread apart).

21.7. A, The mother saying she feels like she needs to have a bowel movement is a normal sensation caused as the infant's head moves into the vagina and pushes against the rectum.

21.8. C, After the baby delivers, you should immediately clear the mouth and nose with gentle suctioning using a bulb aspirator.

SCENARIO TWO

Plan of Action

1. BSI
2. Is the scene safe? Yes. Evaluate nature of illness, number of patients, and need for additional resources.
3. Assess mental status. Ensure an open airway, assess breathing, apply oxygen by non-rebreather mask at 10-15 lpm, assess circulatory status, position patient supine on left side, and prevent loss of body heat.
4. Determine priority, consider ALS.
5. HPI, SAMPLE
6. Focused physical examination
7. Baseline vital signs
8. Transport, perform ongoing assessment, and meet ALS unit.

Rationale

Because the patient is having heavy, painless, bright red vaginal bleeding, she most likely has placenta previa. Call for an ALS unit. Begin treatment for hypovolemic shock. Transport, and meet the ALS unit en route.

21.9. **A,** Heavy, painless, bright red vaginal bleeding during the third trimester of pregnancy indicates the presence of placenta previa—presence of part of the placenta over the cervical opening. Abruptio placentae produces severe abdominal pain; a rigid, tender uterus; and signs and symptoms of shock out of proportion to the amount of visible blood loss. Uterine rupture is characterized by tearing abdominal pain, signs and symptoms of shock, and loss of normal uterine shape. Although small amounts of bleeding sometimes occur during the third trimester, any blood loss greater than that of a normal menstrual period is abnormal and dangerous.

21.10. **A,** A placenta previa occurs when the placenta covers all or part of the cervical opening.

21.11. **C,** Patients in the last half of pregnancy should be placed on their left side to avoid pressure by the uterus against the inferior vena cava.

21.12. **B,** Eclampsia is a disorder of the last half of pregnancy characterized by hypertension, fluid retention, and seizures. Eclampsia does not cause vaginal bleeding.

SCENARIO THREE

Plan of Action

1. BSI
2. Is the scene safe? Yes. Assess nature of illness, number of patients, and need for additional resources.
3. Assess mental status. Ensure an open airway, assess breathing, apply oxygen by non-rebreather mask at 10-15 lpm, assess circulatory status, place patient supine with lower extremities elevated, and prevent loss of body heat.
4. Determine priority, consider ALS.
5. HPI, SAMPLE
6. Focused physical examination
7. Baseline vital signs
8. Transport, perform ongoing assessment, and meet ALS unit.

Rationale

A female patient of child-bearing age who complains of lower abdominal pain or who shows signs of unexplained hypovolemic shock should be suspected of having an ectopic pregnancy. The patient should be treated for hypovolemic shock and transported immediately. Depending on transport time to a facility with surgical capabilities, a meeting with an ALS unit may be appropriate.

21.13. **C,** Any female of child-bearing age with lower abdominal pain or a sudden onset of unexplained shock should be suspected of having a tubal ectopic pregnancy. Bleeding during the first trimester of pregnancy is never normal. Abruptio placentae does not manifest until the third trimester. The left-sided pain and tenderness suggest that this is not just a late, unusually heavy period.

21.14. **A,** A complete spontaneous abortion has occurred when a pregnancy terminates before the 20th week and the uterus discharges all of the products of conception.

21.15. **C,** An incomplete abortion has occurred when a pregnancy terminates before the 20th week and some products of conception remain in the uterus. The uterus is unable to contract, resulting in ongoing blood loss that can lead to shock. Also the tissue retained in the uterus can become infected, possibly leading to sepsis (septic abortion).

21.16. **D,** An ectopic pregnancy is a pregnancy located anywhere outside the uterus. The most common location for an ectopic pregnancy is in the fallopian tube (a tubal ectopic pregnancy). Tubal pregnancies eventually outgrow and rupture the fallopian tube, leading to extensive blood loss.

21.17. **A,** An ectopic pregnancy is a true emergency and requires rapid transport. Rupture of a tubal ectopic pregnancy can cause life-threatening internal blood loss.

SCENARIO FOUR

Plan of Action

1. BSI

2. Is the scene safe? Yes. Assess mechanism of injury/nature of illness, number of patients, and need for additional resources.

3. Assess mental status. Ensure open airway, apply oxygen by non-rebreather mask at 10-15 lpm, and assess circulatory status.

4. Determine priority, consider ALS.

5. Apply cervical collar, rapidly extricate to long spine board, and transport with board tilted to left.

6. Rapid trauma examination

7. Baseline vital signs

8. SAMPLE

9. Do a detailed physical examination during transport if time permits, perform ongoing assessment, and meet ALS unit.

Rationale

The patient probably has either a ruptured uterus or a traumatic abruptio placentae from compression of the uterus by a seat belt. The patient should be treated for hypovolemic shock and transported rapidly. Because she was involved in a high-speed MVC, she should be secured to a long spine board with a cervical collar and cervical immobilizer in place. The board should be tilted to the left to shift the uterus away from the inferior vena cava. Depending on transport time to a facility with surgical capabilities, a meeting with an ALS unit may be appropriate.

21.18. **D,** The patient probably has had a traumatic placental abruption or ruptured uterus caused by the lap belt pressing against the uterus. Abruptio placentae is characterized by severe pain and a uterus that is tender and in continuous spasm. Little or no vaginal bleeding is present, and the patient exhibits signs and symptoms of shock out of proportion to the visible bleeding. Blunt trauma also can cause uterine rupture. However, in uterine rupture the uterus will lose its smooth, rounded shape, and fetal parts sometimes can be felt through the abdominal wall.

21.19. **B,** Placenta previa occurs when a part of the placenta covers a part of or all of the cervical opening, causing excessive vaginal bleeding. Trauma does not cause placenta previa. Very active labor or trauma can cause uterine rupture, particularly in a woman who has a small pelvis that the fetus cannot pass through easily. Blunt trauma also may cause abruptio placentae. Abruptio placentae, separation of the placenta from the uterine wall, presents with a rigid or tender abdomen and little or no vaginal bleeding.

21.20. **C,** Fetal heart tones frequently are difficult to hear in an ambulance with a regular stethoscope. The mother's signs and symptoms are cause for concern, and you should begin care for shock immediately.

21.21. **A,** The problem probably was caused by compression of the uterus by the lap belt.

SCENARIO FIVE

Plan of Action

1. BSI

2. Is the scene safe? Yes. Assess nature of illness, number of patients, and need for additional resources.

3. Assess mental status. Ensure open airway, assess breathing, give oxygen by non-rebreather mask at 10-15 lpm, and assess circulatory status.

4. Determine priority, consider ALS.

5. HPI, SAMPLE

6. Focused physical examination

7. Baseline vital signs

8. Transport, perform ongoing assessment.

Rationale

This patient appears to be in early labor at the end of a full-term, uncomplicated pregnancy. Because this is the patient's first baby, she is unlikely to deliver for several hours. She should be transported with appropriate preparations made to perform a delivery during transport if necessary.

21.22. **D,** There is no need to ask if the pain moves or radiates to another region. Asking about the length of pregnancy, the frequency of the pains, and the number of pregnancies will help determine if she is in labor and whether you need to prepare for an immediate delivery.

21.23. **B,** The first stage of labor begins with the onset of contractions and ends with complete dilation of the cervix.

21.24. **C,** The second stage of labor begins with complete dilation of the cervix and ends with delivery of the baby.

21.25. **C,** Outward bulging of the vaginal area as the baby's head begins to deliver is crowning.

21.26. **A,** Rotation of the head occurs once the head has delivered.

21.27. **C,** The third stage of labor begins when the baby is completely delivered and ends when the placenta is delivered.

SCENARIO SIX

Plan of Action

1. BSI
2. Is the scene safe? Yes. Assess nature of illness, number of patients, and need for additional resources.
3. Assess mental status. Ensure an open airway, assess breathing, give oxygen by blow-by, assess circulatory status, and begin ventilations with BVM and oxygen.
4. Determine priority, consider ALS.
5. HPI, SAMPLE
6. Focused physical examination
7. Baseline vital signs
8. Transport, perform ongoing assessment.

Rationale

Because the infant's heart rate is <100 beats/min, ventilations should be started using a BVM and oxygen. Most infants and small children who have slow heart rates are hypoxic. Supplemental oxygen and assisted ventilations usually will cause the heart rate to increase rapidly.

21.28. C, This infant has an Apgar score of 8 (*A*ppearance = 1; *p*ulse = 2; *g*rimace = 2; *a*ctivity = 1; and *r*espirations = 2).

21.29. A, Guarding against potential heat loss is a critical step in the newborn. Infants have a large body surface compared with their body mass and volume; therefore, they lose heat rapidly. Newborns should be dried and wrapped in warm blankets as soon as possible.

21.30. D, If the heart rate is <100 beats/min, begin bagging the infant with a BVM. Hypoxia usually causes low heart rates in newborns. If you increase the amount of oxygen in the blood, then the heart rate should increase.

22

Pediatric Emergencies

PEDIATRIC DEVELOPMENTAL STAGES

- Neonates (birth to 1 month)
  - Will know parents, but are not upset by being held by others
  - Keep warm, use pacifier
  - Examine on mother's lap
  - Obligate nasal breathers
- Young infants (1 to 5 months)
  - Parents important but usually will accept strangers
  - Examine on mother's lap
  - Keep warm, use pacifier or bottle
- Older infants (6 to 12 months)
  - Often have intense stranger anxiety, may be afraid of being in supine position
  - Ensure parent's presence
  - Examine in parent's arms if possible
  - Examine toe to head
- Toddlers (1 to 3 years)
  - Dislike strange people, situations
  - Strongly assertive, may have temper tantrums
  - Examine on parent's lap if possible
  - Talk to, "examine" parent first
  - Examine toe to head
  - Logic will *not* work
- Preschoolers (3 to 5 years)
  - Totally subjective world view; do not separate fantasy, reality; and think magically
  - Intense fear of pain, disfigurement, and blood loss
  - Talk to child first, then to parent
  - Cover wounds quickly, but assure them the covered area still is there
  - Let them help with examination, treatment
  - Be truthful
  - Examine toe to head
- School age (6 to 12 years)
  - Able to use concepts, make compromises, and think objectively
  - Take the history from the patient, not the parent
  - Explain what is happening
  - Be honest
- Adolescents (12 to 18 years)
  - Fragile self-esteem, acute body image
  - Peer group acceptance can be critical
  - Focus on patient, not parent
  - Talk to them like adults
  - Respect need for modesty
  - Be honest

PEDIATRIC ANATOMICAL DIFFERENCES
General

- Large surface-to-volume ratio, lower tolerance of cold environments
- Thinner skin, burn more easily

Pediatric Respiratory Rates

Age	Rate
Newborn	30 to 50 breaths/min
Infant: 0 to 5 months	25 to 40 breaths/min
Infant: 6 to 12 months	20 to 30 breaths/min
Toddler: 1 to 3 years	20 to 30 breaths/min
Preschool: 3 to 5 years	20 to 30 breaths/min
School age: 6 to 12 years	15 to 30 breaths/min
Adolescent: 12 to 18 years	12 to 20 breaths/min

Pediatric Pulse Rates

Age	Rate
Newborn	120 to 160 beats/min
Infant: 0 to 5 months	90 to 140 beats/min
Infant: 6 to 12 months	80 to 140 beats/min
Toddler: 1 to 3 years	80 to 130 beats/min
Preschool: 3 to 5 years	80 to 120 beats/min
School age: 6 to 12 years	70 to 110 beats/min
Adolescent: 12 to 18 years	60 to 105 beats/min

Pediatric Blood Pressures

Age	Expected	Lower Limit of Systolic
Newborn	74-100 mm Hg systolic 50-68 mm Hg diastolic	<60 mm Hg
Infant	84-106 mm Hg systolic 56-70 mm Hg diastolic	<70 mm Hg
Toddler	98-106 mm Hg systolic 50-70 mm Hg diastolic	<70 mm Hg + (age × 2)
Preschool	98-112 mm Hg systolic 64-70 mm Hg diastolic	<70 mm Hg + (age × 2)
School-age <10 years	104-124 mm Hg systolic 64-80 mm Hg diastolic	<70 mm Hg + (age × 2)
School-age >10 years	104-124 mm Hg systolic 64-80 mm Hg diastolic	>10 years, <90 mm Hg
Adolescent	118-132 mm Hg systolic 70-82 mm Hg diastolic	<90 mm Hg

Airway and Breathing

- Overall airway size smaller than adult's, more easily obstructed
- Tongue relatively larger, placed more posteriorly than adult's, and obstructs airway more easily
- Glottic opening in more superior location than adult's
- Epiglottis larger, less rigid than adult's; overextension of neck may push base of tongue and epiglottis onto glottic opening, causing obstruction.
- Vocal cords placed more superior and anterior than adult's

- Airway narrowest at cricoid cartilage
- Tracheal rings more flexible, collapse more easily, particularly if neck is flexed or hyperextended
- Trachea smaller in diameter
- Accessory muscles weaker
- Ribs more horizontal, decreasing effectiveness of intercostal muscles
- Diaphragm responsible for larger part of ventilation than in adults

Circulation

- Smaller blood volume, smaller amounts of hemorrhage more significant
- Healthy heart and peripheral blood vessels, compensate for blood loss for longer time than adults and then deteriorate quickly

Neurologic

- Mental status more difficult to evaluate in infants, younger patients
- Does patient make eye contact with, follow movements of personnel?
- Does patient recognize parents?

Head and Neck

- Head large in proportion to rest of body, sudden decelerations more likely to cause dislocations of C1 on C2
- Infants have fontanelles (soft spots) in skull, can be used to evaluate for increased intracranial pressure or dehydration.

Chest

- Ribs more flexible than in adults; rib fractures less common but thoracic organs less well protected
- Smaller space allows breath sounds to transmit more easily; listen to lungs in midaxillary line (as far from opposite side as possible).

Abdomen

- Liver and spleen larger, less protected, and more easily injured

Extremities

- Bones more flexible, possibility of greenstick fractures
- Growth plates near ends of long bones, possibility of growth plate fractures leading to abnormal bone growth

PEDIATRIC ASSESSMENT

- Scene size-up
  - Body Substance Isolation (BSI)
  - Is the scene safe?
  - Number of patients?
  - Mechanism of injury/nature of illness?
  - Are available resources adequate to handle problem?
- Initial assessment
  - General impression—*Appearance, Breathing* effort, and *Circulation* to skin (pediatric assessment triangle)

○ *Airway, Breathing, Circulation, Disability,* and *Exposure*
○ Transport decision (stay or go?)
● Focused history and physical examination
○ Performed when mechanism of injury/nature of illness, chief complaint, and history identify the specific body system(s) affected by the illness, injury
● Detailed physical examination
○ Performed when mechanism of injury/nature of illness, chief complaint, and history do not easily identify the specific body system(s) affected by the illness, injury
● Ongoing assessment
○ Performed during transport to hospital
○ Every 5 minutes with critical patients, every 15 minutes with stable patients
○ Components
  ■ Pediatric assessment triangle, ABCDE
  ■ Repeat vital signs
  ■ Reassessment of positive physical examination findings
  ■ Review of effectiveness, safety of treatment

COMMON PEDIATRIC DISEASE PROCESSES
Asthma

● Reactive airway disease
● Reversible narrowing of lower airways by bronchospasm, inflammatory edema, and mucus secretions
● Causes increased work of breathing, dyspnea, tachypnea, anxiety, coughing, and prolonged exhalation with audible wheezing. Fever usually is absent.
● Patients usually >2 years of age
● History of multiple allergies, positive history for asthma common
● Treated with humidified oxygen, nebulized bronchodilators. May require assisted ventilation

Bronchiolitis

● Viral infection of lower respiratory tract
● Patients usually <2 years of age; 90% are <1 year of age.
● History of upper respiratory infection symptoms (fever, runny nose, and nasal congestion), followed by onset of increased work of breathing, dyspnea, tachypnea, coughing, and prolonged exhalation with audible wheezing
● Treated with humidified oxygen. May not respond to nebulized bronchodilators. May require assisted ventilation

Croup

● Also known as laryngotracheobronchitis
● Affects children aged 6 months to 4 years
● Viral infection with slow onset (days), causes swelling of tissues of larynx
● Low-grade fever; mild sore throat; hoarseness; loud, brassy cough (seal bark cough); and nighttime episodes of increased work of breathing, dyspnea, tachypnea, and stridor
● Treated with humidified oxygen. May require assisted ventilation. Advanced life support (ALS) units may give nebulized epinephrine or racemic epinephrine to reduce edema in larynx.

Epiglottitis

- Bacterial infection, inflammation of the epiglottis
- Affects children aged 3 to 7 years. Becoming less common because of vaccination for *Haemophilus influenzae* B (HiB)
- Progresses rapidly (hours)
- High fever, severe sore throat, muffled voice, drooling, increased work of breathing, dyspnea, tachypnea, and stridor
- May lead to respiratory arrest if swollen epiglottis completely obstructs opening to lower airway
- Treated by keeping child in position of comfort, giving oxygen, minimizing agitation, and rapidly transporting to hospital. Do *not* look into or place anything into throat. If patient appears to be losing airway, consider ALS response for endotracheal intubation

Pneumonia

- Bacterial or viral infection of the lower airway and lung tissue
- Most common in infants, toddlers, and preschool-aged children because of immature immune systems
- Fever; pain associated with breathing; cough productive of infected (yellow, green) or bloody sputum; localized crackles, rhonchi, or wheezes; and grunting respirations
- Treated with oxygen and transport to hospital for appropriate antibiotic therapy. Some patients may require assisted ventilation to maintain adequate oxygenation.

Meningitis

- Viral or bacterial infection of the membranes that cover the brain and spinal cord. Bacterial infections are more serious.
- Fever, headache, nausea, vomiting, stiff neck (may be absent in infants and younger children), bulging fontanelles in infants, and seizures
- Some types of bacterial meningitis may be associated with a skin rash consisting of tiny hemorrhages under the skin.
- Treated with support of airway, breathing, and circulation and transport for appropriate antibiotic therapy
- EMS personnel should avoid contact with patient's respiratory secretions and should consider appropriate prophylactic treatment with antibiotics.

REVIEW QUESTIONS
Scenario One

At 2:00 AM you receive a call for a "child with difficulty breathing." The patient is a 4-y.o. male who is sitting upright on the sofa in the tripod position. He is using his accessory muscles to assist his breathing. Intercostal retractions are present; his mouth is open; and his tongue is protruding. The patient's mother says he awoke with this problem. When she took his temperature, it was 104.2° F. When you ask the patient a question, his voice sounds muffled. He is drooling and appears to be having difficulty swallowing. His skin is pale, and his lips are cyanotic. Vital signs are pulse (P)—114, strong, regular; respiration (R)—36, gasping, regular; and blood pressure (BP)—118/76.

Your Plan of Action

Fill in the blank lines with your treatment plan for this patient. Then compare your plan with the questions, answers, and rationale.

1. _____
2. _____
3. _____
4. _____
5. _____
6. _____
7. _____
8. _____
9. _____

Multiple Choice

22.1. Based on your initial findings, your *best* conclusion would be:
  a. this is an emergency and the patient needs rapid transport.
  b. drooling is unusual for age 4 but nothing to be concerned about.
  c. you can go on with the focused history and physical examination.
  d. baseline vital signs should be performed next because the patient is in respiratory distress.

22.2. This patient probably has what problem?
  a. Bronchiolitis
  b. Pneumonia
  c. Epiglottitis
  d. Croup

True/False

22.3. You should call for a paramedic unit because the patient may require endotracheal intubation.
  a. True
  b. False

Multiple Choice

22.4. The *most important* action to take to care for this patient is to:
  a. transport his mother with him but insist she ride up front.
  b. obtain a history of any medications the patient has been taking recently.
  c. place the child on the stretcher in a left lateral recumbent position so if he drools, saliva will run out of his mouth easily.
  d. let the patient's mother give the patient high-concentration oxygen by blow-by while he sits on her lap.

22.5. The normal respiratory rate for a 4-y.o. child is:
   a. 12 to 24 breaths/min.
   b. 20 to 30 breaths/min.
   c. 25 to 40 breaths/min.
   d. 30 to 50 breaths/min.

Scenario Two

You have been called to see a "7-m.o. male with respiratory distress." The patient is alert and very anxious. You can see nasal flaring and slight intercostal retractions. Expiratory wheezing is present. Mom says the baby caught a "cold" last week from an older sibling. He seemed to be recovering but then developed difficulty breathing. Vital signs are R—56, labored, regular with expiratory wheezing; and P—156, weak, regular.

Your Plan of Action

Fill in the blank lines with your treatment plan for this patient. Then compare your plan with the questions, answers, and rationale.

1. _____
2. _____
3. _____
4. _____
5. _____
6. _____
7. _____
8. _____
9. _____

Multiple Choice

22.6. After performing your initial assessment, you should:
   a. give high-concentration oxygen by blow-by, obtain a history, and perform a focused physical examination.
   b. obtain baseline vital signs.
   c. give the child oxygen via nasal cannula at 2 lpm, obtain a history, and perform a focused physical examination.
   d. give high-concentration oxygen by blow-by, perform a detailed head-to-toe examination.
22.7. This patient probably has:
   a. epiglottitis.
   b. asthma.
   c. bronchiolitis.
   d. croup.

22.8. Treating infants and children is different than treating adults because children:
  a. are more trusting than adults.
  b. like to ride in the ambulance with the lights and siren operating.
  c. have no difficulty in communicating because they like to play doctor.
  d. often fear strangers and have difficulty communicating.

22.9. The normal pulse rate range for a 7-m.o. infant is:
  a. 60 to 100 beats/min.
  b. 70 to 110 beats/min.
  c. 80 to 140 beats/min.
  d. 120 to 160 beats/min.

22.10. When performing a detailed physical examination on a 7-m.o. infant, you should:
  a. use a trunk-to-head approach and examination.
  b. try to examine only exposed areas so the child does not become frightened.
  c. use a head-to-toe approach so nothing is missed.
  d. first get a baseline set of vital signs, including BP.

22.11. A 7-m.o. child is considered to be in respiratory arrest when:
  a. the respiratory rate is <6 breaths/min.
  b. the respiratory rate is <10 breaths/min.
  c. the respiratory rate is >44 breaths/min.
  d. the respiratory rate is <20 breaths/min and is accompanied by difficulty breathing.

Scenario Three

You respond to a report of a "child seizing." On arrival you find a 4-y.o. male who is very sleepy. Mom says he has had two generalized seizures in the past 20 minutes, each lasting for approximately 2 minutes. He has no history of a seizure disorder. He has had flu symptoms with a fever for the past week for which he is taking amoxicillin. From across the room, you can tell his respirations are 20, regular, unlabored. His skin appears to be pink and dry.

Your Plan of Action

Fill in the blank lines with your treatment plan for this patient. Then compare your plan with the questions, answers, and rationale.

1. _____
2. _____
3. _____
4. _____
5. _____
6. _____
7. _____
8. _____
9. _____

Multiple Choice

22.12. Which of the following statements about febrile seizures is *correct?*
   a. They usually occur in groups of several seizures in rapid succession.
   b. They occur because of a rapid increase of the child's temperature.
   c. They signify the presence of a serious illness.
   d. They only occur in children <1 year of age.

22.13. The age group that usually is the *most* difficult to evaluate is:
   a. infants.
   b. toddlers.
   c. school-aged children.
   d. adolescents.

22.14. Common causes of seizures in children include all of the following *except:*
   a. fever.
   b. epilepsy.
   c. poisons.
   d. dehydration.

Scenario Four

You respond to a report of an "injured child." The patient is a 10-y.o. female c/o right forearm pain. She says she fell off her bicycle, but no bike is present at the scene. Her right arm is bruised and swollen. You also notice bruises on the patient's face and legs. When you ask her what happened, she insists she fell off her bike. Vital signs are BP—100/72, P—98, strong, regular; and R—22, regular, unlabored. At this point, the patient's father arrives. His speech is slurred; you can smell the odor of beer on his breath; and he is holding a can of beer in his hand.

> **Your Plan of Action**
> *Fill in the blank lines with your treatment plan for this patient. Then compare your plan with the questions, answers, and rationale.*
>
> 1. _____
> 2. _____
> 3. _____
> 4. _____
> 5. _____
> 6. _____
> 7. _____
> 8. _____
> 9. _____

Multiple Choice

22.15. You should suspect a possible fracture of the:
  a. right radius caused by a fall from a bicycle.
  b. right humerus caused by child abuse.
  c. right humerus caused by a fall from a bicycle.
  d. right radius caused by child abuse.

22.16. After completing a focused examination of the patient's right forearm, you should:
  a. call for a paramedic unit because blood loss at the fracture site may cause shock.
  b. obtain a baseline set of vital signs.
  c. continue with ongoing assessment.
  d. reevaluate the ABCs.

22.17. When child abuse is suspected, you should:
  a. refuse to treat the child until the police are on the scene.
  b. report your suspicions to the staff at the emergency room.
  c. advise the parents of what you suspect.
  d. request an immediate response by the police.

22.18. You should suspect possible abuse because:
  a. of the swelling of the right forearm.
  b. the patient did not fall far enough to cause the reported injury.
  c. of the old bruises on the face and legs.
  d. the child is not crying.

Scenario Five

You respond to a report of "a child not breathing." The patient is a 2-y.o. female who is lying beside the family swimming pool. Her mother is trying to perform rescue breathing. A weak pulse is present, but the child is not breathing.

Your Plan of Action

Fill in the blank lines with your treatment plan for this patient. Then compare your plan with the questions, answers, and rationale.

1. _____
2. _____
3. _____
4. _____
5. _____
6. _____
7. _____
8. _____
9. _____

Multiple Choice

22.19. The *most common* cause of death in children is:
  a. drowning.
  b. poisoning.
  c. seizures.
  d. trauma.

22.20. When you open this patient's airway you should:
  a. *not* hyperextend the neck.
  b. do a head-tilt, chin-lift.
  c. keep the body in alignment.
  d. check the pulse before ventilating the patient.

22.21. All of the following statements about rescue breathing for children are correct *except*:
  a. the breaths should be delivered over 1 second.
  b. after opening the airway give only one breath.
  c. limit ventilations to the amount of air needed to just make the chest rise.
  d. the bag-valve mask (BVM) should *not* have pop-off valves.

22.22. After doing rescue breathing for 1 minute, you should:
  a. check for a pulse using the brachial artery.
  b. reposition the head and continue rescue breathing.
  c. check for a pulse using the carotid artery.
  d. apply a cervical collar, spine board, and cervical immobilizer and transport.

22.23. Rescue breathing for children should be performed at a rate of:
  a. 8 to 10 breaths/minute.
  b. 12 to 20 breaths/minute.
  c. 22 to 28 breaths/minute.
  d. 30 to 40 breaths/minute.

Scenario Six

At 2:00 AM you are dispatched to another "child with difficulty breathing." The patient is an 18-m.o. female who is struggling to breathe. Her respirations are 36 breaths/min with intercostal retractions and use of her accessory muscles. According to her mother, the patient has had a cold for the past 3 days and was very hoarse yesterday. The mother also reports that the patient has a "funny cough, like a bark." She has no known allergies.

Your Plan of Action

Fill in the blank lines with your treatment plan for this patient. Then compare your plan with the questions, answers, and rationale.

1. _____
2. _____
3. _____
4. _____
5. _____
6. _____
7. _____
8. _____
9. _____

Multiple Choice

22.24. The childhood illness characterized by a "barking" cough, respiratory stridor, and hoarseness is:
   a. pneumonia.
   b. bronchiolitis.
   c. meningitis.
   d. croup.

True/False

22.25. This patient is in danger of complete airway obstruction.
   a. True
   b. False

Multiple Choice

22.26. All of the following statements about the pediatric respiratory system are correct *except:*
   a. children often use their accessory muscles when they are having difficulty breathing.
   b. a common sign of increased respiratory effort is nasal flaring.
   c. children have a large respiratory reserve.
   d. the pediatric tongue is relatively larger and placed more posteriorly in the airway than the adult tongue.

Answer Key—Chapter 22

SCENARIO ONE

Plan of Action

1. Body Substance Isolation (BSI)

2. Is the scene safe? Yes. Assess nature of illness, number of patients, and need for additional resources.

3. Form general impression by assessing patient's appearance, work of breathing, and circulation to skin (pediatric assessment triangle). Impression—Severe respiratory distress

4. Perform ABCDE assessment—Assess mental status, ensure open airway, assess breathing, apply oxygen at 10-15 lpm by pediatric non-rebreather mask (blow-by if patient will not tolerate mask), and assess circulation.

5. Determine priority, request ALS response because of risk of complete airway obstruction.

6. Transport.

7. History of present illness (HPI), SAMPLE

8. Focused physical examination, but do *not* attempt to visualize or place anything into throat.

9. Baseline vital signs

10. Ongoing assessment, meet ALS unit.

Rationale

The combination of a severe sore throat, respiratory distress, and drooling suggests epiglottitis. The patient is at risk to develop complete airway obstruction from swelling of the epiglottis. He should be kept as calm as possible, given high-concentration oxygen, and transported immediately. Depending on the transport time and the patient's condition, requesting ALS backup may be appropriate. If the patient appears to be in immediate danger of developing a complete obstruction, a paramedic can insert an endotracheal tube to secure the airway.

22.1. A, This is an emergency, and the patient needs rapid transport. Your assessment of the child's appearance, work of breathing, and circulation to skin (the pediatric assessment triangle) indicates severe respiratory distress. The combination of respiratory distress with drooling and difficulty swallowing or a sore throat suggests epiglottitis. Patients with epiglottitis are at risk for complete airway obstruction caused by soft tissue swelling. After giving high-concentration oxygen to the patient, you should transport and perform the rest of the assessment en route to the hospital.

22.2. **C,** This patient has epiglottitis, a bacterial infection of the epiglottis that can lead to complete airway obstruction from soft tissue swelling. Epiglottitis is characterized by a rapid onset (hours), high fever, inspiratory stridor, a severe sore throat that leads to drooling, and respiratory distress. Bronchiolitis is a viral infection of the smaller airways that occurs in infants. Bronchiolitis occurs in children aged <2 years (90% are aged <1 year) and is characterized by wheezing throughout the lung fields. Symptoms of pneumonia include fever; chest pain associated with breathing; a cough that produces yellow, green, or blood-tinged sputum; and crackles, rhonchi, and/or wheezing in the affected areas of the lungs. Croup is a viral illness that affects children aged from 6 months to 4 years. Croup has a slow onset (several days) and is characterized by a low-grade fever, hoarseness, mild sore throat, inspiratory stridor, and a loud, "seal bark" cough.

22.3. **A,** A paramedic unit should be called because this patient may require endotracheal intubation. Children with epiglottitis are at risk for complete airway obstruction caused by swelling of the epiglottis and surrounding soft tissues.

22.4. **D,** Allowing the patient to sit on his mother's lap while she gives him oxygen by blow-by will help keep him calm. Separating this child from his mother is likely to increase his anxiety, increase his demand for oxygen, and possibly lead to struggling that could cause him to obstruct his airway completely. Although a medication history should be obtained, it is not the most important aspect of this child's care. It is unlikely that this patient would tolerate attempts to place him on his left side. Patients in respiratory distress usually prefer to sit up because they can use their respiratory muscles most effectively in that position.

22.5. **B,** The normal respiratory rate for children aged 2 to 6 years is 20 to 30 breaths/min.

SCENARIO TWO

Plan of Action

1. BSI

2. Is the scene safe? Yes. Assess nature of illness, number of patients, and need for additional resources.

3. Form general impression by assessing patient's appearance, work of breathing, and circulation to skin (pediatric assessment triangle). Impression—Moderate respiratory distress

4. Perform ABCDE assessment—Assess mental status, ensure open airway, assess breathing, apply oxygen at 10-15 lpm by pediatric non-rebreather mask (blow-by if patient will not tolerate mask), and assess circulation.

5. Determine priority, consider ALS.

Continued

> **SCENARIO TWO—cont'd**
>
> 6. HPI, SAMPLE
> 7. Focused physical examination of respiratory system
> 8. Baseline vital signs
> 9. Transport.
> 10. Ongoing assessment
>
> **Rationale**
>
> This child has bronchiolitis, a common viral respiratory infection in infants and very young children. He is in moderate respiratory distress but is not in immediate danger. He needs high-concentration oxygen, which probably will need to be given by blow-by. His mother should be allowed to hold him to reduce his anxiety. Continue to observe his respiratory status during transport. If he shows signs of increasing work of breathing or his mental status deteriorates, assisted ventilation will be necessary.

22.6. A, Evaluation of the pediatric assessment triangle (appearance, work of breathing, and circulation to skin) suggests this child is in moderate respiratory distress. He should be given high-concentration oxygen, which can be given by blow-by if he will not tolerate a mask. A history and a physical examination focusing on the respiratory system should then be performed to identify the specific nature of his problem. A nasal cannula would not provide sufficient oxygen to meet this patient's needs. A detailed head-to-toe examination is unnecessary because the history and initial assessment findings indicate this patient has a problem involving his respiratory system.

22.7. C, This patient probably has bronchiolitis. Bronchiolitis is a viral infection of the bronchioles (smallest lower airways) that is most common in infants. After a few days of mild symptoms of upper respiratory infection, bronchiolitis patients develop rapid breathing, respiratory distress, retractions, accessory muscle use, and wheezing. Asthma also produces wheezing; however, it usually occurs in children aged >2 years and is not associated with fever and other signs and symptoms of infection. Epiglottitis has a rapid onset and produces stridor, a high-pitched, crowing inspiratory sound caused by swelling of the tissues in the upper airway. Croup also causes stridor, but it has a slower onset than epiglottitis (days rather than hours) and is associated with a loud, brassy cough (seal bark cough).

22.8. D, Infants and children are often more fearful of strangers and have difficulty communicating with the EMT.

22.9. C, A normal pulse rate for a 7-m.o. infant is 80 to 140 beats/min.

22.10. A, A trunk-to-head approach usually works better for children younger than school age. Young children often are frightened by the head-to-toe examination used for older children and adults because they do not like strangers touching their heads or faces. Children should be undressed when necessary for a complete examination. Blood pressures tend not to be useful for children younger than school age because they are difficult to obtain and interpret.

22.11. B, A 7-m.o. infant who is breathing <10 breaths/min is effectively in respiratory arrest and should be ventilated using a BVM.

Scenario Three

Plan of Action

1. BSI
2. Is the scene safe? Yes. Assess nature of illness, number of patients, and need for additional resources.
3. Form general impression by assessing patient's appearance, work of breathing, and circulation to skin (pediatric assessment triangle). Impression—Altered mental status, no respiratory distress or circulatory impairment
4. Perform ABCDE assessment—Assess mental status, ensure open airway, assess breathing, apply oxygen at 10-15 lpm by pediatric non-rebreather mask, and assess circulation.
5. Determine priority, consider ALS.
6. Rapid head-to-toe examination
7. Assess baseline vital signs.
8. HPI, SAMPLE
9. Transport.
10. Perform detailed examination if time allows, ongoing assessment.

Rationale

This patient appears to be in the postictal phase of a febrile seizure. Febrile seizures occur in infants and children aged <6 years and result from a rapid increase in body temperature. Patients who have febrile seizures usually have only one episode of seizure activity per episode of febrile illness. Febrile seizures are a diagnosis of exclusion. All other possible causes of seizure activity should be excluded before making the conclusion it was only a *febrile* seizure. After ensuring the patient has an adequate airway and is adequately oxygenated, perform a head-to-toe examination and take a history to identify other possible causes of seizure activity such as hypoxia, hypoglycemia, poisoning, or central nervous system infections.

22.12. **B,** Febrile seizures occur because of a rapid increase in the child's body temperature, *not* as a result of a high fever. Typically a child prone to febrile seizures will have one episode of seizure activity during a febrile illness. Febrile seizures do not necessarily indicate presence of serious disease. Febrile seizures can occur in children up to age 6 years.

22.13. **B,** Toddlers are the most difficult age group to evaluate. They do not like being touched, do not like strangers, do not like their clothing being removed, are afraid of needles, and will resist oxygen masks because of the fear of being suffocated.

22.14. **D,** Dehydration is *not* a common cause of pediatric seizures. Fever, epilepsy, and poisoning are all common causes of seizures in children.

SCENARIO FOUR

Plan of Action

1. BSI

2. Is the scene safe? Yes. However, the patient's father should be watched carefully for signs of potential violence. Assess mechanism of injury, number of patients, and need for additional resources.

3. Form general impression by assessing patient's appearance, work of breathing, and circulation to skin (pediatric assessment triangle). Impression—No respiratory distress or circulatory impairment

4. Perform ABCDE assessment—Assess mental status, ensure open airway, assess breathing, and assess circulation.

5. Determine priority, consider ALS.

6. Consider mechanism of injury. Mechanism appears not to be significant.

7. Focused physical examination of injured arm, splint possible fracture.

8. Baseline vital signs

9. SAMPLE

10. Transport, perform ongoing assessment, and report suspicions of child abuse to emergency room staff.

Rationale

This patient appears initially to have isolated extremity trauma associated with a nonsignificant mechanism of injury. However, as the history is taken and the physical examination is performed, inconsistencies are identified. The patient says she was riding her bicycle, but no bike is present. She also has multiple bruises in various stages of healing. Her fracture should be splinted, and she should be transported to the emergency department for treatment. The emergency department staff should be advised that you suspect child abuse. In many states, the law requires EMS personnel who suspect child abuse to directly report their suspicions to a law enforcement or protective services agency. If the patient's father becomes belligerent or refuses to allow you to treat and transport her, a response by the police should be requested.

22.15. **D,** This patient has a fracture of the right radius that you should suspect is the result of child abuse. The patient's injuries are not consistent with the history she is providing, and evidence of repeated previous injury is present.

22.16. **B,** After completing a focused examination of the patient's injured forearm, you should take a set of baseline vital signs. Blood loss at the site of a forearm fracture is unlikely to cause hypovolemic shock. Ongoing assessment is performed after treatment is begun and the patient is en route to the hospital. Because the patient was initially stable and has not shown any change in her condition, reevaluation of the ABCs is not necessary at this time.

22.17. B, As long as the parent remains cooperative and consents to the transport of the child, you should continue care as usual and report your suspicions of child abuse to the staff at the emergency room. Telling the parent you suspect child abuse or immediately calling the police could put you in danger or cause the parent to refuse consent for treatment and transport. If child abuse is suspected and the parents refuse consent, the police should be called so the child can be placed in protective custody.

22.18. C, Multiple injuries in various stages of healing are a warning sign of possible child abuse.

SCENARIO FIVE

Plan of Action

1. BSI
2. Is the scene safe? Yes. Assess nature of illness, number of patients, and need for additional resources.
3. Form initial impression by assessing patient's appearance, work of breathing, and circulation to skin (pediatric assessment triangle). Impression—Respiratory arrest, possible cardiac arrest
4. Perform ABCDE assessment—Assess mental status, ensure open airway, assess breathing, place oral airway, ventilate with BVM and oxygen at 10-15 lpm, and assess circulation.
5. Determine priority, request ALS response.
6. Based on history, consider spinal motion restriction, and transport.
7. Rapid head-to-toe examination
8. Baseline vital signs
9. HPI, SAMPLE
10. Perform detailed examination if time allows, ongoing assessment. Meet ALS unit.

Rationale

This patient is in respiratory arrest secondary to what appears to be a near drowning. An oral airway should be placed, and ventilation with high-concentration oxygen should be started as soon as possible. An ALS unit should be requested in case endotracheal intubation is needed for continuing resuscitation. Depending on transport time to a hospital and response time by the ALS unit, a decision should be made about whether to wait on scene for the ALS unit, meet the ALS unit during transport, or rapidly transport directly to the hospital. A rapid head-to-toe examination should be performed to identify any injuries that might have led to the near drowning or that might have been suffered during the rescue attempt. Care should be taken to open the airway and move the patient's head and neck until presence of a cervical fracture can be ruled out. Even if the patient responds quickly to ventilation with a BVM and begins breathing on her own, she should be transported for evaluation and observation at the hospital.

22.19. D, The number one cause of death in children is trauma. In fact, trauma is the leading cause of death in all patients between ages 1 and 44 years.

22.20. A, Overextension of a small child's neck can cause airway obstruction. This happens because the opening to the child's lower airway is higher in the neck than in adults and the tongue is larger and set farther back in the airway. If the neck is overextended, the back of the tongue presses down on the epiglottis, pushing it over the high glottic opening. Additionally, caution should be used to open the airway of any victim of a near drowning in a swimming pool. Swimming pool near drownings often are caused by patients jumping or diving into shallow water and striking their heads on the bottom or side of the pool. This mechanism of injury can cause a cervical spine fracture.

22.21. B, After opening the airway, *two* rescue breaths should be given initially.

22.22. C, After 1 minute of rescue breathing, the patient's pulse should be reassessed at the carotid artery.

22.23. B, Children are ventilated once every 3 to 5 seconds or 12 to 20 breaths/minute.

SCENARIO SIX

Plan of Action

1. BSI
2. Is the scene safe? Yes. Assess nature of illness, number of patients, and need for additional resources.
3. Form initial impression by assessing patient's appearance, work of breathing, and circulation to skin (pediatric assessment triangle). Impression—Severe respiratory distress
4. Perform ABCDE assessment—Assess mental status, ensure open airway, assess breathing, apply oxygen at 10-15 lpm by pediatric non-rebreather mask (blow-by if patient will not tolerate mask), and assess circulation.
5. Determine priority, request ALS response.
6. Transport.
7. HPI, SAMPLE

Continued

SCENARIO SIX—cont'd

8. <u>Focused physical examination, but do *not* attempt to visualize or place anything into throat.</u>

9. <u>Baseline vital signs</u>

10. <u>Ongoing assessment, meet ALS unit.</u>

Rationale

This patient has croup, a viral infection that causes swelling of the soft tissues of the larynx. Croup is characterized by a slow onset, a mild sore throat, low-grade fever, hoarseness, inspiratory stridor, a barking cough, and difficulty breathing that worsens at night when the patient tries to sleep. Swelling in the larynx increases resistance to air movement in the patient's respiratory tract, increasing the effort required to breathe. Patients with severe croup may become exhausted and develop respiratory failure. This patient should be given high-concentration oxygen. If she begins to tire or her level of consciousness decreases, her ventilations should be assisted with a BVM. Depending on the transport time, a paramedic unit could be called to administer racemic epinephrine, which can decrease the swelling in the larynx. The paramedics also may need to intubate the patient if her respiratory distress worsens.

22.24. **D,** This patient has croup. Croup (laryngotracheobronchitis) is a viral illness characterized by slow onset, low-grade fever, mild sore throat, hoarseness, inspiratory stridor, and a loud, brassy, barking cough (seal bark cough). Respiratory distress from croup usually becomes more severe at night. Pneumonia would be characterized by fever, a productive cough, chest pain associated with breathing, and breath sounds indicating fluid in the lower airway. Symptoms of meningitis include fever, headache, stiff neck, altered mental status, and seizures. Bronchiolitis occurs in infants and presents with fever, difficulty breathing, and expiratory wheezing.

22.25. **B,** Unlike patients with epiglottitis, children with croup are not at risk for complete airway obstruction. However, they can develop severe respiratory distress and are at risk for respiratory failure caused by fatigue from the increased work of moving air past the swelling in their larynx and trachea.

22.26. **C,** Children do not have a large respiratory reserve capacity. They frequently use their accessory muscles when they have difficulty breathing. Nasal flaring is a common response in children who are having trouble moving adequate amounts of air. The pediatric tongue is larger and placed farther back in the airway than an adult's tongue, increasing the risk of obstruction.

23

Geriatric Emergencies

DEMOGRAPHICS OF AGING

- Persons aged >65 years are the fasting-growing age group.
- By 2030, geriatric patients will
    - Comprise 22% of population
    - Account for 70% of ambulance transports

EFFECTS OF AGING

- Cardiovascular system
    - Speed, force of myocardial contraction decrease.
    - Cardiac-conducting system deteriorates.
    - Resistance to peripheral blood flow increases, elevating systolic blood pressure (BP).
    - Blood vessels lose ability to constrict, dilate efficiently.
- Respiratory system
    - Respiratory muscles lose strength; rib cage calcifies, becomes more rigid.
    - Respiratory capacity decreases.
    - Gas exchange across alveolar membrane slows.
    - Cough, gag reflexes diminish, increasing risks of aspiration, lower airway infection.
- Musculoskeletal system
    - Osteoporosis develops, especially in females.
    - Spinal disks narrow, resulting in kyphosis (humpback).
    - Joints lose flexibility, become more susceptible to repetitive stress injury.
    - Skeletal muscle mass decreases.
- Nervous system
    - Brain weight decreases 6% to 7%.
    - Brain size decreases.
    - Cerebral blood flow decreases 15% to 20%.
    - Nerve conduction slows up to 15%.
- Gastrointestinal (GI) system
    - Senses of taste, smell decrease.
    - Gums, teeth deteriorate.
    - Saliva flow decreases.
    - Cardiac sphincter loses tone; esophageal reflux becomes more common.
    - Peristalsis slows.
    - Absorption from GI tract slows.
- Renal system
    - Renal blood flow decreases 50%.
    - Functioning nephrons decrease 30% to 40%.
- Integumentary system
    - Dermis thins by 20%.
    - Sweat glands decrease; sweating decreases.
    - Ability to regulate body temperature by vasoconstriction and dilation decreases.

FACTORS COMPLICATING GERIATRIC ASSESSMENT

- Variability
    - Older people differ from one another more than younger people do.
    - Physiologic age is more important than chronologic age.

- Response to illness
  - Elderly persons seek help for only small part of symptoms.
  - Perceive symptoms as "just getting old"
  - Delay seeking treatment
  - Trivialize chief complaints
- Presence of multiple pathologies
  - 85% have one chronic disease; 30% have three or more.
  - One system's acute illness stresses other's reserve capacity.
  - One disease's symptoms may mask another's.
  - One disease's treatment may mask another's symptoms.
- Altered presentations
  - Decreased, absent pain
  - Depressed temperature regulation
  - Depressed thirst mechanisms
  - Confusion, restlessness, and hallucinations
  - Generalized deterioration
  - Vague, poorly defined complaints
- Communication problems
  - Decreased sight
  - Decreased hearing
  - Decreased mental faculties
  - Depression
  - Poor cooperation, limited mobility
- Polypharmacy
  - Too many drugs!
  - 30% of geriatric hospitalizations are drug induced.

HISTORY TAKING

- Probe for significant complaints
  - Chief complaint may be trivial, nonspecific.
  - Patient may not volunteer information.
- Dealing with communication difficulties
  - Talk to patient before talking to relatives
  - If possible, talk to patient alone
  - Formal, respectful approach
  - Position self near middle of visual field
  - Do not assume deafness or shout
  - Speak slowly, enunciate clearly
  - Do *not* assume confused or disoriented patient is "just senile!"
- Obtain thorough medication history
  - More than one doctor?
  - More than one pharmacy?
  - Multiple medications?
  - Old vs. current medications?
  - Shared medications?
  - Over-the-counter medications?

PHYSICAL EXAMINATION

- Dealing with complications
  - May fatigue easily
  - May have difficulty with positioning required for examination
  - Decreased pain sensation requires thorough examination.
  - Consider modesty
  - Examine in warm area
  - If they say it hurts, it probably *really* hurts! *Examine carefully!*
- Misleading findings
  - Inelastic skin mimics decreased turgor.
  - Mouth breathing gives impression of dehydration.
  - Inactivity, dependent position of feet may cause pedal edema.
  - Crackles in lung bases may be nonpathologic.
  - Peripheral pulses may be difficult to feel.

CARDIOVASCULAR DISEASE

- Acute myocardial infarction (MI)
  - "Silent" MI more common
  - Commonly presents with dyspnea only
  - May present with signs, symptoms of acute abdomen, including tenderness, rigidity
  - Possible vague symptoms
    - Weakness
    - Fatigue
    - Syncope
    - Nausea, vomiting
    - Diaphoresis
    - Incontinence
    - Confusion
    - Transient ischemic attack (TIA)/stroke (10% of strokes are triggered by a cardiac event)
  - If adding "chest pain" to their list of symptoms would make you think MI, it is an MI!
- Congestive heart failure
  - May present as nocturnal confusion caused by hypoxia
  - Large fluid-filled blisters may develop on legs, especially if patient sleeps sitting up.
  - Bed-ridden patients may have fluid over sacral areas rather than feet, legs.

RESPIRATORY DISEASE

- Pulmonary embolism
  - Blockage of branches of pulmonary artery
  - Most common cause is blood clots from lower extremities
  - Suspect in any patient with sudden onset of dyspnea when cause cannot be quickly identified
- Pneumonia
  - Lung infection
  - Common in elderly patients because of aspiration, decreased immune function
  - Possible atypical presentations
    - Absence of cough, fever
    - Abdominal rather than chest pain
    - Altered mental status

- Chronic obstructive pulmonary disease (COPD)
  - Fifth leading cause of death in males aged 55 to 75 years
  - Consider possible spontaneous pneumothorax in COPD patient who *suddenly* decompensates

NEUROPSYCHIATRIC DISEASE

- Dementia or altered mental status
  - Distinguish between acute, chronic onset
  - *Never* assume acute dementia or altered mental status is because of "senility"
  - Ask relatives, other caregivers what baseline mental status is
  - Possible causes
    - Head injury with subdural hematoma
    - Alcohol, drug intoxication, and withdrawal
    - Tumor
    - Central nervous system (CNS) infections
    - Electrolyte imbalances
    - Cardiac failure
    - Hypoglycemia
    - Hypoxia
    - Drug interactions
- Cerebrovascular accident
  - Emboli, thrombi more common than bleeds
  - Stroke/TIA signs often subtle—Dizziness, behavioral change, and altered affect
  - Headache, especially if localized, is significant.
  - TIAs common, one-third progress to a stroke.
  - Strokelike symptoms may be delayed effect of head trauma.
- Seizures
  - *All* first-time seizures in elderly patients are dangerous, indicating serious disease.
  - Possible causes
    - Head injury with subdural hematoma
    - Alcohol, drug intoxication, and withdrawal
    - Tumor
    - CNS infections
    - Electrolyte imbalances
    - Cardiac failure
    - Hypoglycemia
    - Hypoxia
    - Drug interactions
- Syncope
  - Morbidity, mortality higher than in younger persons
  - Consider
    - Cardiogenic causes (MI, arrhythmias)
    - TIA
    - Drug effects (beta blockers, vasodilators)
    - Volume depletion
- Depression
  - Common problem
  - May account for symptoms of "senility"

○ Persons aged >65 years account for 25% of all suicides.
○ Treat as immediate life-threatening problem!

TRAUMA

- Head injury
  ○ More likely, even with minor trauma
  ○ Signs of increased intracranial pressure (ICP) develop slowly.
  ○ Patient may have forgotten injury; delayed presentation may be mistaken for CVA.
- Cervical injury
  ○ Osteoporosis, narrow spinal canal increase injury risk from trivial forces.
  ○ Sudden neck movements may cause cord injury without fracture.
  ○ Decreased pain sensation may mask pain of fracture.
  ○ Positioning and packaging may have to be modified to accommodate physical deformities.
- Hypovolemia and shock
  ○ Decreased ability to compensate
  ○ Progress to irreversible shock rapidly
  ○ Tolerate hypoperfusion poorly, even for short periods
  ○ Hypoperfusion may occur at "normal" pressures.
  ○ Medications (beta blockers) may mask signs of shock.

ENVIRONMENTAL EMERGENCIES

- Tolerate temperature extremes poorly
- Contributing factors
  ○ Cardiovascular disease
  ○ Endocrine disease
  ○ Poor nutrition
  ○ Drug effects
  ○ Low, fixed incomes
- Suspect heat- or cold-related illness in any patient with altered LOC (level of consciousness) or vague presentation in hot or cool environment

GERIATRIC ABUSE AND NEGLECT

- Physical, psychological injury of older person by their children or care providers
- Knows no socioeconomic bounds
- Contributing factors
  ○ Advanced age—Average mid-80s
  ○ Multiple chronic diseases
  ○ Sleep-pattern disturbances leading to nocturnal wandering, shouting
  ○ Family has difficulty upholding commitments.
- Primary findings
  ○ Trauma inconsistent with history
  ○ History that changes with multiple tellings

REVIEW QUESTIONS
Scenario One

An 86-y.o. female complains of lower abdominal pain. As you talk to her, you note she is having difficulty hearing you. She keeps adjusting her glasses, so you also suspect she cannot see well. The pain is located in the lower abdomen and is associated with "burning" when she urinates. She has a past history of angina, hypertension, arthritis, and gout. She is taking numerous medications but refuses to show them to you. Vital signs are BP—168/90; pulse (P)—96, weak, regular; and respirations (R)—16, regular, unlabored.

Your Plan of Action

Fill in the blank lines with your treatment plan for this patient. Then compare your plan with the questions, answers, and rationale.

1. _____
2. _____
3. _____
4. _____
5. _____
6. _____
7. _____
8. _____
9. _____

Multiple Choice

23.1. Common problems to which elderly persons are prone include all of the following *except:*
    a. difficulty with elimination.
    b. difficulty with eyesight.
    c. difficulty with cultural differences.
    d. difficulty in taking medications.

23.2. This patient is *most* likely experiencing:
    a. a urinary tract infection.
    b. a duodenal ulcer.
    c. a lower GI bleed.
    d. dehydration.

23.3. All of the following statements about incontinence are true *except:*
    a. incontinence may cause embarrassment among a patient's family and peers.
    b. incontinence may impair a patient's ability to function socially.
    c. incontinence may lead to an increased bladder capacity.
    d. incontinence may lead to infection as a result of a decreased fluid intake.

True/False

23.4. Elderly patients are at risk for substance abuse.
    a. True
    b. False

Multiple Choice

23.5. All of the following increase the risk of elderly patients for injury *except:*
   a. decreased pain perception.
   b. decreased eyesight and hearing.
   c. decreased bone density.
   d. problems with balance and equilibrium.

Scenario Two

Your patient is a 92-y.o. female who fell at home and cannot get up. She is awake and alert and says she fell yesterday morning—28 hours ago. She is feisty and yells when you try to examine her. The patient says she has no past medical history, but you notice bottles of Nitrostat and Cardizem on the kitchen table. Vital signs are BP—104/78; P—100, weak, regular; and R—18, regular, unlabored.

Your Plan of Action

Fill in the blank lines with your treatment plan for this patient. Then compare your plan with the questions, answers, and rationale.

1. _____
2. _____
3. _____
4. _____
5. _____
6. _____
7. _____
8. _____
9. _____

Multiple Choice

23.6. After completing the scene size-up and initial assessment, you should:
   a. immediately obtain a baseline set of vital signs.
   b. apply a cervical collar, secure the patient to a long spine board, and transport immediately.
   c. do a focused history and physical examination.
   d. do a rapid head-to-toe physical examination.

23.7. If the patient's right leg is shortened and rotated outward, you should suspect a:
   a. pelvic fracture.
   b. fractured hip.
   c. dislocated hip.
   d. midshaft femur fracture.

23.8. A secondary problem that should be suspected in this patient is:
  a. dementia.
  b. hypothermia from being on the floor so long.
  c. a cardiac event.
  d. exhaustion from lack of sleep.

Scenario Three

Your patient is an 83-y.o. female who is lying in bed. Her son-in-law says she has not been feeling well for the past 2 days. However, she denies nausea, vomiting, or abdominal pain and currently is taking some fluids. During your physical examination, you find several large bruises on her forearms and one across her abdomen. She has a past medical history of diabetes controlled by diet, colon cancer that was successfully treated 5 years ago, and a cardiac stent placed 10 years ago. Her medications include furosemide and metoprolol. She has no known drug allergies. Vital signs are BP—106/68; P—98, strong, regular; and R—16, regular, unlabored.

Your Plan of Action

Fill in the blank lines with your treatment plan for this patient. Then compare your plan with the questions, answers, and rationale.

1. _____
2. _____
3. _____
4. _____
5. _____
6. _____
7. _____
8. _____
9. _____

Multiple Choice

23.9. You would consider all of the following pieces of information in your scene size-up *except:*
  a. the patient's bedding is clean and sufficient to keep her warm.
  b. the room is clean and neat.
  c. water is available on the patient's bedside table.
  d. a cat is sleeping at the foot of the bed.

23.10. As you examine the patient, you should be *most* concerned about:
  a. the nausea being related to her cardiac history.
  b. her not having felt well for 2 days.
  c. the bruises on her arms and abdomen.
  d. her past history of diabetes.

23.11. Based on the history and physical examination you should suspect this patient may be experiencing:
   a. an acute MI.
   b. dehydration.
   c. abuse.
   d. hyperglycemia.

Scenario Four

Your patient is a 90-y.o. female who is sitting in a chair in her living room with a dazed look on her face. She tells you the last thing she remembers was walking to the bathroom. Her 92-y.o. husband says she fell suddenly and was unconscious for approximately 1 minute. She is oriented to person and place but does not know exactly what day it is and cannot remember what happened to her. She has chronic osteoarthritis and had cataract surgery 2 months ago. Her skin is warm and dry. Vital signs are BP—112/80; P—70, strong, regular; and R—14, regular, unlabored.

Your Plan of Action

Fill in the blank lines with your treatment plan for this patient. Then compare your plan with the questions, answers, and rationale.

1. _____
2. _____
3. _____
4. _____
5. _____
6. _____
7. _____
8. _____
9. _____

Multiple Choice

23.12. Which of the following types of syncope is caused by the body's inability to compensate when the patient moves from a sitting to a standing position?
   a. Hydrostatic syncope
   b. Orthostatic syncope
   c. Neurogenic syncope
   d. Vasovagal syncope
23.13. All of the following problems are associated with progressive loss of vision in elderly persons *except:*
   a. decreased blood calcium levels.
   b. glaucoma.
   c. cataracts.
   d. diabetes.

23.14. Why should this patient be transported to the hospital?
   a. To make her husband happy
   b. To ensure she does not have a fracture
   c. So she can be evaluated for a possible TIA
   d. So she can be treated for possible hypoglycemia

Scenario Five

You are dispatched to a nonemergency transfer of an 83-y.o. male from the hospital to a nursing home. When you start to move the patient to the stretcher, he becomes combative and begins to yell, "I'm not going anywhere." The only problems noted in his medical record are arthritis and ulcerative colitis. Vital signs are BP—152/92; P—98, strong, regular; and R—18, regular, unlabored.

Your Plan of Action

Fill in the blank lines with your treatment plan for this patient. Then compare your plan with the questions, answers, and rationale.

1. _____
2. _____
3. _____
4. _____
5. _____
6. _____
7. _____
8. _____
9. _____

Multiple Choice

23.15. The *best* approach to dealing with this situation would be to:
   a. ask the patient why he does not want to go.
   b. tell the patient the ride is free and that you are a very safe driver.
   c. tell the patient he will be in trouble with his doctor if he does not go.
   d. ignore the patient's refusal and transport him.
23.16. When the patient continues to refuse transport, you decide to discuss the matter with the nurse. She tells you that you must transport the patient. At this point, you should:
   a. force the patient to go, even if restraints are necessary.
   b. call hospital security.
   c. leave because the patient is competent and has a right to refuse care.
   d. ask the nurse to call the patient's doctor.

True/False

23.17. A patient who has dementia but has *not* been declared legally incompetent may be taken against his will.
  a. True
  b. False

Scenario Six

You are dispatched to a "person down." The patient is an 81-y.o. male who is pulseless and apneic. His wife says he has not been feeling well the past 2 days. After you begin cardiopulmonary resuscitation (CPR), the patient's wife tells you he has a history of terminal colon cancer and hands you a do not resuscitate (DNR) order.

Your Plan of Action

Fill in the blank lines with your treatment plan for this patient. Then compare your plan with the questions, answers, and rationale.

1. _____
2. _____
3. _____
4. _____
5. _____
6. _____
7. _____
8. _____
9. _____

Multiple Choice

23.18. How should you manage this situation?
  a. Call for a paramedic unit after initiating CPR.
  b. Continue CPR, and intubate if protocols allow.
  c. Stop CPR, and call the patient's doctor and the police.
  d. Start CPR, call for a paramedic unit, and intubate if protocols allow.

Scenario Seven

You respond to another "person down." You have been to this address many times in the past. The patient is a 73-y.o. male who has a terminal brain cancer. This time his wife is very excited and is yelling, "He's stopped breathing." The patient is in cardiac arrest. When you ask the wife about a DNR order, she says, "What is a DNR?" You have had several conversations with the patient on other trips to the hospital and know he does not want life-saving measures.

Your Plan of Action

Fill in the blank lines with your treatment plan for this patient. Then compare your plan with the questions, answers, and rationale.

1. _____

2. _____

3. _____

4. _____

5. _____

6. _____

7. _____

8. _____

9. _____

Multiple Choice

23.19. How should you manage this situation?

    a. Call for a paramedic unit after initiating CPR.

    b. Continue CPR, and intubate if protocols allow.

    c. Stop CPR, and call the patient's doctor and the police.

    d. Start CPR, call for a paramedic unit, and intubate if protocols allow.

Scenario Eight

The patient is an 89-y.o. female who fell and was unable to get up because she weighs 350 pounds. She has no other complaints. The house is cluttered with a pile of newspapers close to a wood stove. Dirty dishes and food are on the counters in the kitchen. Her cat is sitting on the kitchen table next to two of her medication bottles. The bottles have tipped over, and because the tops were not on, they are mixed up in a pile. Because it feels very cold in the house, you check the thermostat and find it turned to 55° F. The wood stove was going, but the fire is low. The patient has no injuries. Vital signs are BP—148/88; P—78, weak, regular; and R—12, regular, unlabored.

Your Plan of Action

Fill in the blank lines with your treatment plan for this patient. Then compare your plan with the questions, answers, and rationale.

1. _____
2. _____
3. _____
4. _____
5. _____
6. _____
7. _____
8. _____
9. _____

Multiple Choice

23.20. Your *most immediate* concern should be:
   a. an injury the patient may be unaware of.
   b. the mixed medications on the kitchen table.
   c. the fact the house is poorly heated.
   d. the newspapers piled close to the wood stove.

23.21. The patient refuses to go to the hospital and is willing to sign a refusal form. You should:
   a. call the police so they can transport her.
   b. call the patient's daughter, who lives 75 miles away.
   c. get a signed refusal, return to your station, and call the Department of Social Services.
   d. get a signed refusal, return to your station, and call the sheriff.

23.22. Your *greatest* concern is the fact that this patient:
   a. can no longer care for herself.
   b. poses a danger to her own health.
   c. is not taking her medications as prescribed.
   d. has a mental health problem.

SCENARIO ONE

Plan of Action

1. Body Substance Isolation (BSI)

2. Is the scene safe? Yes. Assess nature of illness, number of patients, and need for additional resources.

3. Assess mental status. Ensure an open airway, assess breathing, and assess circulatory status.

4. Determine priority, consider ALS.

5. History of present illness (HPI), SAMPLE

6. Focused physical examination

7. Baseline vital signs

8. Transport, perform ongoing assessment en route.

Rationale

Elderly patients frequently do not drink adequate amounts of water because their sense of thirst is less intense. Also, some older persons reduce their fluid intake because they have urinary incontinence. Decreased fluid intake increases the risk of dehydration and urinary tract infections.

23.1. **C,** Elderly patients are prone to increased difficulty in elimination, decreased vision, and difficulty taking medications. Tolerance of cultural differences is a learned behavior that is unlikely to change with age.

23.2. **A,** Lower abdominal pain and a burning sensation when urinating suggest this patient has a urinary tract infection.

23.3. **C,** Decreased, not increased, bladder capacity can cause incontinence. Patients with incontinence often are embarrassed by the problem, which interferes with their ability to function socially. Incontinent patients also may decrease their fluid intake, increasing their risk to develop urinary tract infections.

23.4. **A,** Elderly persons are at risk for substance abuse. They may abuse analgesic drugs in an attempt to control chronic pain. They also may abuse alcohol and other drugs to deal with grief or depression.

23.5. A, Decreased pain perception is not a contributing factor for trauma. However, elderly patients may underestimate the severity of injuries because they do not feel pain as intensely as younger persons do.

SCENARIO TWO

Plan of Action

1. BSI
2. Is the scene safe? Yes. Assess nature of illness/mechanism of injury, number of patients, and need for additional resources.
3. Assess mental status. Ensure an open airway, assess breathing, apply oxygen at 10-15 lpm by non-rebreather mask, and assess circulatory status.
4. Determine priority, consider ALS.
5. Rapid head-to-toe examination
6. Baseline vital signs
7. HPI, SAMPLE
8. Transport, do detailed physical examination if time allows, and perform ongoing assessment.

Rationale

Because the patient is unwilling or unable to provide information about locations of possible injuries, a rapid head-to-toe examination is appropriate. The patient could have been injured by the fall. Because she has been lying on the floor for 28 hours she may be hypothermic or dehydrated. Additionally, the medications on her kitchen table suggest a cardiac history. She may have fallen because of a TIA or cardiac event.

23.6. D, Because the patient is not providing information on specific areas that are painful, a rapid head-to-toe physical examination would be most appropriate.

23.7. B, Shortening and external rotation of an elderly person's leg usually indicate a fractured hip.

23.8. B, Because the patient has been lying on the floor for an extended period, she may also be hypothermic.

SCENARIO THREE

Plan of Action

1. BSI
2. Is the scene safe? Yes. Assess nature of illness, number of patients, and need for additional resources.
3. Assess mental status. Ensure an open airway, assess breathing, apply oxygen at 10-15 lpm by non-rebreather mask, and assess circulatory status.
4. Determine priority, consider ALS.
5. HPI, SAMPLE
6. Focused physical examination
7. Baseline vital signs
8. Transport, perform ongoing assessment.

Rationale

This patient needs to be evaluated to determine why she is not feeling well. However, the most immediate concern in this situation is the possibility of abuse indicated by the bruising on her arms and abdomen. With larger numbers of older adults being taken care of at home, the incidence of elder abuse is increasing. The signs and symptoms of elder abuse are similar to those of child abuse. The history does not match the pattern of injuries observed. Multiple injuries in various stages of healing are present, indicating repeated trauma. The history often is vague, incomplete, or subject to change when repeated.

23.9. **D,** The fact that a cat is sleeping at the foot of the bed is not relevant. You should be concerned about the cleanliness of the patient's room, presence of adequate amounts of bedding, and availability of water at the bedside table.

23.10. **C,** The presence of bruises on the patient's arms and abdomen raises concerns about the possibility of her having been abused.

23.11. **C,** Based on the history and physical examination, the patient appears to have been abused.

SCENARIO FOUR

Plan of Action

1. BSI

2. Is the scene safe? Yes. Assess mechanism of injury/nature of illness, number of patients, and need for additional resources.

3. Assess mental status. Ensure an open airway, assess breathing, apply oxygen at 10-15 lpm by non-rebreather mask, and assess circulatory status.

4. Determine priority, consider ALS.

5. Rapid head-to-toe physical examination

6. Baseline vital signs

7. HPI, SAMPLE

8. Transport, do detailed physical examination if time allows, and perform ongoing assessment.

Rationale

Because the patient fell and has altered mental status, she should be examined from head to toe for injuries and signs of a possible cause for her fall. The examination should include a check of her blood glucose level. She should be transported for evaluation of the reason for her fall and continuing altered mental status.

23.12. **B,** Orthostatic syncope occurs when the body is unable to compensate rapidly for shifts in the blood volume that occur when a patient sits up or stands up suddenly. Orthostatic syncope can result from hypovolemia, diabetes, other diseases that affect the nervous system, and the effects of many of the medications used to manage high blood pressure.

23.13. **A,** Decreased blood calcium levels do not affect vision. Glaucoma, cataracts, and diabetes can cause progressive vision loss.

23.14. **C,** This patient needs to be evaluated at the hospital for a possible TIA. Although hypoglycemia can cause altered mental status, this patient's other signs and symptoms (warm, dry skin; normal pulse rate) are not consistent with low blood sugar.

SCENARIO FIVE

Plan of Action

1. BSI
2. Is the scene safe? Yes. Assess nature of illness, number of patients, and need for additional resources.
3. Attempt to determine why the patient is refusing transport, and correct the reasons for the refusal, if possible.
4. Ask that the patient's physician be contacted, so an evaluation can be conducted for possible medical causes for the refusal.
5. Document the events thoroughly.

Rationale

A patient has the right to refuse transport unless he or she has been declared incompetent by a court of law or has been placed in protective custody by a law enforcement officer. For cases in which patients refuse transport, an effort should be made to determine the reason for the refusal. Patients often have legitimate reasons why they do not want to be transported by EMS. If these problems can be resolved, the patient may consent. In this case, the nurse should be asked to call the patient's physician so an evaluation can be conducted for a possible underlying medical cause for the refusal. If leaving without the patient becomes necessary, a report that thoroughly documents the events should be written as soon as possible.

23.15. **A,** If a patient refuses transport, you should try to determine the reason for the refusal. Patients often have legitimate reasons for not wanting to be transported. Once these problems have been addressed, the patient often will consent to transport.

23.16. **D,** A patient cannot be transported against his or her will. However, in this case an evaluation by the patient's physician may disclose a problem that is altering the patient's mental status and leading to the refusal.

23.17. **B,** Until a patient has been declared incompetent by a court of law, he or she has the right to refuse care or transport.

SCENARIO SIX

Plan of Action

1. BSI
2. Is the scene safe? Yes. Assess nature of illness, number of patients, and need for additional resources.

Continued

SCENARIO SIX—cont'd

3. Assess mental status. Ensure an open airway, assess breathing, begin ventilations with bag-valve mask (BVM) and oxygen at 10-15 lpm, assess circulatory status, and begin chest compressions.

4. Assess DNR order for completeness and authenticity.

5. Discontinue CPR.

6. Make appropriate notifications.

7. Ensure family has adequate support, assistance available before leaving the scene.

Rationale

Because a valid DNR order is immediately available, resuscitation can be discontinued. Notification of the death should be provided to local law enforcement, the coroner or medical examiner, and the patient's physician. Before leaving the scene, EMS personnel should ensure that law enforcement officers or other appropriately trained personnel are present to provide assistance and support to the family.

23.18. **C,** Because you have been presented with a properly documented DNR order, you should discontinue care and make the appropriate notifications. Before leaving the scene, be sure someone else is available to support and assist the family.

SCENARIO SEVEN

Plan of Action

1. BSI

2. Is the scene safe? Yes. Assess nature of illness, number of patients, and need for additional resources.

3. Assess mental status. Ensure an open airway, assess breathing, begin ventilations with BVM and oxygen at 10-15 lpm, assess circulatory status, and begin chest compressions.

4. Request response by ALS unit.

5. Attach semi-automated external defibrillator, and deliver shocks as directed.

6. Consider endotracheal intubation or placement of dual-lumen airway if authorized by local protocol.

7. Continue care until ALS unit arrives or transport with continued resuscitation.

Rationale

Because a valid DNR order is not present, resuscitation must be attempted.

23.19. **D,** In the absence of a DNR order, you should begin CPR, intubate if allowed by your protocols, and call for an advanced life support (ALS) unit.

SCENARIO EIGHT

Plan of Action
1. BSI
2. Is the scene safe? No. Take steps to remove immediate hazard caused by papers near stove. Assess nature of illness, number of patients, and need for additional resources.
3. Assess mental status. Ensure open airway, assess breathing, and assess circulatory status.
4. Determine priority.
5. Rapid head-to-toe examination
6. Baseline vital signs
7. HPI, SAMPLE
8. Obtain signed informed refusal from patient.
9. Return to station, document call and patient's living conditions, and notify appropriate social services agencies.

Rationale
This patient appears only to want help getting up from the floor. However, a survey of the scene indicates that she may have a number of medical and economic problems that are creating serious risks to her health. If the patient consents, a head-to-toe examination should be performed to ensure she was not injured by the fall. An attempt should be made to correct the immediate danger posed by the stacks of papers near an open fire. An informed refusal of transport should be obtained from the patient. The patient's situation should be documented thoroughly, and the appropriate social services agency should be notified.

23.20. **D,** Your most immediate concern is moving the newspapers away from the stove so they do not catch fire.

23.21. **C,** Move the papers away from the wood stove, have the patient sign a refusal form, return to your station, and notify the Department of Social Services.

23.22. **B,** Your greatest concern is that this patient may pose a danger to her own health.

24

Communications and Documentation

COMMUNICATIONS
Federal Communications Commission (FCC)
- Controls all radio communications in the United States
- Allocates specific radio frequencies for use
- Licenses base stations and assigns call signs
- Establishes licensing standards and operating specifications
- Establishes limits for transmitter power output
- Monitors radio operations

Frequencies
- Very high frequencies (VHF)
  - "Skip" by bouncing off layers in ionosphere
  - Long range
  - Unpredictable
- Ultrahigh frequencies (UHF)
  - Short ranges (line of sight)
  - Less likely to be interfered with than VHF
  - Work well in urban areas
  - Medical communication
    - 450 to 470 MHz frequency band
    - 800 MHz frequency band

Frequency Use
- Simplex
  - Radios receive, transmit on *same* frequency.
  - Only one party can talk at a time.
- Duplex
  - Radios receive, transmit on *different* frequencies.
  - Both parties can talk at the same time.
  - Transmitting frequency can carry one type of information at a time.
- Multiplex
  - Two or more signals (voice, electrocardiographic [ECG]) on one frequency simultaneously
  - Expensive
  - Loss of some quality in both signals
- Trunking
  - Common in 800-MHz systems
  - Several frequencies are pooled.
  - Computer routes messages to first available frequency.

EMS Communication Components
Base Station
- Transmitter/receiver at fixed location
- Used for dispatch, coordination, and medical control
- Power output is 42 to 275 watts.

Mobile Transmitter/Receivers
- Physically mounted in vehicles
- Power output is 20 to 50 watts.
- Range is 10 to 12 miles over average terrain.
  - Decreases in mountainous areas, areas with large buildings
  - Increases on water or flat terrain

Portable Transmitter/Receivers
- Handheld "walkie-talkie"
- Range limited by low output power

Repeaters
- Extend range of mobile and portable units
- Receive signal on one frequency and retransmit it on second frequency at higher power

Transmitting Information
- Have all information available *before* you start talking
- Report status of ABCs, the chief complaint, and vital signs *early*
- Use standard medical terminology. If you do not know the word, use plain English
- Repeat all orders. If you think an order is incorrect, ask physician to repeat order
- Stop talking every minute to ensure receiving station has copied your transmission
- Use standard format to report patient information
- If a standard format is not used
  - Essential information is not provided.
  - Time is wasted.
  - Patient care is delayed while the hospital attempts to get needed information.
  - Frustration will result.

Presenting Information
- Your unit's identification
- The patient's age and gender
- The patient's chief complaint
- A brief, pertinent history of the present illness (HPI), including scene assessment and mechanism of injury
- Major past illnesses
- The patient's mental status
- The patient's baseline vital signs
- Pertinent findings from your physical examination
- A description of the care you have given
- The patient's response to the care given
- Your estimated time of arrival

Using a Transmitter/Receiver
- Know what you are going to say before you start talking
- Do not waste air time
- Never transmit without monitoring the frequency first

- Wait 2 seconds after keying microphone before talking to allow repeaters to open
- Identify yourself on every transmission
- Speak at close range, directly into microphone
- Do not yell, use normal conversational tone and speed
- Articulate clearly
- Use proper English
- Avoid using codes and signals unless they are understood by everyone
- Be courteous
- Do *not* show emotion
- Do *not* curse or use obscene language
- Do *not* vocalize pauses
- Do *not* unkey your microphone until you have finished talking

Interpersonal Communication

- Make, keep eye contact
- Be confident
- Be respectful
  - Use proper names unless told otherwise
  - Do not speak condescendingly
  - Be conscious of cultural differences
- Be courteous
- Be truthful
- Use terms that the patient and family will understand
- Be careful of what you say about the patient and where you say it
- Be aware of your body language
- Speak slowly and enunciate
- Allow time for patient to answer

Special Patients

- Non–English speaking
  - Use interpreter
  - Use flash cards
  - Do *not* attempt language if unsure
  - Do *not* shout or speak in English slowly
- Hearing impaired
  - Use interpreter
  - Face patient when speaking
    - Allows them to see your lips
    - Allows them to see your facial expression
- Children
  - Get on their "level"
  - Approach slowly
  - Avoid threatening postures
  - Explain everything that you do
  - Do not lie
  - Respect child's modesty
  - Use parents to calm child (if parent is calm)

○ Let parent hold child if not contraindicated
○ Allow child to keep familiar objects
- Elderly patients
  ○ Use last names with appropriate title (Mr., Mrs., Miss) until told otherwise
  ○ Do not use slang
  ○ Do not assume senility, deafness, or infirmities
  ○ Be aware of cultural differences
  ○ Do not rush patient
  ○ Attend to family

DOCUMENTATION
Purpose of Documentation
- Patient care continuity
- Regulatory requirements
- Quality assurance
- Research
- Justification of treatment
- Protection for personnel
- Administration

A Good Medical Record Is...
- Accurate
  ○ Document facts, observations *only*
  ○ Double check numerical entries
  ○ Recheck spellings
  ○ If you make an error in patient care, document it
- Complete
  ○ The lines are there to fill in!
  ○ At least two sets of vitals for *every* patient
  ○ Failure to document implies failure to investigate.
  ○ Document pertinent negative findings
  ○ If it was not documented, it was not done.
- Legible
  ○ In court, documents must "speak for themselves."
  ○ Sloppy report implies sloppy care.
  ○ Recheck spellings
  ○ If the document cannot be deciphered, a jury may ignore it altogether.
- Free of extraneous information
  ○ Avoid labeling patient, report observations
  ○ Preface statements "per the witness" or "per the patient"
  ○ Record hearsay only if applicable
  ○ Do not record hearsay as fact
  ○ Avoid humor. The public does not regard EMS as "funny business."

Documentation Guidelines
- Good documentation reflects good care!
- Write report as soon after run as possible!

- If it needs to be corrected, correct it!
  ○ The earlier the correction, the more reliable the change
  ○ Mark through an error so it is still legible, then make correction and initial it
- For long reports, do not hesitate to add additional pages
- Report only facts, observations
- Avoid using "possible" when observations would have been obvious to anyone
- If you do something, say what you did, why you did it, when you did it, and what the result was
- If something should have been done, but was not, say why
- If you have a prolonged scene time, say why
- If times are to be documented on your report, do so accurately

Documentation of Patient Refusals

- Assess capacity of patient to refuse
- Perform assessment (if patient allows)
- Try to persuade patient to accept treatment, transport (if indicated)
- Explain consequences of refusing treatment, transport
- If the patient still refuses, document
  ○ Patient decision
  ○ Your assessment
  ○ Any attempts made to convince patient to accept treatment, transport
- Document patient refusal, obtain patient signature
- If patient will not sign, have document signed by family, law enforcement, or bystander

REVIEW QUESTIONS

Scenario One

You are transporting a 62-y.o. female who is c/o "squeezing" substernal chest pain. Her vital signs are blood pressure (BP)—118/70; pulse (P)—88, strong, regular; and respirations (R)—18, regular, unlabored. You have applied oxygen and made the patient as comfortable as possible. She has a past history of heart disease and has her own nitroglycerin with her. A paramedic unit is on the way to meet you but is still approximately 15 minutes away.

Multiple Choice

24.1. The UHF radio frequencies typically used by EMS organizations:
  a. fall between 32 and 50 MHz.
  b. fall between 150 and 174 MHz.
  c. fall between 450 and 470 MHz.
  d. are a band of 800 frequencies assigned to public safety agencies by the FCC.

24.2. Which of the following statements about UHF frequencies is *correct?*
  a. They are affected by "skip" more severely than VHF frequencies.
  b. They tend to have short ranges.
  c. They do not work well in urban areas because of interference from buildings.
  d. They are not limited to "line of sight."

24.3. The patient's chest pain would be a:
  a. sign.
  b. symptom.
  c. pertinent positive finding.
  d. pertinent negative finding.

24.4. Calling the emergency department for an order to assist the patient to take her own nitroglycerin would be an example of:

   a. standing orders.

   b. off-line medical control.

   c. on-line medical control.

   d. patient care protocol.

24.5. The radio frequency used by the paramedics to transmit the patient's ECG to the hospital would be:

   a. low band digital.

   b. VHF—low band.

   c. VHF—high band.

   d. UHF.

24.6. Which of the following statements *best* describes a duplex radio system?

   a. Radios can either transmit or receive on a single frequency but cannot transmit and receive at the same time.

   b. Radios can simultaneously transmit two signals (voice, ECG) on a single frequency.

   c. Radios receive on one frequency and transmit on another.

   d. Radios transmit voice on one frequency and ECG telemetry on another.

24.7. When you write your report of this call, which of the following would be an appropriate statement to include?

   a. "The patient was having a heart attack."

   b. "The patient's vital signs were 'normal.'"

   c. "The patient is having chest pain with a severity of 8 on a 1 to 10 scale."

   d. "The patient was very anxious and was exaggerating her pain."

24.8. The next day you remember that you did not document asking the patient about medication allergies when you took her history. You should:

   a. amend the original report to include the updated information, place your initials next to the new information, and date the change.

   b. fill in the missing information, making sure you use the same color pen so the change will not be obvious.

   c. not worry about making the change because this information had no effect on the outcome of the call.

   d. fill out a new run sheet to include the missing information.

Scenario Two

You are called to the main gate of a football stadium 10 minutes before a game is scheduled to start. You find an elderly male in cardiac arrest. After you use an automated external defibrillator (AED) to defibrillate him, a pulse returns, but he still is not breathing. You are having difficulty ventilating the patient with a bag-valve mask (BVM), and your system requires on-line orders to insert a Combitube. After several attempts you are unable to contact on-line medical control, and the patient is becoming increasingly cyanotic. A man steps out of the crowd, identifies himself as a doctor, and gives you an order to place the Combitube. He then accompanies you and the patient to the hospital. Later, when you ask him to sign your report verifying the order, you discover he is not licensed to practice medicine in your state.

Multiple Choice

24.9. Because you need a physician's signature for the orders, you should:

    a. return to the stadium and look for a doctor who is licensed in your state.

    b. have the doctor sign the your form and not document that he is not licensed in your state.

    c. explain the situation to the physician in charge of the emergency department, obtain his signature on the order, and then document the events.

    d. have the doctor sign your form, document the fact that he is not licensed in your state on the run sheet, and hope no one notices.

24.10. Being able to intubate without having to call for an order is an example of:

    a. designated protocols.

    b. quality assurance protocols.

    c. off-line medical control.

    d. standing orders.

24.11. As you call in your report to the emergency department, you should:

    a. use as many 10 codes as possible.

    b. increase your voice volume as you speak into the microphone.

    c. begin speaking immediately after you depress the "transmit" button.

    d. hold the microphone 2 to 3 inches from your mouth.

24.12. Which of the following is the *most* appropriate order in which to relay information to the hospital?

    a. Age, gender, chief complaint, medical history, vital signs, physical examination findings, treatments given, and estimated time of arrival

    b. Age, gender, past medical history, chief complaint, physical examination findings, vital signs, treatments given, and estimated time of arrival

    c. Age, chief complaint, patient's physician, vital signs, physical examination findings, medical history, treatments given, and estimated time of arrival

    d. Gender, age, chief complaint, patient's physician, medical history, vital signs, physical examination findings, treatment given, and estimated time of arrival

24.13. All of the following statements about documentation are true *except:*

    a. documentation prepared by an EMT-Basic may be used later in court.

    b. documentation completed by an EMT-Basic is used in quality assurance programs.

    c. documentation on the run sheet should be available for family members to view if requested.

    d. the EMT-Basic's report is an important part of the hospital's patient care record.

24.14. The *most common* cause of liability for emergency medical technicians is:

    a. breach of confidentiality.

    b. patient refusal of care or transport.

    c. entering too much information on the patient care report.

    d. being exposed to infectious disease.

24.15. What agency has defined the minimum data to be included in all prehospital patient care reports?
   a. National Highway Traffic Safety Administration
   b. Department of Health and Human Services
   c. Department of Transportation
   d. Federal Emergency Management Association

24.16. When you call in a report to the hospital, you should:
   a. always use only the patient's first name.
   b. speak clearly.
   c. use 10 codes as much as possible.
   d. speak clearly and state your opinions near the end of the report.

Answer Key—Chapter 24

24.1. C, The UHF radio frequencies typically used in EMS fall between 450 and 470 MHz.

24.2. B, UHF radios have short ranges that limit them to communicating with radios that are in "line of sight" with their antennas. UHF radios are less affected by "skip" than VHF radios and tend to work better in urban areas.

24.3. B, A symptom is subjective information the patient must tell the EMT about—for example, chest pain, headache, or nausea. A sign is an objective finding the EMT can see, feel, or hear—for example, bruising, cyanosis, crackles, or abdominal rigidity. A pertinent negative finding is a sign or symptom you would expect to be present based on the patient's complaint that is, in fact, not present.

24.4. C, A direct order given by radio or telephone from a physician to an EMT is an example of on-line medical control.

24.5. D, Telemetry is transmitted using UHF frequencies.

24.6. C, Duplex radio systems transmit on one frequency and receive on another. This allows persons using the radios to talk as if they were using a telephone and not have to be concerned about ensuring the other party has completed a transmission before speaking. Simplex systems, which use only one frequency, allow only one radio to transmit at a time. A multiplex system allows two signals (voice, ECG) to be transmitted simultaneously on a single frequency.

24.7. C, Patient care reports should include only objective information about the patient's condition or the management of the call. Describing the patient's pain on a scale of 1 to 10 is an example of this kind of objective information. Until a 12-lead ECG can be performed, it will not be possible to determine that the patient is, in fact, having a myocardial infarction. Use of the term "normal" provides no record of what the patient's condition actually was. Stating that the patient was "very anxious" or was "exaggerating" introduces your subjective opinions into the report.

24.8. A, You should make the new entry, initial it, and date the change so anyone reading the report later can easily determine the addition was made after the original report was written.

24.9. C, The most appropriate response would be to have the physician in charge of the emergency department sign the order and document the events.

24.10. D, When you can perform a task without calling the hospital for permission, you are operating under a standing order. Standing orders often are part of more comprehensive protocols, which detail treatment that should be provided for patients with particular complaints.

24.11. D, When you call in a radio report, you should hold the microphone 2 to 3 inches from your mouth and speak directly into it with a clear voice. The microphone key should be depressed for a couple of seconds before beginning to speak to ensure the first part of your transmission is not cut off. You should not speak more loudly than you do in normal conversation. Codes and signals should not be used unless they are in common use and likely to be understood by everyone who receives a radio transmission.

24.12. **A,** The most appropriate sequence of information in a radio report is age, gender, chief complaint, medical history, vital signs, physical examination findings, treatments given, and estimated time of arrival. Using the same format for every report ensures important information is not omitted.

24.13. **C,** Information on the run sheet is confidential and is not available to family members.

24.14. **B,** The most common cause of liability is patient refusal of care or transport. In these situations, EMS personnel need to document that the patient had the mental capacity to refuse care and transport, was told the potential complications of refusing care, and was advised to call EMS or go to the emergency department if any problems developed later.

24.15. **A,** The National Highway Traffic Safety Administration (NHTSA) has defined a minimum standard set of data to be included in all prehospital patient care reports.

24.16. **B,** Radio transmissions should be made using a clear voice. Patient names should not be included in radio reports. Use of 10 codes should be limited because hospital personnel frequently do not know their meaning. Radio reports should never include opinions. They should include objective information only.

25

Ambulance Operations

AMBULANCE TYPES

- Type I—Conventional cab with modular body, no passageway present between patient compartment and operator compartment
- Type II—Van, usually with a raised roof; patient compartment and operator compartment are an integral unit.
- Type III—Conventional cab with modular body, walkway between patient compartment and operator compartment

AMBULANCE STANDARDS

- KKK—1822 standards
  - Federal government standards for *federally purchased* ambulances
  - Frequently adopted by state and local governments
- Occupational Safety and Health Administration (OSHA) standards
  - Primarily developed for infection control
  - Address ambulance and equipment specifications
- American College of Surgeons Committee on Trauma Minimum Essential Equipment for Ambulances
  - Listing of minimum ambulance equipment developed by American College of Surgeons
  - Frequently used as basis for state and local equipment requirements

EMERGENCY DRIVING LAWS

- Traffic laws in most states allow the driver of an authorized emergency vehicle to
  - *Park or stand* the vehicle where otherwise prohibited
  - *Proceed past a red light or stop signal,* but only after slowing down as may be necessary for safe operation
  - *Exceed the maximum speed* limits as long as the driver does not endanger life or property
  - *Disregard regulations governing direction of movement or turning* in specified directions
- Exemptions from traffic laws granted to an authorized emergency vehicle usually apply only when the vehicle is being operated during an emergency and is making use of *appropriate audible and visual signals.*
- Exemptions from the traffic laws do not relieve the driver of an authorized emergency vehicle from the duty to drive with *due regard for the safety of all persons.*

GOOD DRIVING BASICS

- Wear seat belts
- Practice; become familiar with ambulance
  - Acceleration
  - Deceleration
  - Braking
  - Cornering
  - Fender and bumper clearance
- Hand position on steering wheel
  - 9 o'clock and 3 o'clock positions
  - One hand pulls, the other slides.
  - Neither hand should pass 6 o'clock or 12 o'clock position.
- Keep to the left (other traffic should be to the right)
- Never rely on what another motorist will do

MAINTAINING CONTROL

- Braking
  - Apply brakes slowly, smoothly
  - *Never* brake on curve
  - Brake going into curves, accelerate moving out of them
- Railroads
  - Plan alternate routes for grade crossings
  - Wait out long trains if there is no overpass or underpass within a reasonable distance
- School buses
  - Emergency vehicle exemptions may not apply to laws governing school buses loading and unloading children.
  - If red lights on school bus are flashing, stop and wait until driver motions you on
- Bridges and tunnels
  - Ability to pass may be limited.
  - Consider alternative routes if traffic is heavy
  - Be sure height of roadway will accommodate ambulance
- Traffic patterns
  - Learn traffic flow patterns in your area based on time of day, day of week, and locations
  - Plan for alternative routes through or past specific problem areas
- Road surface
  - Pay attention to irregularities in road surface (bumps, potholes)
  - Inner lanes of multilane highways usually are smoothest
- Hydroplaning
  - Occurs on wet roads at speeds >35 mph
  - Water causes loss of contact between tire and road surface.
  - If you cannot see tread marks of car ahead of you in water on highway, there is risk of hydroplaning.
  - Slow down, lightly tap brakes to ensure dryness
- Backing up
  - *Always* have someone spot for driver while ambulance is backing
  - Move slowly, carefully
- Escorts
  - Extremely dangerous
  - Use only when unfamiliar with location of patient or hospital
  - Allow safe distance between escort vehicle and ambulance

INTERSECTION COLLISIONS

- Most common form of ambulance collision
- Causes
  - Other drivers "timing" lights
  - Emergency vehicles following each other
  - Multiple emergency vehicles converging on same location
  - Motorists going around stopped traffic
  - Vision of pedestrians in crosswalk obstructed by other vehicles
- Slow down at intersections
- Ensure other drivers have seen you and stopped before you proceed

WARNING LIGHTS
- Use at all times when responding to emergency calls
- Turn on headlights during daylight hours
- Use minimal lighting in heavy fog or when parked

SIREN
- Relatively ineffective
- Motorists are less inclined to give the right of way to an ambulance when the siren is used continuously.
- Never pull directly behind a car and blast your siren
- Sirens may affect patients adversely.
- Sirens may cause driver to speed excessively or to take risks.
- Give other drivers time to notice, react to warning devices

POSITIONING AMBULANCE AT SCENE
- Assess scene safety, establish danger zone
- If no fire or hazardous materials, park at least 50 feet away
- If fire present, park at least 100 feet from a wreckage, upwind and uphill (if possible)
- If first on scene, park in front of the wreckage to shield wreck from traffic
- If other emergency vehicles on scene, park beyond wreck so ambulance is shielded from traffic

AEROMEDICAL OPERATIONS
- Why call a helicopter?
  - Access to interventions not available from ground unit (Be sure this is true before calling for this reason.)
  - Rapid patient transport for critically ill or injured patients
  - Most helicopter services will not transport patients who are in cardiac arrest.
- Landing zone (LZ)
  - Flat area clear of obstructions
  - Daytime—60 feet × 60 feet
  - Nighttime—100 feet × 100 feet
  - At least 50 yards from rescue scene to minimize rotorwash effects
  - Remove loose debris, wet down area with water fog to minimize dust
  - On divided highways, stop all traffic in both directions
  - Warn crew of locations of power lines, poles, antennas, and trees
  - At night, mark each corner of LZ with a light; put a fifth light on the upwind side
  - *Never* point any kind of light at a helicopter on approach at night
  - Move bystanders back at least 200 feet
  - Keep emergency personnel 100 feet away during landing
  - No smoking within 50 feet of aircraft
- Communications with crew
  - Describe your location in terms of the ship's location, not yours
  - For example, "Medivac 1, we have you in sight. We are at your 10 o'clock position."
- Operations near helicopters
  - Secure all loose items, including hats and stretcher sheets
  - Never approach until pilot signals you to

- ○ Approach from front, keeping pilot in sight
- ○ Approach from downhill if ship is on incline
- ○ *Never* cross behind or underneath the ship
- ○ Crouch when approaching, leaving ship
- ○ *Never* attempt to open a door or operate other equipment on the ship
- ○ Follow *all* crew instructions exactly
- ○ By federal law, the pilot has absolute command over the ship.
- ○ He or she has final authority to determine whether to attempt a mission or a maneuver.
- ○ Highest priority always is given to the safety of the ship and its crew.

REVIEW QUESTIONS

Scenario One

It is 11:15 PM on a cold day in January. You are transporting a patient who has been drinking and is c/o chest pain. Your ambulance is passing through a green traffic signal when it is struck broadside by a car traveling at approximately 50 mph.

Multiple Choice

25.1. How many feet away from the collision should responding units park?
- **a.** 25
- **b.** 50
- **c.** 75
- **d.** 100

25.2. All of the following statements about ambulance operations are correct *except:*
- **a.** an ambulance on an emergency call should have its lights and siren operating.
- **b.** intersections are the most common location for ambulance collisions.
- **c.** ambulances must come to a full stop even if the light is green.
- **d.** the driver should look left, then right, and then left again before crossing an intersection.

25.3. As rescuers arrive on the scene their *first* concern should be:
- **a.** extricating any patients using appropriate spinal precautions.
- **b.** ensuring no hazards are present.
- **c.** calling for air transport as quickly as possible.
- **d.** requesting any additional emergency vehicles needed.

25.4. The rescue vehicles should park:
- **a.** downhill from the wreckage.
- **b.** in the nearest parking lot.
- **c.** on the sidewalk.
- **d.** upwind from the wreckage.

25.5. All of the following statements about using the siren are correct *except:*
- **a.** motorists are less likely to yield when the siren is used continuously.
- **b.** the siren should be used at intersections as little as possible.
- **c.** continuous siren use may worsen a patient's condition.
- **d.** you should assume that some motorists will be unable to hear the siren.

Scenario Two

You have been dispatched to a motor vehicle collision (MVC). En route, the dispatcher tells you two other ambulances, the fire department, and law enforcement also are responding. On arrival you find two cars have been involved. The first vehicle is resting on its top and has extensive structural damage. The second vehicle is on fire. The driver of the first vehicle is lying in the roadway with a piece of metal protruding from his upper right chest. He is having difficulty breathing, and his lips are cyanotic. Breath sounds are diminished in the right side of his chest. A passenger is trapped inside the first vehicle. She has her seat belt on, is alert and oriented, and says she is not in any distress. Bystanders have removed the driver of the second vehicle from the burning wreckage. He has burns on his arms, hands, and face. He is alert and oriented and has severe pain.

Multiple Choice

25.6. Which of the following statements about air transport is *correct?*
   a. Helicopters are able to operate effectively in any type of terrain.
   b. The LZ should be at least 300 feet × 300 feet at night.
   c. A 68-y.o. trauma patient in cardiac arrest is a good candidate for air transport.
   d. When communicating with the helicopter, give directions relative to its location: for example, "Air One, we are at your 3 o'clock position."

25.7. A landing zone should slope:
   a. <8 degrees.
   b. <10 degrees but >5 degrees.
   c. at least 8 degrees.
   d. at least 10 degrees.

25.8. Which of the following statements is *most* correct?
   a. The burn patient should be flown.
   b. The patient with the penetrating object in his chest should be flown.
   c. The burn patient and the patient with the penetrating object in his chest should be flown.
   d. All three patients should be flown.

25.9. The *most* dangerous area near a helicopter is the:
   a. approach area.
   b. area under the main rotor.
   c. rear of the aircraft near the tail rotor.
   d. area downhill from where the helicopter lands.

25.10. One advantage of using a helicopter is its:
   a. lack of altitude limitations.
   b. ability to access remote areas.
   c. ability to fly regardless of environmental conditions.
   d. ability to land on steep slopes.

25.11. An ambulance with conventional cab, a modular body, and no passageway from the patient area to the driver's area is a:
   a. type I ambulance.
   b. type II ambulance.
   c. type III ambulance.
   d. type IV ambulance.

25.12. What is the duration of the "golden hour"?
   a. From the time EMS arrives until the patient is in the emergency department
   b. From the time the patient is injured until the patient arrives at the emergency department
   c. From the time the patient is injured until the patient is in the operating room
   d. From the time the call is dispatched until the patient is given advanced care

Scenario Three

While you are responding to single-car MVC, your ambulance comes up behind an 85-y.o. female who is driving at 15 mph. The oncoming traffic is very heavy.

Multiple Choice

25.13. All of the following statements about road safety are true *except:*
   a. excessive speed may cause loss of vehicle control.
   b. anticipating other drivers' actions may result in an accident.
   c. failure to obey traffic lights and signals may result in an accident.
   d. inadequate dispatch information may result in unsafe driving.

25.14. As you approach the scene what should be your *highest* priority?
   a. Using kinematics to determine if the patients may be critically injured
   b. Deciding whether fire-rescue is needed
   c. Identifying any hazards that may be present
   d. Determining if the patients will need air transport

25.15. The recommended list of equipment and supplies that should be carried on all basic life support ambulances was developed by the:
   a. American College of Surgeons Committee on Trauma.
   b. U.S. Department of Transportation.
   c. American College of Emergency Physicians.
   d. U.S. Department of Health and Human Services.

25.16. What are protocols?
   a. Guidelines that allow EMTs to treat patients without having to contact on-line medical control
   b. Guidelines that provide EMTs with standardized patient care procedures
   c. Procedures for paramedics to follow when giving medications so they do not have to contact medical control
   d. Suggestions for EMTs to follow when treating patients

Scenario Three—cont'd

At the scene you find an 18-y.o. female with multiple lacerations and abrasions suffered when her car skidded off the road and struck a tree. After bandaging her injuries, you place her in a Kendrick extrication device (KED), extricate her to a long spine board, and place the spine board on an ambulance stretcher.

Multiple Choice

25.17. How many rescuers should be present when a wheeled ambulance stretcher is moved over rough terrain?
   a. At least six
   b. Two, one at the foot and one at the head facing forward
   c. Four, one on each end and one on each side facing each other
   d. Four, one on each corner of the stretcher

25.18. Which statement about rolling a wheeled ambulance stretcher over level ground is *correct?*
   a. The stretcher should be pushed from the head end.
   b. The stretcher should be moved by at least three rescuers.
   c. The EMTs should stand at the sides of the stretcher while it is moving.
   d. The stretcher should be pulled from the foot end.

25.19. When you receive an order from medical control, you should *immediately:*
   a. carry out the order, and then document the treatment provided.
   b. document the order and the time it was issued.
   c. relay the order to the rest of your crew so they can assist you.
   d. repeat the order to the physician.

25.20. The radio at the hospital is a _____ _____, whereas the radio you carry with you is a _____ _____.
   a. base radio, mobile radio
   b. fixed radio, portable radio
   c. base radio, portable radio
   d. high-power transmitter, low-power transmitter

Answer Key—Chapter 25

25.1. B, If no fire or hazardous materials are present, emergency vehicles should park at least 50 feet away from the scene.

25.2. C, If the traffic light is green, the driver should slow, look in both directions, and then proceed. If the light is red, the driver should stop, look in both directions, and then proceed cautiously.

25.3. B, The EMT's first concern is to ensure no hazards are present.

25.4. D, If fire or hazardous materials may be present, vehicles should be parked upwind and uphill from the scene.

25.5. B, The siren should be used at intersections to ensure crossing traffic is aware an emergency vehicle is present. Motorists are less inclined to give the right of way to an ambulance when the siren is used continuously. Continuous use of a siren may cause the patient to become more anxious, worsening his or her condition. Some motorists may not be able to hear the siren because of hearing impairment or design features of their vehicles.

25.6. D, Directions to the helicopter should be given relative to its position, not the EMT's. LZs must be ~100 × 100 feet with <8-degree slope. Helicopters may be unable to land if the terrain is steep or uneven. Patients in cardiac arrest are not good candidates for air transport because the small patient care area limits the crew's ability to provide appropriate care for them.

25.7. A, The ground at a LZ should slope <8 degrees.

25.8. C, The burn patient and the patient with penetrating chest trauma are candidates for air transport.

25.9. C, The most dangerous area near a helicopter is the rear of the aircraft where the tail rotor is spinning so fast it cannot be seen. Never approach a helicopter from the rear.

25.10. B, Helicopters can access remote areas and provide rapid transport. However, helicopters have altitude and weather limitations and cannot land on steep slopes.

25.11. A, A type I ambulance has a conventional cab with a modular body and no passageway present between the patient and driver compartments. A type II ambulance is a van with a raised roof. A type III ambulance has a conventional cab with a modular body and a passageway between the patient and driver compartments.

25.12. C, The "golden hour" begins when a patient is injured and ends when the patient is in the operating room. A seriously injured patient who reaches the operating room within the "golden hour" has a greater probability of survival.

25.13. B, Always anticipate the possibility of inappropriate responses by other drivers when they realize an emergency vehicle is approaching. Anticipating improper or erratic moves by other drivers reduces your risk of having an accident by allowing you to plan ahead and respond quickly.

25.14. C, As you approach a scene, your highest priority should be to identify any hazards that may be present.

25.15. A, The American College of Surgeons Committee on Trauma developed the essential equipment list for ambulances.

25.16. B, Protocols are guidelines that provide EMTs with standardized patient care procedures. A portion of a protocol that may be carried out without contacting on-line medical control is a standing order.

25.17. D, A minimum of four rescuers, one for each corner of the stretcher, should be present when a wheeled ambulance cot is moved over rough terrain.

25.18. A, When a wheeled stretcher is being rolled over level ground it should be pushed from the head end while the rescuer at the foot guides. When a stretcher is being rolled, the patient will be more comfortable if he or she is facing the direction of movement.

25.19. D, When you receive an order on-line from a physician, always immediately repeat the order back to the doctor word for word.

25.20. C, The hospital has a base radio, and the radio you carry is a portable radio.

26

Extrication and Rescue

GENERAL PRINCIPLES

- Successful rescues are based on planning, practice.
- Know what your community's target hazards are
- Have plans for managing these hazards
- Know who you will be working with; train with them.
- Know what kinds of help are available
- Do *not* be afraid to call for help if you need it!
- All rescue operations include seven basic stages:
  - Size-up
  - Hazard control
  - Gaining access
  - Life-saving care
  - Disentanglement
  - Preparation for removal
  - Removal
- Use the seven stages to form a mental picture of how the operation will be carried out

SIZE-UP

- Begins at moment of dispatch, continues throughout rescue
- En route
  - Think through the seven stages
  - Decide what you are going to do first
- When you arrive
  - Avoid being caught up in the situation
  - Step back, survey scene for
    - Safety
      - Are there potential hazards to you?
      - Are bystanders at risk?
      - Is the patient in danger?
    - Outside help
      - Is additional assistance needed?
      - If you need something, call for it!
      - Stay ahead of the situation
      - If you routinely work with other agencies, have plan of operations worked out in advance
    - Significant information
      - What kinds of vehicles?
      - How many?
      - What kind of collision?
      - How many patients?
      - Any potential for hazardous materials?
      - Anyone ejected?

HAZARD CONTROL

- Traffic
  - Park on same side of highway as collision
  - Park up highway, beyond scene if possible
  - Have someone spotting traffic at all times

○ Wear reflective clothing at night
○ Provide clear visual signals to drivers *well in advance* of reaching scene
- Power lines
  ○ Consciously look for lines on ground
  ○ Use particular caution when vehicle has struck utility pole or tree
  ○ Tell patients to stay in vehicle
  ○ Call the power company!
- Gasoline or fuel spillage
  ○ Shut off vehicle ignition keys
  ○ Remove all ignition sources from area, use caution with flares
  ○ Ask fire department to get a charged hose line on the ground
  ○ Disconnect battery cable—Weigh risks vs. benefits
- "Loaded" bumpers
  ○ Impact-absorbing bumpers may be locked in compressed position by impact.
  ○ During extrication operations compressed bumpers may be released, causing them to spring out and strike rescuers.
  ○ Identify loaded bumpers and ensure they are appropriately secured or avoid working in front of them
- Air bags
  ○ May deploy during rescue attempts, striking rescuers
  ○ Disconnecting battery does *not* immediately deactivate air bags because of charge stored in capacitors.
- Unstable vehicles
  ○ Any vehicle that does not have all four wheels touching the pavement is unstable!
  ○ Never push back into position
  ○ Stabilize as found
  ○ Maximize number of contact points with ground, spread over as wide an area as possible
  ○ Tools for stabilizing vehicles
    - Wood wedges, cribbing
    - Air bags
    - Come-along tool
    - Hydraulic rams
    - Jacks, hydraulic jacks
    - Chains
- Hazardous materials
  ○ Assume presence at all incidents until proven otherwise
  ○ Base decision to attempt rescue on best available information about product(s) and on expert advice
- Appropriate protective clothing
  ○ At least helmet, gloves
  ○ Eye protection
  ○ Work boots
  ○ Turnout coat

GAINING ACCESS

- Objective is to get to patient to provide care, *not* to remove patient
- Try before you pry!

- Work from simple to complex
  - Simple access—Does not require equipment
  - Complex access—Requires specialized equipment
- Residences
  - Check for open windows, doors
  - Ask if anyone else (neighbor, relative) has key
  - If a window is open, cut through screen
  - If no windows are open, break smallest window through which access can be obtained
- Upright vehicle
  - Enter through doors
  - When you open door, be sure patient is not against it
  - If door is locked, ask patient if he or she can open it
  - If door will not open, break furthest window away from patient to gain access
- Vehicle on side
  - Stabilize vehicle
  - Enter through top door
  - If door will not open, break rear window
- Vehicle upside down
  - Gain access through windows
  - Doors may be supporting vehicle body.
  - Careless door opening, removal may cause vehicle to collapse.
- Breaking vehicle windows
  - Tempered glass (side, rear windows) can be broken quickly and effectively with a sharp blow to the corner of a window approximately 2 inches from the edge of the glass.
  - Safety glass (windshields) contains a plastic laminate between two layers of glass, which resists breaking.

LIFE-SAVING CARE

- Rapidly evaluate patient's condition
- Immediate threats are
  - Hypoxia
  - Shock
- At this point, *why* the patient is not oxygenating or perfusing is irrelevant.
- If the ABCs are compromised, correct the problem!
- If you cannot correct problem
  - Support oxygenation, ventilation
  - Extricate patient to long board as quickly as possible
  - Rapidly transport

DISENTANGLEMENT

- Patient-centered process
- Remove vehicle from patient, *not* patient from vehicle!
- Keep someone with patient to
  - Monitor condition
  - Ensure attack on vehicle does not endanger patient
- Protect patient at all times
  - Cover with blanket for protection

○ Explain what is happening
- Do *not* do anything to vehicle unless you know *exactly* what the result will be

PREPARATION FOR REMOVAL

- Packaging—Preparing patient for removal as unit
- All injuries stabilized
- Patient moves as single unit through route of egress.
- Any lower extremity injury can be stabilized temporarily by securing it to other extremity.
- Any upper extremity injury can be stabilized temporarily by securing it to the chest.
- Kendrick extrication devices (KEDs) are used to keep head-neck-torso in line during extrication; patient must be extricated onto a long board.
- Do *not* attempt complete packaging of patients with compromised ABCs

REMOVAL

- Through *doors* if vehicle is *upright*
- Through *roof* if vehicle is on *side*
- Through *window* if vehicle is *overturned*

REVIEW QUESTIONS
Scenario One

You have been dispatched to a motor vehicle collision (MVC) involving multiple vehicles. Three cars are involved. The first car is upside down in a drainage ditch with access obstructed from either side. The next five questions concern this vehicle.

Multiple Choice

26.1. Which of the following actions should be performed *first?*
    a. Perform initial assessments on all patients
    b. Gain entry through the windshield
    c. Gain entry through the back window
    d. Stabilize the vehicle

26.2. The following are potential hazards *except:*
    a. the fact the vehicle is upside down in the ditch.
    b. the gasoline that has spilled from the gas tank and engine.
    c. the broken glass around the perimeter of the vehicle.
    d. the fact the ignition is shut off.

True/False

26.3. The presence of spectators is a hazard.
    a. True
    b. False

Multiple Choice

26.4. Accessing the vehicle through the rear window would be an example of:
    a. simple access.
    b. disentanglement.
    c. complex access.
    d. rapid access.

True/False

26.5. The rescue crew should place safety flares at the scene.
  a. True
  b. False

Scenario One—cont'd

The second vehicle is a small passenger automobile that rolled over but now is sitting upright on all four wheels. The vehicle has major damage to its front end, and its sides appear to be crushed in.

Multiple Choice

26.6. The rescuers should *first:*
  a. stabilize the vehicle, then attempt to open the doors.
  b. attempt to pry open the doors.
  c. stabilize the vehicle, then attempt to gain entry through the rear window.
  d. stabilize the vehicle, then attempt to gain entry through the side windows.

True/False

26.7. Removing a vehicle's roof is a quick, efficient means of gaining access.
  a. True
  b. False

Multiple Choice

26.8. All of the following are advantages of removing a vehicle's roof *except:*
  a. removing the roof makes the vehicle's entire interior accessible.
  b. rescuers are able to kneel next to the vehicle while carrying out patient care.
  c. a large opening is created to rapidly remove patients with life-threatening injuries.
  d. removing the roof provides fresh air for the patients.

26.9. The best place for EMTs to park ambulances as they arrive on the scene would be:
  a. as close as possible.
  b. within 50 feet of the accident so equipment is readily available.
  c. on the opposite side of the road, at least 25 feet away.
  d. on the same side of the road at least 50 feet away.

Scenario One—cont'd

The third vehicle is a sport utility vehicle that is lying on its side across the roadway.

26.10. The crew needs to:
  a. begin rapid extrication of the patient inside.
  b. gain access through the rear window.
  c. gain access through one of the side doors.
  d. stabilize the vehicle.

26.11. Vehicle windshields are made of:
  a. blunt glass.
  b. tempered reinforced glass.
  c. safety glass.
  d. unbreakable tempered glass.

26.12. The part of the vehicle that separates the engine compartment from the passenger compartment is the:
   a. firewall.
   b. support post.
   c. rocker wall.
   d. safety wall.

26.13. What is the function of the Nader pin?
   a. It limits how much glass breaks when a windshield is struck.
   b. It prevents car doors from flying open when the vehicle is involved in a collision.
   c. It automatically cuts off the ignition when the vehicle is involved in a collision.
   d. It separates the engine from the passenger compartment.

26.14. The side and back windows of a vehicle are made of:
   a. blunt glass.
   b. tempered glass.
   c. safety glass.
   d. unbreakable tempered glass.

26.15. All of the following statements about MVC management are correct *except:*
   a. an airbag is unlikely to deploy after a crash.
   b. unstable vehicles are an uncommon hazard in rescue operations.
   c. ordinary fire extinguishers can be used to put out vehicle fires.
   d. the car battery generally should be left connected.

26.16. The *best* way to remove a patient from the drainage ditch to the ambulance would be with a:
   a. wheeled stretcher carried by at least six rescuers.
   b. basket stretcher carried by four rescuers.
   c. basket stretcher carried by six rescuers.
   d. spine board placed in a basket stretcher with at least four rescuers carrying the stretcher.

Scenario Two

After clearing the multicar MVC, you receive another call for a plane down in a swamp. On arrival at the staging area, you find local fire-rescue personnel preparing to walk 2 miles to the plane's location. At the crash site you find a small twin-engine aircraft lying upside down. One wing is missing, and both doors are crushed. Two victims are inside the plane. Both appear to be unconscious.

Multiple Choice

26.17. The *first* action you should take is:
   a. attempting to open the aircraft's doors.
   b. observing the ground around the plane for spilled fuel.
   c. observing the ground for other victims.
   d. attempting entry through the front window.

26.18. The *greatest* hazard in this situation is:
   a. broken glass.
   b. collapse of the plane's roof.
   c. being overcome by fumes.
   d. fire caused by spilled fuel.

Scenario Three

A 36-y.o. male fell 8 feet into a silo, landing on a pile of silage. Fire-rescue personnel are preparing to remove him. His only complaints are back pain and right lower leg pain. Vital signs are not available because no one has reached him yet.

Multiple Choice

26.19. The *most* common danger associated with confined spaces is that:
  a. rescuers have limited access caused by structural problems.
  b. they are difficult for the rescuer to crawl through.
  c. they often are oxygen deficient.
  d. they frequently contain hazardous materials.

26.20. All of the following statements about confined spaces are correct *except:*
  a. confined spaces may contain toxic or explosive chemicals.
  b. confined spaces may pose difficult extrication problems.
  c. there always is the danger of being entrapped in machinery.
  d. equipment in confined spaces may contain stored energy, creating a potential for electrocution.

Answer Key—*Chapter 26*

26.1. D, Before attempting to enter the vehicle or assess the patients, you should ensure the vehicle is stabilized. An unstable vehicle could shift position, injuring you or causing further injury to the patients.

26.2. D, The ignition being off is not a hazard. However, it may create difficulty opening electric windows and door locks.

26.3. A, Spectators are a hazard because they may become injured or interfere with rescue operations.

26.4. C, Breaking a window or forcing a door to gain entry is complex access. Simple access would be to roll down the window or unlock the door.

26.5. A, Flares are placed around the accident scene to give rescuers a perimeter to work in, to warn approaching motorists, and to keep spectators out of the area. Flares should be used cautiously because they may ignite spilled fuel.

26.6. A, After stabilizing the vehicles, rescuers should attempt simple access by trying to open all of the vehicle's doors. If a door will not open, breaking a window or using power tools to pry open a door can be done to achieve complex access.

26.7. A, Sometimes removing the roof is the quickest way to gain access.

26.8. B, When the roof is removed rescuers are *not* able to kneel next to the vehicle to provide patient care.

26.9. D, Position the ambulance at least 50 feet from the wreckage on the same side of the road as the collision. If the ambulance is the first vehicle on the scene, park behind the wreckage. If not, then park ahead of the wreckage. Always try to position the vehicle so it protects the scene and at the same time provides the least amount of disruption to the traffic flow.

26.10. D, The vehicle must be stabilized before attempts are made to gain access.

26.11. C, Windshields are made of safety glass. The side and back windows of vehicles are made of tempered glass. Safety glass consists of two layers of glass with a layer of plastic laminate between.

26.12. A, The firewall separates the engine compartment from the passenger compartment.

26.13. B, The Nader pin prevents car doors from flying open during collisions.

26.14. B, The side and back windows of vehicles are made of tempered glass. When tempered glass breaks, it shatters into small cubes.

26.15. B, Unstable vehicles are a common hazard in rescue operations.

26.16. D, The patient should be secured to a long spine board and then placed in a basket stretcher for removal from the drainage ditch.

26.17. B, Scene safety should be ensured including determining whether fuel has spilled from the plane. After any hazards are corrected, attempts to gain access can begin.

26.18. D, The greatest danger in this situation is the potential for a fire caused by spilled fuel.

26.19. C, The most common danger associated with confined spaces is lack of adequate oxygen levels to sustain life.

26.20. C, Confined spaces do not always contain machinery.

27

Biological and Chemical Terrorism

CHEMICAL AGENTS
Categories
- Nerve agents (neurotoxins)
- Blood agents (chemical asphyxiants)
- Blister agents (skin irritants)
- Choking agents (pulmonary irritants)
- Others (anhydrous ammonia, sulfur dioxide, sulfuric acid, and hydrogen fluoride)

Nerve Agents
- Toxicology
  - Related to organophosphate pesticides but several times more deadly
  - Nerve agents enter the body primarily through inhalation but can also be absorbed, ingested, or injected (including entering through open wounds). VX and tabun (GA) can persist in liquid form for extended periods and pose a contact hazard.
  - Bind to and inactivate enzyme acetylcholinesterase
  - Cause buildup of excess acetylcholine
- Examples, military designations, and characteristics
  - Tabun (GA)—Colorless to brown liquid with fruity odor, gives colorless vapor
  - Sarin (GB)—Colorless, odorless liquid
  - Soman (GD)—Yellow-brown liquid with camphor odor (industrial product) or colorless liquid with fruity odor (pure product)
  - VX—Amber-colored oily, odorless liquid
- Signs and symptoms
  - Eyes and nose—Miosis (constricted pupils), tearing, conjunctivitis, dim or blurred vision, pain, and rhinorrhea (runny nose)
  - Respiratory—Difficulty breathing, cough, bronchospasms, chest tightness, and excessive secretions
  - Gastrointestinal—Increased bowel activity, cramps, nausea, vomiting, and diarrhea
  - Central nervous system—Restlessness, anxiety, tachycardia, respiratory and circulatory depression, and coma
  - Somatic—Weakness, paralysis, general muscle twitching, and seizures
- Treatment
  - Remove patient from environment
  - Remove clothing, wash with diluted hypochlorite solution, soap, and water
  - Maintain open airway, give high-concentration oxygen, and assist ventilations as needed
  - Advanced life support (ALS)
    - Atropine 2 mg every 5 minutes until excessive secretions stop
    - Pralidoxime (2-PAM chloride) 600 mg every 5 minutes for a total of 1600 mg
    - Valium (diazepam) for seizures

Blood Agents (Chemical Asphyxiants)
- Toxicology
  - Interfere with ability of cells to use oxygen
  - Enter body through inhalation
- Examples, military designations, and characteristics
  - Cyanide chloride (CK)—Colorless gas or liquid

○ Hydrogen cyanide (AC)—Colorless gas with odor of bitter almonds
- Signs and symptoms
  ○ Respiratory—Tachypnea progressing to bradycardia, deep breathing, dyspnea, bradypnea, respiratory depression, and respiratory failure
  ○ Cardiovascular—Heart palpitations, flushing of skin, headache, tachycardia, cherry red skin, bright red venous blood, hypertension progressing to hypotension, and cardiac arrest
  ○ Gastrointestinal—Nausea, vomiting
  ○ Central nervous system—Dizziness, giddiness, restlessness, anxiety, seizures, and coma
  ○ Causes almost no effects with brief exposure to low concentrations
  ○ High concentrations can cause death within minutes.
- Treatment
  ○ Remove patient from contaminated environment
  ○ Remove clothing, wash with water
  ○ Maintain open airway, give high-concentration oxygen, and assist ventilations as needed
  ○ ALS
    - Amyl nitrite by inhalation 15 to 30 seconds every minute until IV line established; if patient is apneic, hold amyl nitrite perles over bag-valve mask (BVM) intake port
    - Sodium nitrite 300 mg slow IV push
    - Nitrites may cause hypotension secondary to vasodilation.
    - Sodium thiosulfate 12.5 g slow IV push

Blister Agents

- Toxicology
  ○ Enter body through absorption
  ○ Produce damage to skin, eyes, and mucous membranes
  ○ Absorbed mustard will damage bone morrow, causing anemia, inability to clot, and inability to fight infection.
  ○ Absorbed Lewisite will produce systemic effects of arsenic toxicity.
- Examples, military designations, and characteristics
  ○ Distilled mustard (HD)—Light yellow to brown oily liquid with odor of garlic, mustard, or onions
  ○ Nitrogen mustard (HN)—Colorless to pale yellow oily liquid with faint fishy or musty odor
  ○ Sulfur mustard (H)—Light yellow to brown oily liquid with odor of garlic, mustard, or onions
  ○ Lewisite (L)—Amber to dark brown liquid with geranium-like odor
  ○ Phosgene oxime (CX)—Colorless liquid or crystalline solid with intense, disagreeable, and penetrating odor
- Signs and symptoms
  ○ Blister agents
    - Skin—Redness in 2 to 24 hours; large, dome-shaped, and thin-walled yellowish blisters
    - Eyes—Reddening, conjunctivitis, sensitivity to light, eyelid spasm, pain, and corneal damage
    - Pulmonary—Hoarseness, productive cough, fever, dyspnea, rhonchi, and crackles
    - Gastrointestinal—Nausea, vomiting, pain, diarrhea, and hypovolemic shock
  ○ Lewisite
    - Skin—Immediate pain, reddening within 30 minutes, and blistering in 13 hours
    - Eyes—Immediate pain, loss of sight unless decontaminated within 1 minute
    - Pulmonary—Pulmonary edema
    - Systemic—Restlessness, weakness, subnormal body temperature, and hypotension

- ○ Phosgene oxime
  - Skin—Skin blanching within 30 seconds, followed by skin necrosis
  - Eyes—Extreme pain, permanent loss of sight if not decontaminated
  - Pulmonary—Upper airway irritation, pulmonary edema
  - Gastrointestinal—Inflammation, hemorrhage
- Treatment
  - ○ Remove patient from contaminated environment
  - ○ Remove clothing, wash with water. Bleach solution for mustard and Lewisite
  - ○ Maintain open airway, give high-concentration oxygen, and assist ventilations as needed
  - ○ Irrigate eyes with large amounts of water
  - ○ Cover injured skin areas with dry, sterile dressings
  - ○ Bronchodilators for bronchospasms, wheezing
  - ○ ALS
    - Endotracheally intubate patients at risk of airway obstruction
    - Positive end-expiratory pressure (PEEP) for pulmonary edema
    - Analgesics for pain
    - Fluid loss from blister agent exposure is *not* of same magnitude as with thermal burns. Massive fluid infusion is *not* necessary.
    - Lewisite exposure can be treated with British anti-Lewisite agent (BAL)

Choking Agents (Pulmonary Irritants)

- Toxicology
  - ○ Damage airway mucosa and alveolar walls
  - ○ Produce pulmonary edema
- Examples, military designations, and characteristics
  - ○ Phosgene (CG)—Colorless gas with odor of freshly cut grass or corn
  - ○ Chlorine (CL)—Greenish-yellow gas with irritating "swimming pool" odor
- Signs and symptoms
  - ○ Phosgene
    - Eyes—Increased tear production
    - Pulmonary—Choking, coughing, chest tightness, delayed pulmonary edema (approximately 4 hours after exposure), crackles and rhonchi, and hypoxia
    - Gastrointestinal—Nausea, vomiting
    - Systemic—Hypotension
  - ○ Chlorine
    - Eyes—Redness, increased tear production
    - Pulmonary—Choking, coughing, irritation and swelling of upper airway mucosa, chest tightness, hemoptysis (coughing up blood), pulmonary edema, and hypoxia
    - Gastrointestinal—Abdominal pain, hematemesis (vomiting blood)
    - Systemic—Hypotension
- Treatment
  - ○ Remove patient from contaminated environment
  - ○ Remove clothing, wash with water
  - ○ Maintain open airway, give high-concentration oxygen, and assist ventilations as needed
  - ○ For chlorine exposure, flush eyes with large amounts of water
  - ○ Bronchodilators for bronchospasms, wheezing
  - ○ ALS

- Endotracheally intubate patients at risk of airway obstruction
- PEEP for pulmonary edema

BIOLOGICAL AGENTS
Categories
- Bacteria—Single-celled microorganisms without an organized nucleus
  - Anthrax
  - Cholera
  - Plague
  - Tularemia
  - Salmonella
- Viruses—Protein-enclosed DNA or RNA chains. Must use host cells to reproduce themselves
  - Smallpox
  - Venezuelan equine encephalitis
- Toxins—Poisonous substances produced by microorganisms, plants, or animals
  - Botulinum toxin
  - Ricin
  - Staphylococcal enterotoxin

Anthrax
- Type and name of agent
  - Bacterium
  - *Bacillus anthracis*
- Mode of transmission
  - Handling of contaminated wool, hides, or tissues of infected animals
  - Inhalation or ingestion of bacterial spores
- Signs and symptoms
  - Cutaneous (skin) anthrax—Black sores and blisters on hands and forearms
  - Inhalation anthrax—Nonspecific "chest cold" or "flu" symptoms followed by respiratory distress, diaphoresis, stridor, cyanosis, and death
  - Gastrointestinal anthrax (rare in humans)—Intense abdominal pain, bowel obstruction, dehydration, diarrhea, sepsis, and death
- Incubation period
  - 1 to 7 days
  - Most cases within 48 hours
- Treatment
  - Intubation
  - Assisted ventilation
  - Antibiotics—Ciprofloxacin, doxycycline, and penicillin

Plague
- Type and name of agent
  - Bacterium
  - *Yersinia pestis*
- Mode of transmission
  - Bites from infected fleas
  - Inhalation of droplets from coughing of patients with pneumonic plague

- Signs and symptoms
  - Bubonic plague—Malaise; high fever; and tender, enlarged lymph nodes (buboes). May progress to septicemia with spread to the spleen, lungs, and meninges
  - Pneumonic plague—High fever, chills, headache, hemoptysis (coughing up blood), dyspnea, cyanosis, respiratory failure, and death
- Incubation period
  - Bubonic plague—2 to 10 days
  - Pneumonic plague—2 to 3 days
- Treatment
  - Respiratory and circulatory support as needed
  - Strict isolation for patients with pneumonic plague
  - Antibiotics—Streptomycin, doxycycline, ciprofloxacin, and chloramphenicol

Cholera

- Type and name of agent
  - Bacterium
  - *Vibrio cholerae*
- Mode of transmission
  - Contaminated water
- Signs and symptoms
  - Vomiting
  - Headache
  - Little or no fever
  - Intestinal cramping
  - Painless, massive diarrhea (rice water diarrhea) with fluid losses of up to 10 L/day
- Incubation period
  - Hours to 5 days, usually 2 to 3 days
- Treatment
  - Fluid and electrolyte replacement
  - Antibiotics—Tetracycline

Tularemia (rabbit fever, deerfly fever)

- Type and name of agent
  - Bacterium
  - *Francisella tularensis*
- Mode of transmission
  - Handling tissues of infected animals, particularly rabbits
  - Bites of infected deerflies, mosquitoes, and ticks
  - Inhalation of contaminated dust or ingestion of contaminated food, water (typhoidal tularemia)
  - *Francisella tularensis* is *very* infective. A single organism has the potential to infect a human. A biological weapons attack using an aerosol would cause an infection rate approaching 100% in unprotected persons.
- Signs and symptoms
  - Ulceroglandular tularemia—Local ulcer at site of exposure, local lymph node swelling, fever, chills, headache, and malaise

○ Typhoidal tularemia—Fever, headache, fatigue, weight loss, nonproductive cough, and substernal chest discomfort
- Incubation period
  ○ 2 to 10 days, average 3 days
- Treatment
  ○ Antibiotics—Streptomycin, gentamicin, and doxycycline
  ○ Isolation of patients not required

Salmonella
- Type and name of agent
  ○ Bacterium
  ○ Various *Salmonella* species
- Mode of transmission
  ○ Contaminated food
- Signs and symptoms
  ○ Gastrointestinal—Abdominal pain, diarrhea, headache, and fever
  ○ Possible progression to pericarditis, endocarditis, pneumonia, or meningitis if not treated
- Incubation period
  ○ 8 to 48 hours
- Treatment
  ○ Fluid and electrolyte replacement
  ○ Antibiotics for severe cases—Chloramphenicol, ampicillin

Smallpox
- Type of agent
  ○ Virus
- Mode of transmission
  ○ Droplets produced by coughing of infected persons
  ○ Contact with fluids from skin lesions
- Signs and symptoms
  ○ Severe fever, red rash progressing to red papules that then form fluid-filled pustules, bleeding of skin and mucous membranes, vomiting, weakness, headache, and backache
  ○ Rash appears first on face, forearms, and hands, and then spreads to trunk. This centripetal (extremities to body) spread of the rash distinguishes smallpox from chicken pox, which has a similar rash that has a centrifugal (body to extremities) spread.
- Incubation period
  ○ 7 to 17 days, typically 10 to 12 days before onset of illness with 2 to 4 more days to onset of rash
- Treatment
  ○ Smallpox vaccine can be given prophylactically within 1 week of exposure.
  ○ Care of active cases is supportive and must include steps to prevent secondary bacterial infections of open skin lesions.
  ○ Infection may be transmitted from the first appearance of the rash until the last scab falls off.

Venezuelan Equine Encephalitis
- Type of agent
  ○ Virus
- Mode of transmission

    ○ Bites of infected mosquitoes
- Signs and symptoms
  - ○ Sudden onset of illness with generalized malaise, spiking fever, chills, severe headache, light sensitivity, and muscle pain in the legs and back
  - ○ Nausea, vomiting, sore throat, and diarrhea
  - ○ Prolonged weakness and lethargy lasting up to 2 weeks
  - ○ Approximately 4% of patients experience seizures, coma, and paralysis.
- Incubation period
  - ○ 1 to 5 days
- Treatment
  - ○ Supportive care only

Botulinum Toxin

- Type of agent
  - ○ Toxin
- Natural source
  - ○ Bacterium
  - ○ *Clostridium botulinum*
- Signs and symptoms
  - ○ Dry mouth, drooping of the eyelids, difficulty speaking, difficulty swallowing, blurred vision, double vision, and dilated pupils
  - ○ Dyspnea, shortness of breath, and apnea from paralysis of diaphragm and intercostal muscles
- Rate of action
  - ○ 1 to 12 hours
- Treatment
  - ○ Intubation and ventilatory support
  - ○ Administration of antitoxin

Ricin

- Type of agent
  - ○ Toxin
- Natural source
  - ○ Castor bean
  - ○ *Ricinus communis*
  - ○ A byproduct of the processing of castor beans to make castor oil
- Signs and symptoms
  - ○ Inhalation—Cough, tightness in chest, difficulty breathing, nausea, muscle aches, severe inflammation of airway, cyanosis, and death in 36 to 48 hours
  - ○ Ingestion—Nausea, vomiting, internal bleeding from stomach and intestines, and failure of liver, spleen, and kidney
- Rate of action
  - ○ Inhaled—1 to 12 hours
  - ○ Ingested—5 minutes to 1 hour
- Treatment
  - ○ Inhaled—Supportive care, including management of pulmonary edema
  - ○ Ingested—Gastric lavage, activated charcoal, and cathartics
  - ○ There is no antidote or antitoxin for ricin.

Staphylococcal Enterotoxin B

- Type of agent
  - ○ Toxin
- Natural source
  - ○ Bacterium
  - ○ *Staphylococcus aureus*
- Signs and symptoms
  - ○ Inhalation—Fever, chills, headache, muscle pain, and nonproductive cough lasting for 1 to 4 weeks
  - ○ Ingestion—Fever, chills, nausea, vomiting, and diarrhea
- Rate of action
  - ○ 3 to 12 hours after exposure
- Treatment
  - ○ Ventilatory support for inhalation exposure
  - ○ Fluid and electrolyte replacement

REVIEW QUESTIONS

Scenario One

At 7:30 PM you are called to see two people with difficulty breathing at a catered church supper. On arrival you find there now are four patients. They are short of breath and are having difficulty speaking. One complains of double vision, and all are complaining of unusually dry mouths. All have drooping eyelids. After you begin treatment, three more patients present with similar symptoms.

Multiple Choice

27.1. The patients probably have been exposed to what agent?
- **a.** Botulism
- **b.** Sarin
- **c.** Mustard gas
- **d.** Cyanide

27.2. All of the following statements about botulism are correct *except:*
- **a.** symptoms will begin within 1 to 12 hours.
- **b.** excessive secretions will be present.
- **c.** botulism is one of the most lethal poisons that can be ingested.
- **d.** botulism is not contagious.

27.3. What kind of agent is sarin?
- **a.** A neurotoxin
- **b.** A blister agent
- **c.** A respiratory (choking) agent
- **d.** A blood agent

27.4. Blister agents cause which of the following signs and symptoms?
- **a.** Overproduction of secretions
- **b.** Weakness and seizures
- **c.** Flushing and hypotension
- **d.** Possible airway obstruction and crackles in the lung fields

True/False

27.5. Organophosphate neurotoxins inactivate acetylcholinesterase.
  a. True
  b. False

27.6. The patients in Scenario One need to be decontaminated.
  a. True
  b. False

Multiple Choice

27.7. Treatment for botulism includes all of the following *except:*
  a. airway management.
  b. atropine.
  c. antitoxin.
  d. assisted ventilations.

27.8. A key factor to identify the problem in Scenario One is the:
  a. patients being gathered together in one location.
  b. presence of dry mouth, difficulty swallowing, and dyspnea.
  c. presence of dyspnea.
  d. patients all needing treatment at the same time.

27.9. Which of the following are nerve agents?
  a. Botulinum and ricin
  b. Lewisite and mustard
  c. Tabun and sarin
  d. Ebola and encephalitis

Scenario Two

At 8:30 AM on a Thursday morning, several small canisters exploded in a bus station. Later in the day, many of the people who were present at the time of the explosion developed shortness of breath, muscle pain, and chest pain. The hazard materials (Hazmat) team has determined the canisters contained ricin.

Multiple Choice

27.10. What kind of agent is ricin?
  a. A bacterium
  b. A virus
  c. A toxin
  d. A blister agent

True/False

27.11. Ricin is produced from castor beans.
  a. True
  b. False

Multiple Choice

27.12. All of the following statements about ricin are correct *except:*
  a. inhaled ricin attacks the respiratory system, causing pneumonia and pulmonary edema.
  b. ingested ricin causes gastrointestinal bleeding, which can lead to death.
  c. ricin can be produced in an aerosolized form and solid form.
  d. symptoms of ricin toxicity begin 48 to 72 hours after exposure.

27.13. Signs and symptoms of ricin exposure include:
  a. dry mouth, difficulty speaking, and double vision.
  b. tissue necrosis, pneumonia, internal bleeding, and vascular collapse.
  c. generalized weakness, numbness, photophobia, and headache.
  d. fever, vomiting, weakness, and pustular rash.

True/False

27.14. Secondary inhalation of ricin vapors is not a concern for EMS personnel; however, the patient's skin should be decontaminated with hypochlorite solution, soap, and water.
  a. True
  b. False

Scenario Three

Three days after a college football game attended by >100,000 people, patients complaining of fever, chills, headache, and swollen lymph nodes overwhelm EMS and area hospitals. An investigation by state and federal law enforcement and public health authorities identifies the agent as tularemia, which was dispersed in an aerosol.

Multiple Choice

27.15. All of the following statements about tularemia are true *except:*
  a. tularemia also is known as "rabbit fever" or "deerfly fever."
  b. tularemia is caused by virus.
  c. tularemia may be transmitted by tick or mosquito bites.
  d. inhaled tularemia causes symptoms in approximately 2 to 10 days.

27.16. Which of the following are signs and symptoms of tularemia?
  a. Fever, chills, fatigue, and deep skin ulcers
  b. Fever, headache, skin and mucous membrane hemorrhages, and glandular swelling
  c. Vomiting, diarrhea, loss of body fluids, and severe muscle cramps
  d. Fever, headache, skin rash with rose-colored spots, constipation or diarrhea, and abdominal pain

True/False

27.17. Tularemia has an incubation period of 2 to 10 days with an average of 3 days.
  a. True
  b. False

Multiple Choice

27.18. All of the following statements about tularemia are true *except:*
  a. tularemia is transmitted easily from one individual to another, so strict isolation procedures must be followed.
  b. tularemia may persist for weeks in soil, water, or animal hides.
  c. tularemia may remain in frozen rabbit meat for years.
  d. the death rate of tularemia is usually approximately 5%.

True/False

27.19. Because tularemia is not easily transmitted, use of gloves and other personal protective equipment is unnecessary.
   a. True
   b. False

Scenario Four

Patients in several communities present to EMS or the local emergency department with fever, vomiting, and weakness. Within 2 to 4 days they develop a rash consisting of red papules that later form vesicles. The state health department determines that all of the patients recently received free samples of a new aerosol air freshener.

Multiple Choice

27.20. These patients have been exposed to:
   a. encephalitis.
   b. viral hemorrhagic fever.
   c. smallpox.
   d. staphylococcal enterotoxin.
27.21. Smallpox is caused by a:
   a. bacterium.
   b. virus.
   c. toxin.
   d. blister agent.

True/False

27.22. Smallpox was eradicated as a naturally occurring disease in 1980.
   a. True
   b. False

Multiple Choice

27.23. Which of the following signs and symptoms characterize smallpox?
   a. Fever, chills, fatigue, and deep skin ulcerations
   b. Fever, headache, skin and mucous membrane hemorrhages, and glandular swelling
   c. Vomiting, constipation, loss of body fluids, and severe muscle cramps
   d. Fever, headache, vomiting, backache, and a vesicular rash
27.24. All of the following statements about smallpox are true *except:*
   a. it could infect thousands of people in a short time, overwhelming the health care system.
   b. the rash appears first on the extremities and face.
   c. symptoms typically begin 3 to 5 days after exposure.
   d. exposed persons must be quarantined for 16 to 17 days.

Scenario Five

Three weeks before Christmas, large numbers of people begin to collapse at a shopping mall. EMS, the fire department Hazmat team, and the police respond. The Hazmat team determines cyanide was introduced into the mall's heating/air conditioning system.

Multiple Choice

27.25. Cyanide is a:
   a. blister agent.
   b. nerve agent.
   c. pulmonary (choking) agent.
   d. blood agent.
27.26. All of the following statements about cyanide are correct *except:*
   a. two forms of cyanide are used in chemical warfare: hydrogen cyanide and cyanogen chloride.
   b. cyanide causes severe respiratory distress, abdominal pain, and a rash.
   c. cyanide prevents cells from using oxygen.
   d. death may occur within 10 minutes.

True/False

27.27. Hydrocyanic acid and cyanogen chloride evaporate quickly.
   a. True
   b. False
27.28. Cyanide may cause dyspnea, respiratory depression, apnea, hypotension, and acidosis.
   a. True
   b. False

Scenario Six

A number of persons eating in the cafeteria of a 600-bed hospital developed difficulty breathing, watering eyes, runny noses, and blurred or dim vision. By the time EMS and the fire department arrived, several individuals had collapsed and were seizing. The FBI and state police later determined that tabun had been dispersed onto the cafeteria tables, leaving a deadly residue. More than 100 deaths occurred, and decontamination of the hospital took several weeks.

Multiple Choice

27.29. Which of the following best describes tabun's odor?
   a. Fruit
   b. Camphor
   c. Sulfur
   d. Odorless
27.30. What kind of agent is tabun?
   a. A neurotoxin
   b. A blister agent
   c. A respiratory (choking) agent
   d. A blood agent

True/False

27.31. Chemical terrorism agents may be delivered as solids, liquids, or gases.
   a. True
   b. False

Scenario Seven

A 32-y.o.male and his 28-y.o. wife are complaining of headache and a cough. A rash consisting of reddened areas surrounding small, fluid-filled blisters is present on their arms, legs, and faces and is beginning to appear on their chests. They spent the last month traveling with a tour group in the Middle East. The male patient's vital signs are pulse (P)—112, strong, regular; blood pressure (BP)—124/82; respiration (R)—18, regular, unlabored; and temperature (T)—102.6° F. The female patient's vital signs are P—118, strong, regular; BP—108/76; R—22, regular, unlabored; and T—103.2° F.

Multiple Choice

27.32. These patients *most* likely have:
  a. meningitis.
  b. smallpox.
  c. measles.
  d. chicken pox.

27.33. Smallpox is spread by:
  a. contaminated food.
  b. droplets produced by sneezing or coughing.
  c. mosquitoes.
  d. sexual contact.

27.34. The signs and symptoms of smallpox are similar to those of:
  a. measles.
  b. meningitis.
  c. botulism.
  d. chicken pox.

27.35. The incubation period of smallpox is:
  a. 2 to 4 days.
  b. 7 to 17 days.
  c. 21 to 30 days.
  d. 24 to 48 hours.

27.36. Smallpox is contagious:
  a. from the time the rash develops until the scabs are gone.
  b. only until the rash begins to appear.
  c. from 1 week before the rash develops until the scabs are formed.
  d. within 24 hours of first coming into contact with the virus.

True/False

27.37. The smallpox virus remains on contaminated clothing and bedding.
  a. True
  b. False

Multiple Choice

27.38. On this call you should:
  a. not do an initial assessment.
  b. call for additional help.
  c. do a scene size-up, quarantine the scene, and call for additional help.
  d. not be concerned if you were vaccinated when you were a child.

27.1. A, The patients' unusually dry mouths, drooping eyelids, and double vision suggest they have been exposed to botulinum toxin.

27.2. B, Botulinum toxin blocks release of acetylcholine from nerve endings, causing a *decrease* in secretions.

27.3. A, Sarin is a neurotoxin.

27.4. D, In addition to skin damage, exposure to blister agents can cause pulmonary edema and airway swelling that can progress to obstruction.

27.5. A, Organophosphate neurotoxins bind with acetylcholinesterase, inactivating it. The neurotransmitter acetylcholine accumulates in excessive amounts, stimulating overproduction of body secretions and causing paralysis of skeletal muscles.

27.6. B, The botulinum toxin usually is spread through contaminated food. You should take normal body substance isolation (BSI) precautions. Patients with skin exposure to botulinum toxin should be undressed and washed with diluted bleach solution, soap, and water.

27.7. B, Atropine is not given to manage exposure to botulinum toxin.

27.8. B, The patients' dry mouths, difficulty swallowing, and dyspnea suggest exposure to botulinum toxin.

27.9. C, Tabun (GA) and sarin (GB) are nerve agents. Botulinum and ricin are biological toxins. Lewisite and mustard are blister agents. Ebola and encephalitis are viruses.

27.10. C, Ricin is a toxin isolated from castor beans.

27.11. A, Ricin is a potent toxin that can be isolated from the "mash" that remains after castor beans are processed to make castor oil. Two to four castor beans contain enough ricin to kill an adult. Ingestion of one castor bean can be lethal to a child.

27.12. D, Ricin's effects begin in 1 to 12 hours.

27.13. B, Ricin causes tissue necrosis, pneumonia, internal bleeding, and vascular collapse.

27.14. A, Ricin is not volatile; therefore, secondary inhalation is not a hazard. However, skin contact should be avoided, and the patient should be washed with diluted bleach solution, soap, and water.

27.15. B, Tularemia is caused by a bacterium, not a virus.

27.16. A, Tularemia caused by skin and mucous membrane exposure causes fever, chills, headache, fatigue, swollen lymph nodes, and deep skin ulcerations.

27.17. A, Tularemia causes symptoms in 2 to 10 days, with 3 days being the average.

27.18. A, Tularemia is *not* easily passed from one individual to another; therefore, strict isolation is not necessary, although blood and body fluid precautions must be taken. It is transmitted through the bite of an infected deerfly, tick, or mosquito. The organism may persist for weeks in soil, water, and animal hides. It is resistant to freezing and may exist in frozen rabbit or deer meat for years.

27.19. B, The patient does not have to be isolated. However, health care personnel should wear appropriate personal protective equipment to prevent contact with body fluids. Equipment can be decontaminated with bleach solution.

27.20. **C,** The signs and symptoms suggest smallpox. Smallpox is characterized by a rash consisting of red bumps (papules) that begins on the face and extremities and spreads to the trunk. The papules progress to fluid- and pus-filled vesicles that may bleed and that heal leaving deep scars.

27.21. **B,** Smallpox is a virus.

27.22. **A,** Smallpox was eradicated as a naturally occurring disease in 1980 through the use of strict quarantine and vaccinations. However, it is suspected that a number of countries have maintained the virus in laboratory settings for potential use as a biological weapon.

27.23. **D,** Smallpox is characterized by fever, headache, vomiting, backache, and a vesicular (blisterlike) rash that begins on the face and extremities and spreads to the trunk.

27.24. **C,** Symptoms of smallpox typically begin 7 to 17 days after exposure.

27.25. **D,** The military classifies cyanide as a "blood" agent. Cyanide is toxic because it prevents metabolic use of oxygen, causing asphyxiation at the cellular level.

27.26. **B,** Cyanide does not cause abdominal pain or a rash. Cyanosis causes signs and symptoms of severe hypoxia. However, the patient does not become cyanotic, and a pulse oximeter will not show decreased hemoglobin saturation.

27.27. **A,** Hydrocyanic acid and cyanogen chloride are highly volatile and evaporate quickly. The vapors of hydrocyanic acid are lighter than air and disperse rapidly. Cyanogen chloride vapor is heavier than air and will sink into low-lying areas.

27.28. **A,** Cyanide interferes with the body's ability to use oxygen at the cellular level and causes dyspnea, respiratory depression, apnea, hypotension, and acidosis.

27.29. **A,** Tabun has a fruity odor.

29.30. **A,** Tabun is a neurotoxin.

27.31. **A,** Chemical terrorism agents may be in solids, liquids, or gases.

27.32. **B,** These patients probably have smallpox. Meningitis causes a headache, but the rash that occurs with some types of meningitis looks like pinpoint hemorrhages under the skin surface. Measles causes headache and upper respiratory infection symptoms, but the rash consists of reddened, slightly raised spots. Smallpox and chicken pox produce similar lesions; however, the lesions of chicken pox appear on the trunk first and then spread to the extremities.

27.33. **B,** Coughing and sneezing transmit the smallpox virus.

27.34. **D,** The signs and symptoms of smallpox are similar to those of chicken pox. In chicken pox, the rash appears first on the trunk and spreads to the extremities. In smallpox, the rash begins on the extremities and spreads to the trunk.

27.35. **B,** The incubation period for smallpox is 7 to 17 days with an average of 12 days. Exposed persons should be quarantined for a minimum of 17 days following exposure.

27.36. **A,** Smallpox is contagious from the time the rash develops until the last scab falls off.

27.37. **A,** The smallpox virus is present in the fluid that fills the skin lesions and remains on contaminated clothing and bedding.

27.38. **C,** You should do a scene size-up, quarantine the scene, and call for additional help from law enforcement and the health department. Your principal objective at this point is to prevent the spread of smallpox from these patients to others in the community. Investigators from the health department can begin the process of identifying contacts of these patients to locate other possible cases and of tracing the origin of the infection. Because smallpox does not occur naturally, this event possibly is the result of terrorist activity. Law enforcement should be involved to begin an investigation to identify the parties responsible for the smallpox outbreak. Protection from smallpox vaccination lasts 3 to 10 years. After this time booster doses should be given if exposure has occurred. Vaccination is effective up to 1 week after exposure.

28

Advanced Airway Management

ENDOTRACHEAL INTUBATION

- Insertion of tube into trachea to provide controlled breathing with bag-valve mask (BVM) or ventilator
- Indications
  - Patients cannot protect their own airway (no gag flex).
  - Patient is at risk of losing airway (trauma, allergic reactions, or airway burns).
  - Prolonged assisted ventilations are necessary.
  - Patient cannot be ventilated effectively using a BVM or pocket mask.
- Advantages
  - Complete control of airway
  - Decreased risk of aspiration
  - Improved oxygenation and ventilation
  - Route for suctioning trachea and bronchi
- Disadvantages
  - Extensive training required
  - Special equipment required
  - Vocal cords must be visualized to place tube properly.
- Complications
  - Intubation of esophagus, leading to inadequate ventilation and anoxia
  - Prolonged time to perform procedure, leading to hypoxia
  - Injury to soft tissues of mouth and throat, leading to bleeding
  - Vomiting and aspiration
  - Damage to teeth
  - Damage to vocal cords
  - Spasms of vocal cords (laryngospasm)
  - Laryngeal edema
  - Intubation of right mainstem bronchus, leading to hypoxia, hypoventilation, or pneumothorax
  - Bradycardia as a result of stimulating airway
- Equipment
  - Laryngoscope handle and blades
    - Curved blade (Macintosh)—Inserted into vallecula
    - Straight blade (Miller)—Positioned under epiglottis
  - Endotracheal (ET) tube
    - Standard sizes
      - Adult males—7.5 to 8.5 mm
      - Adult females—7.0 to 8.0 mm
      - Children aged >1—(Child's age in years divided by 4) + 4; cuffed if aged ≥ 8 years, uncuffed if aged <8 years
      - Infant—3.5 to 4.0 mm (uncuffed)
      - Newborn—3.0 to 3.5 mm (uncuffed)
      - Premature infant—2.5 to 3.0 mm (uncuffed)
  - Stylette
    - Helps maintain tube stiffness
    - Should be recessed at least ½ inch from distal end of tube to prevent trauma
  - Other equipment
    - Water-soluble lubricant

- 10-mL syringe
- Tube-securing device
- Suction unit
- Towels or padding
- Stethoscope
- BVM
- Oxygen source
- Secondary confirmation device (end-tidal CO_2 detector or esophageal intubation detection device)
- Procedure
  - Body substance isolation (BSI) precautions
  - Open airway, insert oral airway, and preoxygenate with BVM and oxygen
  - Check ET tube cuff by inflating with 10-mL syringe
  - Insert stylette, form ET tube into desired shape
  - Lubricate tube
  - Assemble laryngoscope blade and handle, check light
  - Prepare suction unit
  - Position head in "sniffing position"
  - Stop ventilating, remove oral airway
  - Holding laryngoscope in left hand, insert blade in right side of mouth
  - Sweep tongue to left, advance laryngoscope blade to base of tongue
  - Lift at 45-degree angle on laryngoscope handle to move mandible and tongue, visualize glottic opening
  - Insert ET tube into glottic opening, advance ½ to 1 inch past vocal cords. Do not let go of tube until it is secured
  - Inflate cuff with 5 to 10 mL of air
  - Ventilate through ET tube with BVM, observe chest rise
  - Auscultate over epigastrium to check for misplacement of tube in esophagus
  - Auscultate for breath sounds over both lung fields to check tube placement, check for misplacement of tube in mainstem bronchus
  - Use end-tidal CO_2 detector to confirm tube placement
  - Check for condensation in ET tube to confirm placement
    - Secure tube in place; note depth of tube insertion by checking markings on tube. (Proper depth of insertion, in centimeters, is approximately the tube size × 3. For example, a 7.0-mm tube should be inserted to 7.0 × 3 = 21 cm.)
    - Monitor patient
- Important considerations
  - The patient should never go unventilated for >30 seconds during ET intubation.
  - The laryngoscope handle should be used to lift *up*. Prying back with the laryngoscope can result in breaking of teeth.
  - The *best* way to confirm proper ET tube placement is to *see* the tube pass through the vocal cords.
  - If breath sounds are absent or diminished over one of the lung fields, the tube probably is in one of the mainstem bronchi. Although ET tubes typically enter the right mainstem bronchus because it is shorter and straighter, tubes can enter the left mainstem bronchus. The cuff should be deflated, and the tube should be pulled out slowly until breath sounds equalize. If breath sounds continue to be diminished over one of the lung fields after the tube is repositioned, the possibility of a pneumothorax should be considered.

COMBITUBE

- Double-lumen airway device
- Advantages
  - No visualization required for insertion
  - Device is properly placed whether it is in esophagus or trachea.
  - Pharyngeal cuff prevents ventilations from escaping through mouth and nose, eliminating need to maintain mask seal.
  - If device is placed in esophagus, gastric contents can be suctioned.
  - Can be used for trauma patients because the neck can remain in neutral position during insertion and use
- Disadvantages
  - Requires accurate assessment of tracheal vs. esophageal intubation
  - Difficult to place ET tube once Combitube is in place
  - Cannot be used for patients with gag reflex
  - Cannot be used to suction trachea if device is in esophagus
  - Cannot be used for patients aged <16 years or for those <5 feet tall
- Contraindications
  - Patient has gag reflex.
  - Patient is aged <16 years.
  - Patient is <5 feet tall.
  - Patient has swallowed a corrosive substance (acid or alkali).
  - Esophageal disease is present.
- Procedure
  - BSI
  - Open airway, insert oral airway, and preoxygenate with BVM and oxygen
  - Check cuffs on Combitube for leaks, lubricate distal end of tube
  - Place patient's head and neck in neutral position
  - Perform tongue-jaw lift, insert device until teeth are between two black rings on the tube
  - Inflate pharyngeal cuff (blue pilot balloon marked #1) with 100 mL of air
  - Inflate distal cuff (white pilot balloon marked #2) with 15 mL of air
  - Attach BVM to tube #1 and ventilate; watch for chest rise, auscultate over epigastrium, and auscultate over lung fields. If chest rise is seen, breath sounds are heard in both lung fields, and no sounds are heard over the epigastrium, continue to ventilate through tube #1.
  - If gurgling is heard over the epigastrium and no chest rise is observed, ventilate through tube #2; watch for chest rise, auscultate over the epigastrium, and auscultate over lung fields. If chest rise is seen, breath sounds are heard in both lung fields, and no sounds are heard over the epigastrium, continue to ventilate through tube #2.
  - Monitor patient

PHARYNGOTRACHEAL LUMEN AIRWAY (PTL)

- Advantages
  - Cannot be improperly placed
  - Mask seal not required because large pharyngeal cuff seals upper airway
  - Insertion does not require visualization of vocal cords.
  - Head and neck do not have to be moved during insertion.
  - Pharyngeal cuff protects lower airway from oral or nasal secretions or bleeding.

- Disadvantages
  - Patient must be completely unresponsive with no gag reflex.
  - Patient must be aged >16 years and >5 feet tall.
  - Device must be removed if patient becomes responsive or regains a gag reflex.
  - If pharyngeal tube deflates and longer tube is in esophagus, the device loses its effectiveness.
  - Device requires accurate assessment of tracheal vs. esophageal placement.
- Contraindications
  - Patient is responsive or has gag reflex.
  - Patient is aged <16 years.
  - Patient is <5 feet tall.
  - Patient has swallowed a corrosive substance (acid or alkali).
  - Esophageal disease is present.
- Procedure
  - BSI
  - Open airway, insert oral airway, and preoxygenate with BVM and oxygen
  - Check equipment
  - Stop ventilating, remove oral airway, and move head and neck to neutral position
  - Insert device into patient's mouth until flange rests at teeth
  - Loop white strap around patient's head, secure it
  - Inflate both distal cuffs using white inflation port marked #1. Close white cap
  - Deliver breath into shorter (green) tube marked #2; if chest rises longer tube is in esophagus; continue to ventilate
  - If chest does not rise, longer tube is in trachea; remove stylette from longer clear tube marked #3, attach BVM, and ventilate
  - Observe for rise and fall of chest, listen for breath sounds in both lung fields, and check for absence of sound over epigastrium
  - Monitor patient

END-TIDAL CARBON DIOXIDE DETECTION

- Measurement of exhaled CO_2 levels
- Capnography provides a numeric reading of CO_2 levels plus a digital signal similar to an ECG tracing on the monitor screen
- Clinical applications
  - Confirm ET tube placement
  - Provide continuous monitoring of the ET tube position
  - Confirm bronchospasms in patients with asthma or chronic obstructive pulmonary disease (COPD)
  - Early recognition of pulmonary edema
  - Monitor perfusion status and give an early warning of impending shock
  - Detection of hypoventilation

REVIEW QUESTIONS
Scenario One

You are dispatched to a report of a patient with "respiratory distress." The patient is a 29-y.o. female who is struggling to breathe. Her lips and oral mucosa are cyanotic. Her mother tells you the patient has a history of asthma and began having difficulty breathing approximately 4 hours ago. She has used her inhalers several times; however, her mother is unsure of exactly how many. She has no other past medical history. Her medications include a Brethine inhaler and an Azmacort inhaler. Vital signs are blood pressure (BP)—102/72; pulse (P)—124, strong, regular; and respirations (R)—36, regular, labored with decreased lung sounds over both lung fields. As you assess the patient, she loses consciousness, and her breathing slows.

Your Plan of Action

Fill in the blank lines with your treatment plan for this patient. Then compare your plan with the questions, answers, and rationale.

1. _____
2. _____
3. _____
4. _____
5. _____
6. _____
7. _____
8. _____
9. _____

Multiple Choice

28.1. What is your *most immediate* concern with this patient?
   a. The BP of 102/72
   b. The pulse rate of 124 beats/min
   c. The labored respirations at 36 breaths/min
   d. The decreased lung sounds and cyanosis

28.2. All of the following statements about the Combitube are true *except:*
   a. it is a double-lumen airway with a partition separating the two lumens.
   b. before air is placed in the second cuff, the patient should be ventilated.
   c. the larger cuff rests in the posterior pharynx.
   d. if the tube is placed in the trachea, ventilations will be delivered directly into the trachea.

28.3. Complications that may occur while intubating the patient include:
   a. hypoxia.
   b. bradycardia.
   c. hypoxia and tachycardia.
   d. hypoxia and bradycardia.

True/False

28.4. A 100-mL syringe, a 10- to 15-mL syringe, and a laryngoscope are needed to properly insert a Combitube.
   a. True
   b. False

Multiple Choice

28.5. How many milliliters of air are placed in the Combitube's *large* cuff?
   a. 25
   b. 50
   c. 75
   d. 100

28.6. Contraindications to inserting the Combitube include all of the following persons *except* an unconscious patient who is:
   a. age 20 years and 5 feet tall.
   b. age 12 years who appears to have been sniffing paint in his garage.
   c. age 21 years who has ingested a corrosive substance.
   d. age 58 years with a history of chronic alcohol abuse.

28.7. When you ventilate through the tube marked "#1," the chest rises and no sounds are heard over the epigastrium. This means the tube is in the:
   a. esophagus.
   b. trachea.

28.8. The Combitube would be *most* beneficial in which of the following situations?
   a. A 45-y.o. female who is semiconscious with extreme shortness of breath from pulmonary edema
   b. A 17-y.o. male involved in a motor vehicle collision (MVC) who is unresponsive and is vomiting
   c. An 81-y.o. female who is unresponsive with severe epistaxis
   d. A 16-y.o. male who accidentally swallowed drain cleaner and now is unresponsive

Scenario Two

You are dispatched to a report of an "unconscious person." When you arrive, you find the fire department doing cardiopulmonary resuscitation (CPR) on a 4-y.o. male. He has no past medical history and takes no medications. However, his mother found some pills lying on his bedside table. No one knows what they are.

Your Plan of Action

Fill in the blank lines with your treatment plan for this patient. Then compare your plan with the questions, answers, and rationale.

1. _____
2. _____
3. _____
4. _____
5. _____
6. _____
7. _____
8. _____
9. _____

Multiple Choice

28.9. As you prepare to intubate this patient you choose a curved laryngoscope blade, also known as a:

    a. Macintosh blade.

    b. Miller blade.

28.10. Which of the following is an advantage of the ET tube over the Combitube?

    a. The ET tube is easier to place than the Combitube.

    b. Breaths sounds are easier to hear when an ET tube is used.

    c. The ET tube allows for better oxygenation and ventilation.

    d. The ET tube decreases the possibility of laryngeal injury.

28.11. As you prepare to intubate, in what position should you place the patient's head?

    a. The neutral in-line position

    b. The hyperflexed position

    c. The hyperextended position

    d. The sniffing position

28.12. What size and type of tube would be most appropriate to use with this patient?

    a. Size 5, uncuffed

    b. Size 5, cuffed

    c. Size 7, uncuffed

    d. Size 7, cuffed

28.13. To what depth would the ET tube be inserted with this patient?

    a. 11 cm

    b. 15 cm

    c. 19 cm

    d. 21 cm

28.14. What will a capnometer tell you?

    a. The percentage of oxygen inhaled

    b. The percentage of oxygen being ventilated and the amount of CO_2 being exhaled

    c. The amount of CO_2 exhaled

    d. The percentage of oxygen exhaled and the amount of CO_2 remaining in the system

28.15. What structure forms the lower border of the larynx?

    a. Cricoid cartilage

    b. Septum

    c. Vallecula

    d. Inferior laryngeal cartilage

28.16. Why do you hold the laryngoscope in your left hand?

    a. The tongue must be swept to the right.

    b. The tube is inserted on the left side of the mouth.

    c. It is easier to visualize the vocal cords from the right side.

    d. The light and flange are on the left side of the blade.

28.17. What should you do *immediately* after inserting the ET tube?

    a. Check for breath sounds bilaterally and observe for chest rise

    b. Ventilate the patient with two slow breaths by mouth

    c. Secure the tube in place using a tube holder

    d. Fill the cuff with air

28.18. All of the following indicate esophageal intubation *except:*
- **a.** failure to hear breath sounds bilaterally.
- **b.** a gurgling sound over the epigastrium.
- **c.** improved skin color.
- **d.** a low CO_2 level on the capnometer.

28.19. Which of the following blades is recommended for pediatric intubation?
- **a.** Macintosh
- **b.** Miller

Scenario Three

You are dispatched to an MVC. On arrival you find a 19-y.o. male whose face struck the steering wheel. He has massive facial trauma, is unresponsive, and is breathing at a rate of 6 breaths/min.

Your Plan of Action

Fill in the blank lines with your treatment plan for this patient. Then compare your plan with the questions, answers, and rationale.

1. _____
2. _____
3. _____
4. _____
5. _____
6. _____
7. _____
8. _____
9. _____

Multiple Choice

28.20. To ensure an adequate airway for the patient you should:
- **a.** ventilate the patient and prepare for ET intubation.
- **b.** suction the patient before intubating.
- **c.** provide high-flow oxygen at 15 lpm.
- **d.** use a double-lumen airway.

28.21. To intubate a trauma patient, you should:
- **a.** keep the head and neck in a neutral position.
- **b.** perform a chin-lift, then suction.
- **c.** intubate, then apply a cervical collar.
- **d.** fully immobilize the patient first.

28.22. During intubation, Sellick's maneuver is used to:
- **a.** increase the size of the glottic opening.
- **b.** assist in maintaining an open airway.
- **c.** reduce the risk of aspiration.
- **d.** lift the epiglottis.

Scenario Four

A 78-y.o. female has severe respiratory distress. She has been having difficulty breathing for 4 days that has worsened rapidly during the past 3 hours. She has a history of congestive heart failure (CHF), asthma, and emphysema. She is allergic to Ceclor and ibuprofen. Vital signs are BP—192/108; P—138, weak, regular; R—44, shallow, labored; and SaO_2—85%. During the next 5 minutes the patient becomes increasingly cyanotic and begins to lapse in and out of consciousness.

Your Plan of Action

Fill in the blank lines with your treatment plan for this patient. Then compare your plan with the questions, answers, and rationale.

1. _____
2. _____
3. _____
4. _____
5. _____
6. _____
7. _____
8. _____
9. _____

Multiple Choice

28.23. As you prepare to intubate the patient, she begins to vomit. The two common types of suction catheters used in prehospital care are the:
   a. tonsil tip and the standard tip.
   b. tonsil tip and the Yankauer tip.
   c. whistle tip and the French.
   d. whistle tip and the Yankauer tip.

28.24. After you intubate the patient, breath sounds are decreased on the right. What should you do?
   a. Push the tube in a little farther because it is resting just above the trachea
   b. Remove the tube, use the BVM to ventilate
   c. Suction because secretions have plugged the tube
   d. Reposition the tube, recheck lung sounds to see if they are equal

28.25. Which of the following would indicate ET tube displacement?
   a. An increased reading of CO_2 in the CO_2 detector
   b. Noticeable abdominal distension
   c. Increased secretions in the oropharynx
   d. Moisture inside the lumen of the ET tube

Answer Key—*Chapter 28*

SCENARIO ONE

Plan of Action

1. Body Substance Isolation (BSI)
2. Is the scene safe? Yes. Assess nature of illness, number of patients, and need for additional resources.
3. Assess mental status. Ensure an open airway, assess breathing, begin assisting the patient's ventilations with a BVM and oxygen at 10-15 lpm, and assess circulatory status.
4. Determine priority, consider advanced life support (ALS).
5. History of present illness (HPI), SAMPLE
6. Focused physical examination
7. Baseline vital signs
8. Transport, perform ongoing assessment, and meet ALS unit.

Rationale

This patient has respiratory failure caused by bronchospasms that have increased resistance to airflow in her lower airways. Her ventilations should be assisted with a BVM and oxygen, and an ALS unit should be requested to begin bronchodilator therapy. If the patient's level of consciousness continues to decrease and you are unable to adequately ventilate her with a BVM and oxygen, placement of an advanced airway such as a Combitube may be indicated.

28.1. **D,** The decreased lung sounds indicate there is little air movement in the lungs. The presence of cyanosis indicates the patient is severely hypoxic. This patient has respiratory failure and is at risk of having a respiratory arrest.

28.2. **B,** For the Combitube to function properly, *both* cuffs must be inflated before ventilations are attempted. The Combitube is a dual-lumen airway with two cuffs: one that seals the pharynx and one that inflates in the esophagus or trachea. If the tube enters the esophagus, air enters the trachea through openings in the part of the tube located in the pharynx. If the tube enters the trachea, then ventilations are delivered directly into the trachea.

28.3. **D,** Common complications during intubation include hypoxia, caused by taking too long to perform the procedure, and bradycardia, caused by hypoxia or reflex stimulation of the vagus nerve from insertion of the tube into the patient's throat.

28.4. B, A laryngoscope is *not* needed to insert a Combitube. A 100-mL syringe and a 10- to 15-mL syringe are needed to inflate the Combitube's cuffs.

28.5. D, The large cuff is filled with 100 mL of air, and the smaller one is filled with 15 mL of air.

28.6. A, The Combitube is contraindicated for patients aged <16 years, patients <5 feet tall, patients who have ingested corrosive substances, and patients with known esophageal or liver disease.

28.7. A, Chest rise and absence of sounds over the epigastrium when ventilating through tube #1 indicate the tube is in the esophagus. If the chest does not rise and sounds are heard over the epigastrium when ventilating through tube #1, the tube is in the trachea. The patient then should be ventilated through tube #2, and proper tube placement should be confirmed by chest rise, breath sounds in both lung fields, and absence of epigastric sounds.

28.8. B, The Combitube would be most useful for the unresponsive 17-y.o. patient from the MVC. The 45-y.o. female is semiconscious and probably would vomit if the tube were placed. Patients with bleeding from the nasal cavity or nasopharynx are at risk of aspirating blood when a Combitube is placed because the tube does not protect the airway effectively from bleeding in the nasal cavity or nasopharynx. Attempted insertion of a Combitube in a patient who has ingested a corrosive agent such as drain cleaner can cause esophageal perforation.

SCENARIO TWO

Plan of Action

1. BSI
2. Is the scene safe? Yes. Evaluate nature of illness, number of patients, and need for additional resources.
3. Assess mental status. Ensure an open airway, assess breathing, continue to ventilate with BVM and oxygen, assess circulatory status, and continue chest compressions.
4. Determine priority, consider ALS.
5. Consider placing advanced airway if patient cannot be ventilated adequately with BVM.
6. Rapid physical examination
7. HPI, SAMPLE
8. Transport, perform ongoing assessment, and meet ALS unit.

Rationale

This patient is in cardiac arrest. Because a 4-y.o. is too small for use of a semi-automated external defibrillator (SAED), the only option is to continue CPR, transport, and meet an ALS unit. If the patient cannot be ventilated adequately with a BVM and oxygen, placement of an ET tube is indicated. A double-lumen (blind insertion) airway device would not be appropriate because of the child's age and size.

28.9. **A,** The *Macintosh blade* is a curved blade that is inserted directly into vallecula to lift the tongue and epiglottis and to visualize vocal cords or glottic opening. The *Miller blade* is a straight blade that is placed under the epiglottis to expose the vocal cords or glottic opening.

28.10. **C,** The ET tube provides better oxygenation and ventilation than other airway devices because it allows direct ventilation of the lower airway. The ET tube is more difficult to place than the Combitube because it requires direct visualization of the vocal cords. Breath sounds can be heard when a patient is being ventilated adequately with any of the airway devices. During ET intubation there is a greater risk of laryngeal injury because the tube must be passed through the vocal cords.

28.11. **D,** The head should be placed in the "sniffing" position when placing an ET tube.

28.12. **A,** If the patient's age is known, the proper tube size can be selected by using the formula (age/4) + 4. A 4-y.o. child requires a 5.0-mm tube. For children aged <8 years, tubes should be uncuffed because the cricoid cartilage is the narrowest part of the airway and forms a functional cuff on the tube.

28.13. **B,** If the patient is 4 y.o., the ET tube should be inserted to 15 cm at the teeth. The correct depth of insertion, in centimeters, can be determined from multiplying the size of the ET tube × 3.

28.14. **C,** A capnometer tells you the amount of CO_2 being exhaled by the patient.

28.15. **A,** The cricoid cartilage forms the inferior border of the larynx.

28.16. **D,** The laryngoscope is held in the left hand because the flange and light are on the left side of the blade. This allows the tongue to be moved to the left and the tube to be inserted on the right side of the mouth.

28.17. **A,** After you see the tube pass through the vocal cords, you should ventilate by attaching a bag-valve device to the tube and confirm proper tube placement by observing chest rise and hearing breath sounds bilaterally.

28.18. **C,** Improved skin color indicates the tube is correctly placed in the trachea. Absence of breath sounds bilaterally, gurgling over the epigastrium, or a low CO_2 reading on the capnometer indicates the tube is in the esophagus.

28.19. **B,** The Miller (straight) blade is indicated for pediatric intubation. The pediatric epiglottis tends to be narrower and softer than the adult epiglottis and is easier to control with a straight blade.

SCENARIO THREE

Plan of Action

1. BSI

2. Is the scene safe? Yes. Assess mechanism of injury, number of patients, and need for additional resources.

3. Manually control head and neck, assess mental status, open airway using jaw-thrust technique, assess breathing, assist breathing using BVM and oxygen, and assess circulatory status.

4. Determine priority, consider ALS.

Continued

SCENARIO THREE—cont'd

5. Apply cervical collar, rapidly extricate patient to long spine board, apply straps and cervical immobilizer, and consider intubation if patient cannot be ventilated adequately with BVM and oxygen or if patient is at risk of losing airway patency.
6. Transport.
7. Rapid physical examination
8. Baseline vital signs
9. HPI, SAMPLE
10. Perform ongoing assessment, detailed examination if time permits, and meet ALS unit.

Rationale

Patients with maxillofacial trauma are at risk for losing airway patency because of soft tissue swelling or bleeding into the airway. Early placement of an ET tube may be needed to ensure that the patient can continue to ventilate. Patients with significant facial trauma should always be suspected of having associated head or cervical spine injuries.

28.20. **A,** An ET tube provides the best control over the airway, particularly for patients with trauma to the face or neck when swelling may restrict airflow. Before ET intubation is attempted, patients should be hyperoxygenated using a BVM.

28.21. **A,** During intubation of a trauma patient with possible spinal injuries, the head and neck should be kept in a neutral position.

28.22. **C,** Sellick's maneuver (pushing the cricoid cartilage toward the body's posterior surface) reduces the risk of aspiration during intubation by partially closing the esophagus.

SCENARIO FOUR

Plan of Action

1. BSI
2. Is the scene safe? Yes. Assess nature of illness, number of patients, and need for additional resources.
3. Assess mental status. Ensure an open airway, assess breathing, apply oxygen by non-rebreather mask at 10-15 lpm, consider assisting ventilations with BVM and oxygen, and assess circulatory status.

Continued

SCENARIO FOUR—cont'd

4. Determine priority, consider ALS.

5. If patient's mental status continues to deteriorate, consider ET intubation, particularly if patient cannot be ventilated adequately with BVM and oxygen.

6. HPI, SAMPLE

7. Focused physical examination

8. Baseline vital signs

9. Transport, perform ongoing assessment, and meet ALS unit.

Rationale

This patient is not oxygenating or ventilating adequately. Her decreasing mental status indicates that she has respiratory failure. Her ventilations should be assisted with a BVM and oxygen. If she cannot be ventilated adequately with a BVM, intubation should be considered.

28.23. D, The two common types of suction catheters used are the whistle tip or flexible suction catheter and the Yankauer or tonsil-tip catheter. The Yankauer catheter is rigid and less easily obstructed; therefore, it should be used to clear the mouth and pharynx of secretions. Flexible catheters are better suited for suctioning airway adjuncts such as ET tubes.

28.24. D, If breath sounds are decreased in one of the lung fields, the tube probably is in one of the mainstem bronchi. You should pull the tube back slightly, then recheck the lung sounds to see if they are equal on both sides. Although ET tubes most commonly enter the right mainstem bronchus, which is shorter and straighter, they can enter the left.

28.25. B, Noticeable abdominal distension indicates possible displacement of the ET tube. Moisture inside the lumen and an increased reading of CO_2 in the $ETCO_2$ detector indicate correct tube placement. Increased airway secretions have no relationship to proper or improper tube placement.

Appendix: National Registry Skills Sheets*

AIRWAY, OXYGEN AND VENTILATION SKILLS
UPPER AIRWAY ADJUNCTS AND SUCTION

Start Time: _____

Stop Time: _____　Date: _____

Candidate's Name: _____

Evaluator's Name: _____

OROPHARYNGEAL AIRWAY	Points Possible	Points Awarded
Takes, or verbalizes, body substance isolation precautions	1	
Selects appropriately sized airway	1	
Measures airway	1	
Inserts airway without pushing the tongue posteriorly	1	
Note: The examiner must advise the candidate that the patient is gagging and becoming conscious		
Removes the oropharyngeal airway	1	

SUCTION

Note: The examiner must advise the candidate to suction the patient's airway		
Turns on/prepares suction device	1	
Assures presence of mechanical suction	1	
Inserts the suction tip without suction	1	
Applies suction to the oropharynx/nasopharynx	1	

NASOPHARYNGEAL AIRWAY

Note: The examiner must advise the candidate to insert a nasopharyngeal airway		
Selects appropriately sized airway	1	
Measures airway	1	
Verbalizes lubrication of the nasal airway	1	
Fully inserts the airway with the bevel facing toward the septum	1	
Total:	13	

Critical Criteria

_____ Did not take, or verbalize, body substance isolation precautions

_____ Did not obtain a patent airway with the oropharyngeal airway

_____ Did not obtain a patent airway with the nasopharyngeal airway

_____ Did not demonstrate an acceptable suction technique

_____ Inserted any adjunct in a manner dangerous to the patient

BAG-VALVE-MASK
APNEIC PATIENT

Start Time: _____

Stop Time: _____ Date: _____

Candidate's Name: _____

Evaluator's Name:	Points Possible	Points Awarded
Takes, or verbalizes, body substance isolation precautions	1	
Voices opening the airway	1	
Voices inserting an airway adjunct	1	
Selects appropriately sized mask	1	
Creates a proper mask-to-face seal	1	
Ventilates patient at no less than 800 ml volume **(The examiner must witness for at least 30 seconds)**	1	
Connects reservoir and oxygen	1	
Adjusts liter flow to 15 liters/minute or greater	1	
The examiner indicates arrival of a second EMT. The second EMT is instructed to ventilate the patient while the candidate controls the mask and the airway		
Voices re-opening the airway	1	
Creates a proper mask-to-face seal	1	
Instructs assistant to resume ventilation at proper volume per breath **(The examiner must witness for at least 30 seconds)**	1	
Total:	11	

Critical Criteria

_____ Did not take, or verbalize, body substance isolation precautions

_____ Did not immediately ventilate the patient

_____ Interrupted ventilations for more than 20 seconds

_____ Did not provide high concentration of oxygen

_____ Did not provide, or direct assistant to provide proper volume/breath
(more than two (2) ventilations per minute are below 800 ml)

_____ Did not allow adequate exhalation

BLEEDING CONTROL/SHOCK MANAGEMENT

Start Time: _____

Stop Time: _____ Date: _____

Candidate's Name: _____

Evaluator's Name: _____	Points Possible	Points Awarded
Takes, or verbalizes, body substance isolation precautions	1	
Applies direct pressure to the wound	1	
Elevates the extremity	1	
Note: The examiner must now inform the candidate that the wound continues to bleed.		
Applies an additional dressing to the wound	1	
Note: The examiner must now inform the candidate that the wound still continues to bleed. The second dressing does not control the bleeding.		
Locates and applies pressure to appropriate arterial pressure point	1	
Note: The examiner must now inform the candidate that the bleeding is controlled		
Bandages the wound	1	
Note: The examiner must now inform the candidate the patient is now showing signs and symptoms indicative of hypoperfusion		
Properly position the patient	1	
Applies high concentration oxygen	1	
Initiates steps to prevent heat loss from the patient	1	
Indicates the need for immediate transportation	1	
Total:	10	

Critical Criteria

_____ Did not take, or verbalize, body substance isolation precautions

_____ Did not apply high concentration oxygen

_____ Applied a tourniquet before attempting other methods of bleeding control

_____ Did not control hemorrhage in a timely manner

_____ Did not indicate a need for immediate transportation

CARDIAC ARREST MANAGEMENT/AED

Start Time: _____

Stop Time: _____ Date: _____

Candidate's Name: _____

Evaluator's Name: _____

	Points Possible	Points Awarded
ASSESSMENT		
Takes, or verbalizes, body substance isolation precautions	1	
Briefly questions the rescuer about arrest events	1	
Directs rescuer to stop CPR	1	
Verifies absence of spontaneous pulse **(skill station examiner states "no pulse")**	1	
Directs resumption of CPR	1	
Turns on defibrillator power	1	
Attaches automated defibrillator to the patient	1	
Directs rescuer to stop CPR and ensures all individuals are clear of the patient	1	
Initiates analysis of the rhythm	1	
Delivers shock (up to three successive shocks)	1	
Verifies absence of spontaneous pulse **(skill station examiner states "no pulse")**	1	
TRANSITION		
Directs resumption of CPR	1	
Gathers additional information about the arrest event	1	
Confirms effectiveness of CPR (ventilation and compressions)	1	
INTEGRATION		
Verbalizes or directs insertion of a simple airway adjunct (oral/nasal airway)	1	
Ventilates, or directs ventilation of the patient	1	
Assures high concentration of oxygen is delivered to the patient	1	
Assures CPR continues without unnecessary/prolonged interruption	1	
Re-evaluates patient/CPR in approximately one minute	1	
Repeats defibrillator sequence	1	
TRANSPORTATION		
Verbalizes transportation of the patient	1	
Total:	21	

Critical Criteria

_____ Did not take, or verbalize, body substance isolation precautions

_____ Did not evaluate the need for immediate use of the AED

_____ Did not direct initiation/resumption of ventilation/compressions at appropriate times

_____ Did not assure all individuals were clear of patient before delivering each shock

_____ Did not operate the AED properly (inability to deliver shock)

_____ Prevented the defibrillator from delivering indicated stacked shocks

IMMOBILIZATION SKILLS
JOINT INJURY

Start Time: _____

Stop Time: _____ Date: _____

Candidate's Name: _____

Evaluator's Name: _____	Points Possible	Points Awarded
Takes, or verbalizes, body substance isolation precautions	1	
Directs application of manual stabilization of the shoulder injury	1	
Assesses motor, sensory and circulatory function in the injured extremity	1	
Note: The examiner acknowledges "motor, sensory and circulatory function are present and normal."		
Selects the proper splinting material	1	
Immobilizes the site of the injury	1	
Immobilizes the bone above the injured joint	1	
Immobilizes the bone below the injured joint	1	
Reassesses motor, sensory and circulatory function in the injured extremity	1	
Note: The examiner acknowledges "motor, sensory and circulatory function are present and normal."		
Total:	8	

Critical Criteria

_____ Did not support the joint so that the joint did not bear distal weight

_____ Did not immobilize the bone above and below the injured site

_____ Did not reassess motor, sensory and circulatory function in the injured extremity before and after splinting

IMMOBILIZATION SKILLS
LONG BONE INJURY

Start Time: _____

Stop Time: _____ Date: _____

Candidate's Name: _____

Evaluator's Name: _____	Points Possible	Points Awarded
Takes, or verbalizes, body substance isolation precautions	1	
Directs application of manual stabilization of the injury	1	
Assesses motor, sensory and circulatory function in the injured extremity	1	
Note: The examiner acknowledges "motor, sensory and circulatory function are present and normal"		
Measures the splint	1	
Applies the splint	1	
Immobilizes the joint above the injury site	1	
Immobilizes the joint below the injury site	1	
Secures the entire injured extremity	1	
Immobilizes the hand/foot in the position of function	1	
Reassesses motor, sensory and circulatory function in the injured extremity	1	
Note: The examiner acknowledges "motor, sensory and circulatory function are present and normal"		
Total	10	

Critical Criteria

_____ Grossly moves the injured extremity

_____ Did not immobilize the joint above and the joint below the injury site

_____ Did not reassess motor, sensory and circulatory function in the injured extremity before and after splinting

IMMOBILIZATION SKILLS
TRACTION SPLINTING

Start Time: _____

Stop Time: _____ Date: _____

Candidate's Name: _____

Evaluator's Name: _____	Points Possible	Points Awarded
Takes, or verbalizes, body substance isolation precautions	1	
Directs application of manual stabilization of the injured leg	1	
Directs the application of manual traction	1	
Assesses motor, sensory and circulatory function in the injured extremity	1	
Note: The examiner acknowledges "motor, sensory and circulatory function are present and normal"		
Prepares/adjusts splint to the proper length	1	
Positions the splint next to the injured leg	1	
Applies the proximal securing device (e.g..ischial strap)	1	
Applies the distal securing device (e.g..ankle hitch)	1	
Applies mechanical traction	1	
Positions/secures the support straps	1	
Re-evaluates the proximal/distal securing devices	1	
Reassesses motor, sensory and circulatory function in the injured extremity	1	
Note: The examiner acknowledges "motor, sensory and circulatory function are present and normal"		
Note: The examiner must ask the candidate how he/she would prepare the patient for transportation		
Verbalizes securing the torso to the long board to immobilize the hip	1	
Verbalizes securing the splint to the long board to prevent movement of the splint	1	
Total:	14	

Critical Criteria

_____ Loss of traction at any point after it was applied

_____ Did not reassess motor, sensory and circulatory function in the injured extremity before and after splinting

_____ The foot was excessively rotated or extended after splint was applied

_____ Did not secure the ischial strap before taking traction

_____ Final immobilization failed to support the femur or prevent rotation of the injured leg

_____ Secured the leg to the splint before applying mechanical traction

Note: If the Sagar splint or the Kendricks Traction Device is used without elevating the patient's leg, application of manual traction is not necessary. The candidate should be awarded one (1) point as if manual traction were applied.

Note: If the leg is elevated at all, manual traction must be applied before elevating the leg. The ankle hitch may be applied before elevating the leg and used to provide manual traction.

MOUTH TO MASK WITH SUPPLEMENTAL OXYGEN

Start Time: _____

Stop Time: _____ Date: _____

Candidate's Name: _____

Evaluator's Name: _____

	Points Possible	Points Awarded
Takes, or verbalizes, body substance isolation precautions	1	
Connects one-way valve to mask	1	
Opens patient's airway or confirms patient's airway is open (manually or with adjunct)	1	
Establishes and maintains a proper mask to face seal	1	
Ventilates the patient at the proper volume and rate (800-1200 ml per breath/10-20 breaths per minute)	1	
Connects the mask to high concentration or oxygen	1	
Adjusts flow rate to at least 15 liters per minute	1	
Continues ventilation of the patient aT the proper volume and rate (800-1200 ml per breath/10-20 breaths per minute)	1	
Note: The examiner must witness ventilations for at least 30 seconds		
Total:	8	

Critical Criteria

_____ Did not take, or verbalize, body substance isolation precautions

_____ Did not adjust liter flow to at least 15 liters per minute

_____ Did not provide proper volume per breath
(more than 2 ventiliations per minute were below 800 ml)

_____ Did not ventilate the patient at a rate of 10-20 breaths per minute

_____ Did not allow for complete exhalation

OXYGEN ADMINISTRATION

Start Time: _____

Stop Time: _____ Date: _____

Candidate's Name: _____

Evaluator's Name: _____	Points Possible	Points Awarded
Takes, or verbalizes, body substance isolation precautions	1	
Assembles the regulator to the tank	1	
Opens the tank	1	
Checks for leaks	1	
Checks tank pressure	1	
Attaches non-rebreather mask to oxygen	1	
Prefills reservoir	1	
Adjusts liter flow to 12 liters per minute or greater	1	
Applies and adjusts the mask to the patient's face	1	
Note: The examiner must advise the candidate that the patient is not tolerating the non-rebreather mask. The medical director has ordered you to apply a nasal cannula to the patient.		
Attaches nasal cannula to oxygen	1	
Adjusts liter flow to six (6) liters per minute or less	1	
Applies nasal cannula to the patient	1	
Note: The examiner must advise the candidate to discontinue oxygen therapy		
Removes the nasal cannula from the patient	1	
Shuts off the regulator	1	
Relieves the pressure within the regulator	1	
Total:	15	

Critical Criteria

_____ Did not take, or verbalize, body substance isolation precautions

_____ Did not assemble the tank and regulator without leaks

_____ Did not prefill the reservoir bag

_____ Did not adjust the device to the correct liter flow for the non-rebreather mask
(12 liters per minute or greater)

_____ Did not adjust the device to the correct liter flow for the nasal cannula
(6 liters per minute or less)

Patient Assessment/Management - Medical

Start Time: _____

Stop Time: _____ Date: _____

Candidate's Name: _____

Evaluator's Name: _____

	Points Possible	Points Awarded
Takes, or verbalizes, body substance isolation precautions	1	
SCENE SIZE-UP		
Determines the scene is safe	1	
Determines the mechanism of injury/nature of illness	1	
Determines the number of patients	1	
Requests additional help if necessary	1	
Considers stabilization of spine	1	
INITIAL ASSESSMENT		
Verbalizes general impression of the patient	1	
Determines responsiveness/level of consciousness	1	
Determines chief complaint/apparent life threats	1	

Assesses airway and breathing	Assessment	1	
	Indicates appropriate oxygen therapy	1	
	Assures adequate ventilation	1	
Assesses circulation	Assesses/controls major bleeding	1	
	Assesses pulse	1	
	Assesses skin (color, temperature and condition)	1	

	Points Possible	Points Awarded
Identifies priority patients/makes transport decisions	1	
FOCUSED HISTORY AND PHYSICAL EXAMINATION/RAPID ASSESSMENT		
Signs and symptoms (Assess history of present illness)	1	

Respiratory	Cardiac	Altered Mental Status	Allergic Reaction	Poisoning/ Overdose	Environmental Emergency	Obstetrics	Behavioral
*Onset? *Provokes? *Quality? *Radiates? *Severity? *Time? *Interventions?	*Onset? *Provokes? *Quality? *Radiates? *Severity? *Time? *Interventions?	*Description of the episode. *Onset? *Duration? *Associated Symptoms? *Evidence of Trauma? *Interventions? *Seizures? *Fever?	*History of allergies? *What were you exposed to? *How were you exposed? *Effects? *Progression? *Interventions?	*Substance? When did you ingest/become exposed? *How much did you ingest? *Over what time period? *Interventions? *Estimated weight?	*Source? *Environment? *Duration? *Loss of consciousness? *Effects-general or local?	*Are you pregnant? *How long have you been pregnant? *Pain or contractions? *Bleeding or discharge? *Do you feel the need to push? *Last menstrual period?	*How do you feel? *Determine suicidal tendencies. *Is the patient a threat to self or others? Is there a medical problem? Interventions?

	Points Possible	Points Awarded
Allergies	1	
Medications	1	
Past pertinent history	1	
Last oral intake	1	
Event leading to present illness (rule out trauma)	1	
Performs focused physical examination (assesses affected body part/system or, if indicated, completes rapid assessment)	1	
Vitals (obtains baseline vital signs)	1	
Interventions (obtains medical direction or verbalizes standing order for medication interventions and verbalizes proper additional intervention/treatment)	1	
Transport (re-evaluates the transport decision)	1	
Verbalizes the consideration for completing a detailed physical examination	1	
ONGOING ASSESSMENT (verbalized)		
Repeats initial assessment	1	
Repeats vital signs	1	
Repeats focused assessment regarding patient complaint or injuries	1	
Critical Criteria Total:	30	

Critical Criteria

_____ Did not take, or verbalize, body substance isolation precautions when necessary

_____ Did not determine scene safety

_____ Did not obtain medical direction or verbalize standing orders for medical interventions

_____ Did not provide high concentration of oxygen

_____ Did not find or manage problems associated with airway, breathing, hemorrhage or shock (hypoperfusion)

_____ Did not differentiate patient's need for transportation versus continued assessment at the scene

_____ Did detailed or focused history/physical examination before assessing the airway, breathing and circulation

_____ Did not ask questions about the present illness

_____ Administered a dangerous or inappropriate intervention

Patient Assessment/Management - Trauma

Start Time: _____

Stop Time: _____ Date: _____

Candidate's Name: _____

Evaluator's Name: _____

		Points Possible	Points Awarded
Takes, or verbalizes, body substance isolation precautions		1	
SCENE SIZE-UP			
Determines the scene is safe		1	
Determines the mechanism of injury		1	
Determines the number of patients		1	
Requests additional help if necessary		1	
Considers stabilization of spine		1	
INITIAL ASSESSMENT			
Verbalizes general impression of the patient		1	
Determines responsiveness/level of consciousness		1	
Determines chief complaint/apparent life threats		1	
Assesses airway and breathing	Assessment	1	
	Initiates appropriate oxygen therapy	1	
	Assures adequate ventilation	1	
	Injury management	1	
Assesses circulation	Assesses/controls major bleeding	1	
	Assesses pulse	1	
	Assesses skin (color, temperature and conditions)	1	
Identifies priority patients/makes transport decision		1	
FOCUSED HISTORY AND PHYSICAL EXAMINATION/RAPID TRAUMA ASSESSMENT			
Selects appropriate assessment (**focused or rapid assessment**)		1	
Obtains, or directs assistance to obtain, baseline vital signs		1	
Obtains S.A.M.P.L.E. history		1	
DETAILED PHYSICAL EXAMINATION			
Assesses the head	Inspects and palpates the scalp and ears	1	
	Assesses the eyes	1	
	Assesses the facial areas including oral and nasal areas	1	
Assesses the neck	Inspects and palpates the neck	1	
	Assesses for JVD	1	
	Assesses for tracheal deviation	1	
Assesses the chest	Inspects	1	
	Palpates	1	
	Auscultates	1	
Assesses the abdomen/pelvis	Assesses the abdomen	1	
	Assesses the pelvis	1	
	Verbalizes assessment of genitalia/perineum as needed	1	
Assesses the extremities	1 point for each extremity includes inspection, palpation, and assessment of motor, sensory and circulatory function	4	
Assesses the posterior	Assesses thorax	1	
	Assesses lumbar	1	
Manages secondary injuries and wounds appropriately **1 point for appropriate management of the secondary injury/wound**		1	
Verbalizes re-assessment of the vital signs		1	
	Total:	40	

Critical Criteria

_____ Did not take, or verbalize, body substance isolation precautions

_____ Did not determine scene safety

_____ Did not assess for spinal protection

_____ Did not provide for spinal protection when indicated

_____ Did not provide high concentration of oxygen

_____ Did not find, or manage, problems associated with airway, breathing, hemorrhage or shock (hypoperfusion)

_____ Did not differentiate patient's need for transportation versus continued assessment at the scene

_____ Did other detailed physical examination before assessing the airway, breathing and circulation

_____ Did not transport patient within (10) minute time limit

SPINAL IMMOBILIZATION
SEATED PATIENT

Start Time: _____

Stop Time: _____ Date: _____

Candidate's Name: _____

Evaluator's Name: _____

	Points Possible	Points Awarded
Takes, or verbalizes, body substance isolation precautions	1	
Directs assistant to place/maintain head in the neutral in-line position	1	
Directs assistant to maintain manual immobilization of the head	1	
Reassesses motor, sensory and circulatory function in each extremity	1	
Applies appropriately sized extrication collar	1	
Positions the immobilization device behind the patient	1	
Secures the device to the patient's torso	1	
Evaluates torso fixation and adjusts as necessary	1	
Evaluates and pads behind the patient's head as necessary	1	
Secure the patient's head to the device	1	
Verbalizes moving the patient to a long board	1	
Reassesses motor, sensory and circulatory function in each extremity	1	
Total:	**12**	

Critical Criteria

_____ Did not immediately direct, or take, manual immobilization of the head

_____ Released, or ordered release of, manual immobilization before it was maintained mechanically

_____ Patient manipulated, or moved excessively, causing potential spinal compromise

_____ Device moved excessively up, down, left or right on the patient's torso

_____ Head immobilization allows for excessive movement

_____ Torso fixation inhibits chest rise, resulting in respiratory compromise

_____ Upon completion of immobilization, head is not in the neutral position

_____ Did not assess motor, sensory and circulatory function in each extremity after voicing immobilization to the long board

_____ Immobilized head to the board before securing the torso

SPINAL IMMOBILIZATION
SUPINE PATIENT

Start Time: _____

Stop Time: _____ Date: _____

Candidate's Name: _____

Evaluator's Name: _____	Points Possible	Points Awarded
Takes, or verbalizes, body substance isolation precautions	1	
Directs assistant to place/maintain head in the neutral in-line position	1	
Directs assistant to maintain manual immobilization of the head	1	
Reassesses motor, sensory and circulatory function in each extremity	1	
Applies appropriately sized extrication collar	1	
Positions the immobilization device appropriately	1	
Directs movement of the patient onto the device without compromising the integrity of the spine	1	
Applies padding to voids between the torso and the board as necessary	1	
Immobilizes the patient's torso to the device	1	
Evaluates and pads behind the patient's head as necessary	1	
Immobilizes the patient's head to the device	1	
Secures the patient's legs to the device	1	
Secures the patient's arms to the device	1	
Reassesses motor, sensory and circulatory function in each extremity	1	
Total:	14	

Critical Criteria

_____ Did not immediately direct, or take, manual immobilization of the head

_____ Released, or ordered release of, manual immobilization before it was maintained mechanically

_____ Patient manipulated, or moved excessively, causing potential spinal compromise

_____ Patient moves excessively up, down, left or right on the device

_____ Head immobilization allows for excessive movement

_____ Upon completion of immobilization, head is not in the neutral position

_____ Did not assess motor, sensory and circulatory function in each extremity after immobilization to the device

_____ Immobilized head to the board before securing the torso

VENTILATORY MANAGEMENT
DUAL LUMEN DEVICE INSERTION FOLLOWING
AN UNSUCCESSFUL ENDOTRACHEAL INTUBATION ATTEMPT

Start Time: _____

Stop Time: _____ Date: _____

Candidate's Name: _____

Evaluator's Name: _____

	Points Possible	Points Awarded
Continues body substance isolation precautions	1	
Confirms the patient is being properly ventilated with high percentage oxygen	1	
Directs the assistant to hyper-oxygenate the patient	1	
Checks/prepares the airway device	1	
Lubricates the distal tip of the device (may be verbalized)	1	
Note: the examiner should remove the OPA and move out of the way when the candidate is prepared to insert the device		
Positions the patient's head properly	1	
Performs a tongue-jaw lift	1	

USES COMBITUBE	USES THE PTL		
Inserts device in the mid-line and to the depth so that the printed ring is at the level of the teeth	Inserts the device in the mid-line until the bite block flange is at the level of the teeth	1	
Inflates the pharyngeal cuff with the proper volume and removes the syringe	Secures the strap	1	
Inflates the distal cuff with the proper volume and removes the syringe	Blows into tube #1 to adequately inflate both cuffs	1	
Attaches/directs attachment of BVM to the first (esophageal placement) lumen and ventilates		1	
Confirms placement and ventilation through the correct lumen by observing chest rise, auscultation over the epigastrium and bilaterally over each lung		1	
Note: The examiner states, "You do not see rise and fall of the chest and hear sounds only over epigastrium"			
Attaches/directs attachment of BVM to the second (endotracheal placement) lumen and ventilates		1	
Confirms placement and ventilation through the correct lumen by observing chest rise, auscultation over the epigastrium and bilaterally over each lung		1	
Note: The examiner states, "You see rise and fall off the chest, there are no sounds over the epigastrium and breath sounds are equal over each lung"			
Secures device or confirms that the device remains properly secured		1	
Total:		15	

Critical Criteria

_____ Did not take or verbalize body substance isolation precautions
_____ Did not initiate ventilations within 30 seconds
_____ Interrupted ventilations for more than 30 seconds at any time
_____ Did not hyper-oxygenate the patient prior to placement of the dual lumen airway device
_____ Did not provide adequate volume per breath (maximum 2 errors/minute permissable)
_____ Did not ventilate the patient at a rate of at least 10 breaths per minute
_____ Did not insert the dual lumen airway device at a proper depth or at the proper place within 3 attempts
_____ Did not inflate both cuffs properly
_____ **Combitube** - Did not remove the syringe immediately following inflation of each cuff
_____ **PTL** - Did not secure the strap prior to cuff inflation
_____ Did not confirm, by observing chest rise and auscultation over the epigastrium and bilaterally over each lung that the proper lumen of the device was being used to ventilate the patient
_____ Inserted any adjunct in a manner that was dangerous to the patient

VENTILATORY MANAGEMENT
ENDOTRACHEAL INTUBATION

Start Time: _____

Stop Time: _____   Date: _____

Candidate's Name: _____

Evaluator's Name: _____

Note: If a candidate elects to initially ventilate the patient with a BVM attached to a reservoir and oxygen, full credit must be awarded for steps denoted by "*" provided first ventilation is delivered within the initial 30 seconds	Points Possible	Points Awarded
Takes, or verbalizes, body substance isolation precautions	1	
Opens the airway manually	1	
Elevates the patient's tongue and inserts a simple airway adjunct (Oropharyngeal/nasopharyngeal airway)	1	
Note: The examiner must now inform the candidate "no gag reflex is present and the patient accepts the airway adjunct"		
**Ventilates the patient immediately using a BVM device unattached to oxygen	1	
**Hyperventilates the patient with room air	1	
Note: The examiner must now inform the candidate that ventilation is being properly performed without difficulty		
Attaches the oxygen reservoir to the BVM	1	
Attaches the BVM to high flow oxygen (15 liter per minute)	1	
Ventilates the patient at the proper volume and rate (800-1200 ml/breath and 10-20 breaths/minute)	1	
Note: After 30 seconds, the examiner must auscultate the patient's chest and inform the candidate that breath sounds are present and equal bilaterally and medical direction has ordered endotracheal intubation. The examiner must now take over ventilation of the patient.		
Directs assistant to hyper-oxygenate the patient	1	
Identifies/selects the proper equipment for endotracheal intubation	1	
Checks equipment — Checks for cuff leaks	1	
Checks laryngoscope operation and bulb tightness	1	
Note: The examiner must remove the OPA and move out of the way when the candidate is prepared to intubate the patient.		
Positions the patient's head properly	1	
Inserts the laryngoscope blade into the patient's mouth while displacing the patient's tongue laterally	1	
Elevates the patient's mandible with the laryngoscope	1	
Introduces the endotracheal tube and advances the tube to the proper depth	1	
Inflates the cuff to the proper pressure	1	
Disconnects the syringe from the cuff inlet port	1	
Directs assistant to ventilate the patient	1	
Confirms proper placement of the endotracheal tube by auscultation bilaterally and over the epigastrium	1	
Note: The examiner must ask, "If you had proper placement, what would you expect to hear?"		
Secures the endotracheal tube (may be verbalized)	1	
Total:	21	

Critical Criteria

_____ Did not take or verbalize body substance isolation precautions when necessary

_____ Did not initiate ventilation within 30 seconds after applying gloves or interrupts ventilations for greater than 30 seconds at a time

_____ Did not voice or provide high oxygen concentrations (15 liter/minute or greater)

_____ Did not ventilate the patient at a rate of at least 10 breaths per minute

_____ Did not provide adequate volume per breath (maximum of 2 errors per minute permissible)

_____ Did not hyper-oxygenate the patient prior to intubation

_____ Did not successfully intubate the patient within 3 attempts

_____ Used the patient's teeth as a fulcrum

_____ Did not assure proper tube placement by auscultation bilaterally over each lung **and** over the epigastrium

_____ The stylette (if used) extended beyond the end of the endotracheal tube

_____ Inserted any adjunct in a manner that was dangerous to the patient

_____ Did not immediately disconnect the syringe from the inlet port after inflating the cuff

VENTILATORY MANAGEMENT
ESOPHAGEAL OBTURATOR AIRWAY INSERTION FOLLOWING
AN UNSUCCESSFUL ENDOTRACHEAL INTUBATION ATTEMPT

Start Time: _____

Stop Time: _____ Date: _____

Candidate's Name: _____

Evaluator's Name:	Points Possible	Points Awarded
Continues body substance isolation precautions	1	
Confirms the patient is being ventilated with high percentage oxygen	1	
Directs the assistant to hyper-oxygenate the patient	1	
Identifies/selects the proper equipment for insertion of EOA	1	
Assembles the EOA	1	
Tests the cuff for leaks	1	
Inflates the mask	1	
Lubricates the tube (may be verbalized)	1	
Note: The examiner should remove the OPA and move out of the way when the candidate is prepared to insert the device		
Positions the head properly with the neck in the neutral or slightly flexed position	1	
Grasps and elevates the patient's tongue and mandible	1	
Inserts the tube in the same direction as the curvature of the pharynx	1	
Advances the tube until the mask is sealed against the patient's face	1	
Ventilates the patient while maintaining a tight mask-to-face seal	1	
Directs confirmation of placement of EOA by observing for chest rise and auscultation over the epigastrium and bilaterally over each lung	1	
Note: The examiner must acknowledge adequate chest rise, bilateral breath sounds and absent sounds over the epigastrium		
Inflates the cuff to the proper pressure	1	
Disconnects the syringe from the inlet port	1	
Continues ventilation of the patient	1	
Total:	17	

Critical Criteria

_____ Did not take or verbalize body substance isolation precautions

_____ Did not initiate ventilations within 30 seconds

_____ Interrupted ventilations for more than 30 seconds at any time

_____ Did not direct hper-oxygenation of the patient prior to placement of the EOA

_____ Did not successfully place the EOA within 3 attempts

_____ Did not ventilate at a rate of at least 10 breaths per minute

_____ Did not provide adequate volume per breath (maximum 2 errors/minute permissible)

_____ Did not assure proper tube placement by auscultation bilaterally and over the epigastrium

_____ Did not remove the syringe after inflating the cuff

_____ Did not successfully ventilate the patient

_____ Did not provide high flow oxygen (15 liters per minute or greater)

_____ Inserted any adjunct in a manner that was dangerous to the patient

Index

A

Abandonment, 37
Abdomen
  in children, 460
  physical examination of, 261
  trauma assessment, 140
Abduction, 11
Abnormal deliveries, 442–443
Abortion, spontaneous, 439
Abrasion, 203
Abruptio placentae, 440
Absorbed poison, 371
Abuse, elderly, 483
Acquired immunodeficiency syndrome (AIDS), 27–28
Actidose, 371
Activated charcoal, 371
Acute mountain sickness, 396
Acute myocardial infarction, 316
  in elderly, 481
Acute pulmonary edema, 289
Addiction, 372
Adduction, 11
Adequate breathing, 121
Adolescents
  blood pressure of, 459t
  breathing rate, 121
  development of, 458
  pulse rates of, 459t
  respiratory rates of, 459t
Adrenal glands, 52
Advanced airway management, 545–559
Aeromedical operations, 513–514
Aging
  demographics of, 479
  effects of, 479
Agonal breathing, 121
AIDS. See Acquired immunodeficiency syndrome (AIDS)
Air bags, 522
Air embolism, 395
Air sacs, 120
Airway, 98
  adjuncts, 122
  advanced management, 545–559
  assessment of, 286
  in children, 459–460
  lower, 120, 285
    burns, 399
  nasopharyngeal, 122

Airway (Continued)
  obstruction, 287
  opening, 122
  oropharyngeal, 122
  pharyngotracheal lumen, 548–549
  reactive disease in children, 461
  upper, 120, 285
    burns, 399
Alcohol, 372
Alcoholics, 393
Altered mental status, 349–368
Altitude, 395–396
Alveoli, 50, 120
Ambulance
  control, 512
  operations, 510–519
  positioning at scene, 513
  standards, 511
  types, 511
American College of Surgeons Committee on Trauma Minimum Essential equipment for Ambulances, 511
Ammonia
  anhydrous, 530
Amniotic sac, 439
Amphetamines, 372
Amputations, 203
Anaphylactic shock, 206, 230
Anatomy, 47–65
  definitions, 10–11, 47
  position, 10, 10f
  structure, 47
Angina pectoris, stable, 316
Anhydrous ammonia, 530
Ankle, 157
Anterior, 10
Anthrax, 533
Anxiety, 422
Aorta, 50
Apgar score, 442t
Appendicular skeleton, 156
Arachnoid, 178
Arc burns, 400
Arterial bleeding, 204
Arteries, 100, 315
Artificial ventilation devices, 123
Assault, 37
Asthma, 288
  in children, 461

Page references followed by "f" indicate figures and by "t" indicate tables.

Asystole, 319f
Atherosclerosis, 316
Athletes, exertional heat stroke, 393
Atropine, 530
Avulsions, 203
Axial skeleton, 156

B

Bacillus anthracis, 533
Back, trauma assessment, 140
Backing up, 512
Bag-valve mask (BVM), 123
Bandages, 204
Barbiturates, 372
Barrel chest, 288
Base station, 500
Basket stretcher, 84
Battery, 37
Behavior, 422
Behavioral emergencies, 421–437
    assessment, 424–425
Bends, 396
Benzodiazepines, 372
Biological agents, 533–534
Biological and chemical terrorism, 529–544
Bipolar disorder, 422
Birth canal, 439
Blanket drag, 75, 77f
Bleeding control, 205
Blister agents, 530, 531–532
Blood
    agents, 530–531
    glucose level, 350
    pathway through heart, 315
Blood pressure, 100
    in adolescents, 459t
    in children, 459t
    in elderly, 479
Blood vessels, 50, 51
Blood volume, 204
Body mechanics, 74
Body temperature, 392
    in elderly, 479
Bones, 156
Botulinum toxin, 536
Bourdon gauge, 123
Bradypnea, 121
Brain, 52, 178
Brain stem, 178
Braking, 512
Breathing, 98
    adequate, 121
    agonal, 121
    assessment of, 121, 286

Breathing (*Continued*)
    in children, 459–460
    control, 121
    inadequate, 121
    rate, 121
Breech delivery, 442
Bridges, 512
Bronchi, 50
Bronchioles, 120
Bronchiolitis in children, 461
Bronchitis, chronic, 288
Bruise, 202
Bubonic plague, 534
Burnout, 23
Burns, 396–400
    arc, 400
    carpet, 203
    chemical, 399–400
    children, 397
    electrical, 400
    flame, 400
    lower airway, 399
    upper airway, 399
Buses, school, 512
BVM. *See* Bag-valve mask (BVM)

C

Caffeine, 372
Calcaneus, 157
Cannabis, 373
Capillaries, 315
    bleeding, 204
    refill, 100
Carbon dioxide detection, 549
Carbon monoxide, 399
Cardiac muscle, 48, 156
Cardiac output, 315
Cardiac volume, 315
Cardiogenic shock, 206, 230
Cardiovascular disease, 316–317
    in elderly, 481
Cardiovascular emergencies, 315–348
Cardiovascular system, 50–51
    in elderly, 479
Carpals, 156
Carpet burns, 203
Carrying devices, 83–84
Cartilage, 156
Caudad, 10
Cell, 47, 47f
Central nervous system, 52, 178
Cephalad, 10
Cerebellum, 178
Cerebral contusions and lacerations, 179

Cerebrovascular accident in elderly, 482
Cerebrum, 178
Cervical collars, 181
Cervical injury in elderly, 483
Cervical spine, 156, 178
Cervix, 439
Charcoal, activated, 371
Chemical agents, 530
Chemical asphyxiants, 530–531
Chemical burns, 399–400
Chemicals in eyes, 400
Chemical terrorism, 529–544
Chest
    barrel, 288
    in children, 460
    penetrating injuries of, 203
    physical examination of, 261
    silent, 288
    trauma assessment, 140
Children
    abdomen, 460
    airway, 459–460
    anatomical differences, 458–460
    assessment of, 460–461
    asthma, 461
    blood pressure, 459t
    breathing, 459–460
    breathing rate, 121
    bronchiolitis, 461
    burns, 397
    chest, 460
    circulation, 460
    communication with, 502–503
    croup, 461
    developmental stages, 458
    emergencies, 457–477
    epiglottitis, 462
    exertional heat stroke, 393
    extremities, 460
    head and neck, 460
    laryngotracheobronchitis, 461
    meningitis, 462
    neurologic system, 460
    physical examination, 461
    pneumonia, 462
    pulse rates, 459t
    reactive airway disease, 461
    respiratory rates, 459t
    school age
        blood pressure of, 459t
        development of, 458
        pulse rates of, 459t
        respiratory rates of, 459t
    unconscious with foreign body airway obstruction, 287

Chloral hydrate, 372
Chlorine, 532
Choking agents, 530, 532
Cholera, 534
Chronic bronchitis, 288
Chronic obstructive pulmonary disease (COPD), 482
Circulation, 98
    in children, 460
Circulatory system, 50–51, 50f
Clavicle, 156
Closed extremity injury, 157
Clostridium botulinum, 536
Clot busters, 317
Clothing
    drag, 74, 74f
    protective, 522
Coarse ventricular fibrillation, 319f
Cocaine, 372
Coccygeal spine, 156, 178
Codeine, 372
Cold illness, 392
Collarbone, 156
Combitube, 548
Communicable disease, 25–26
Communication, 499–509
    with elderly, 480, 503
    interpersonal, 502
    radio, 500
    with special patients, 502
Compensated shock, 231
Concussion, 179
Confidentiality, 37
Congestive heart failure, 317, 393
    in elderly, 481
Connective tissue, 47
Conscious infant, foreign body airway obstruction, 287
Conscious patient, foreign body airway obstruction, 287
Construction workers, exertional heat stroke, 393
Contusion, 202
    cerebral, 179
COPD. *See* Chronic obstructive pulmonary disease (COPD)
Countrecoup, 179
Coup, 179
Cradle carry, 76
Cranium, 48, 156, 178
Critical incident stress, 24–25
Croup in children, 461
Crush injury, 202
Cyanide chloride, 530

D
Danger zones, 97
Death and dying, 23

Decompensated shock, 231
Decompression sickness, 396
Deep, 11
Deerfly fever, 534–535
Delirium tremens, 372
Delivery complications, 442–443
Dementia, 482
Depressants, 372
Depression, 422
    in elderly, 482–483
Dermis, 54, 202
Designated agent, 3
Developmental stages, 458
Diabetes, 350
Diaphoresis, 317
Diaphragm, 50
Diaphysis, 156
Diastole, 315
Diazepam. *See* Valium (diazepam)
Digestive system, 51
Dilation, 441
Direct carry, 82, 83f
Direct ground lift, 82, 82f
Direct pressure, 205
Disentanglement, 523
Dislocation, 157
Distal, 11
Distilled mustard, 531
DMT, 372
Documentation, 499–509
DOM, 372
Dorsal, 10
Draw sheet method, 80, 81f
Dressings, 204
Driving basics, 511
Drowning, 394–395
Drug abuse, 372
Dry lung, 394
Duplex frequency, 500
Dura mater, 178
Duty to act, 37
Dying, 23

E

Ear drum rupture, 395
Eclampsia, 440
Ectopic pregnancy, 440
Elderly
    abuse and neglect, 483
    acute myocardial infarction, 481
    anatomical differences, 479
    blood pressure, 479
    body temperature, 479
    cardiovascular disease, 481

Elderly (*Continued*)
    cardiovascular system, 479
    cerebrovascular accident, 482
    cervical injury, 483
    chronic obstructive pulmonary disease (COPD),
        482
    communication with, 503
    congestive heart failure, 481
    dementia, 482
    depression, 482–483
    emergencies, 478–498
    environmental emergencies, 483
    factors complicating assessment, 479–480
    gastrointestinal system, 479
    head injury, 483
    heat stroke, 393
    history taking, 480
    hypovolemia, 483
    integumentary system, 479
    musculoskeletal system, 479
    nervous system, 479
    neuropsychiatric disease, 482
    physical examination, 481
    pneumonia, 481
    pulmonary embolism, 481
    renal system, 479
    respiratory disease, 481
    respiratory system, 479
    seizures, 482
    shock, 483
    silent MI, 481
    stroke, 481
    syncope, 482
    transient ischemic attack (TIA), 481
    trauma, 483
Electrical burns, 400
Elevation, 205
Emancipated minor, 37
Emergency care, emotional aspects of, 23
Emergency driving laws, 511
Emergency moves, 74–79
Emotional aspects of emergency care, 23
Emphysema, 288
EMS system, 2–8
EMS training, 2
EMT-Basic, 2
    traits of, 2
    well-being of, 23–35
EMT-Intermediate, 3
EMT responsibilities, 2
Endocrine system, 52, 53f
Endotracheal intubation, 546–547
Endotracheal tube, 546
End-tidal carbon dioxide detection, 549

Environmental emergencies, 391–420
  in elderly, 483
Ephedrine, 372
Epidermis, 54, 202
Epidural hematoma, 179
Epidural space, 178
Epiglottis, 50, 120
Epiglottitis in children, 462
Epiphysis, 156
Epithelial tissue, 47
Escorts, 512
Esophagus, 51
Evisceration, 203
Exertional heat stroke, 393
Exhalation, 120
Expiration, 285
Expressed consent, 37
Expulsion, 441
Extension, 11
External, 11
External bleeding, 204–205
Extremities
  in children, 460
  physical examination of, 261
  trauma assessment, 140
Extremity carry, 79–80
Extremity lift, 81f
Extrication and rescue, 520–528
  hazard control, 521–522
  size-up, 521
Eyes
  chemicals in, 400
  sockets, 178

F

Face, 48, 156, 178
Fallopian tubes, 439
False imprisonment, 37
Federal Communications Commission (FCC), 500
Female reproduction, 439
Femur, 157
Fentanyl, 372
Fibula, 157
Fine ventricular fibrillation, 319f
Fingers, 156
Firefighter's carry, 77–78, 79, 80f
Firefighter's drag, 74, 75f
First responder, 2
Flame burns, 400
Flexible stretcher, 84
Flexion, 11
Flow-restricted oxygen-powered ventilation device, 124
Foot, 157
Foot drag, 74, 76f

Force, 425
Foreign body airway obstruction, 287
Fowler's, 11
Fracture, 157
  skull, 178–179
Francisella tularensis, 534
Frostbite, 393–394
Fuel spillage, 522

G

Gaining access, 522–523
Gallbladder, 51
Gasoline spillage, 522
Gastrointestinal system, 51, 51f
  in elderly, 479
Geriatric. *See* Elderly
Glucose, 350
Gonads, 52
Grand mal seizure, 352
Grief, 23
Gynecologic emergencies, 438–456

H

Haemophilus influenzae B (HiB), 462
Hallucinogens, 372
Hashish, 373
Hazardous materials, 97, 522
Head
  in children, 460
  injuries, 178–181
    in elderly, 483
  physical examination of, 260
  trauma assessment, 140
Hearing impaired, 502
Heart, 50, 315
Heart attack, 316
Heat/cold illness, 392
Heat cramps, 392
Heat exhaustion, 392–393
Heat stroke, 393
Helicopters, 513–514
Hematoma, 202
  epidural, 179
  intracerebral, 180
  subdural, 180
Hemorrhagic shock, 206, 230–231
Hemorrhagic stroke, 353
Hepatitis A, 26
Hepatitis B, 26
Hepatitis C, 26
Hepatitis D, 26
Hepatitis E, 26
Heroin, 372
HiB. *See Haemophilus influenzae* B (HiB)

High altitude sickness, 396
History
    in elderly, 480
    of present illness, 260
    of respiratory disease, 286
HIV. *See* Human immunodeficiency syndrome (HIV)
Homeostasis, 47
Human immunodeficiency syndrome (HIV), 27–28
Humerus, 156
Humpback, 479
Hydrocodone, 372
Hydrogen cyanide, 531
Hydrogen fluoride, 530
Hydroplaning, 512
Hyperglycemia, 351
Hypoglycemia, 350
Hypoperfusion, 206
Hypothermia, 394
Hypovolemia in elderly, 483
Hypovolemic shock, 206, 230

I

Impaled objects, 203
Implied consent, 37
Imprisonment, false, 37
Inadequate breathing, 121
Incline (bent-arm) drag, 74, 76f
Infants
    blood pressure of, 459t
    breathing rate, 121
    foreign body airway obstruction, 287
    premature, 443
    pulse rates of, 459t
    respiratory rates of, 459t
Infectious disease, 25
Inferior, 10
Information, presenting, 501
Informed consent, 37
Ingested poison, 370
Inhalants, 372–373
Inhalation, 120
Inhalation injury, 399
Inhaled poison, 370
Initial assessment, 98–99
Injected poison, 371
Inspiration, 285
InstaChar, 371
Integumentary system, 53–54, 53f
    in elderly, 479
Intercostal muscles, 50
Internal, 11
Internal bleeding, 205
Interpersonal communication, 502
Intersection collisions, 512

Intracerebral hematoma, 180
Intracranial injuries, 179–180
Intubation, endotracheal, 546–547
Involuntary muscle, 48
Irreversible shock, 231
Ischemia, 316
Ischemic stroke, 352–353
Islet of Langerhans, 52

J

Jaw, 178
Joints, 156

K

Kendrick extrication devices (KED), 524
Kidneys, 54
KKK-1822 standards, 511
Kneecap, 157
Kyphosis, 479

L

Labor, 441
Lacerations, 203
    cerebral, 179
Landing zone, 513–514
Large intestine, 51
Laryngopharynx, 120
Laryngoscope handle and blades, 546
Laryngotracheobronchitis in children, 461
Larynx, 50, 120
Lateral, 10
Lateral rotation, 11
Left lateral recumbent, 11
Legal issues, 37–45
    defined, 37–38
Lewisite, 531
Libel, 37
Life-saving care, 523
Lifting patients, 74–95
Ligaments, 156
Limb presentation, 442–443
LiquiChar, 371
Liver, 51
Loaded bumpers, 522
Long spine board, 83
Lower airway, 120, 285
    burns, 399
Lower extremities, 48, 157
LSD, 372
Lumbar spine, 156, 178

M

Mandible, 178
Manic-depressive disorder, 422

Marijuana, 373
Maxilla, 178
MDA, 372
Meconium, 443
Medial, 10
Medial rotation, 11
Medical assessment, 258–283, 259f
Medical control, 3
Medical direction, 3
Medical director, 3
Medical-legal issues, 37–45
    defined, 37–38
Medical records, 503–504
Medical terminology, 10–21
Meningeal spaces, 178
Meninges, 178
Meningitis
    in children, 462
    meningococcal, 27
Meningococcal meningitis, 27
Mental status, 98
    altered, 349–368
Metabolism, 392
Metacarpals, 156
Metaphysis, 156
Metatarsals, 157
Methadone, 372
Methylphenidate, 372
Midaxillary line, 11
Midclavicular line, 11
Midline, 10
Military recruits, exertional heat stroke,
    393
Minute volume, 120
Mobile receiver, 501
Mobile transmitter, 501
Morphine, 372
Motor vehicle crashes, 97
Mouth, 50, 120
Movements, 11
Moving and lifting patients, 74–95
Multiple births, 443
Multiplex frequency, 500
Muscles, 156
Muscle tissue, 47
Muscular system, 49f
Musculoskeletal system
    anatomy of, 156
    in elderly, 479
    injuries of, 156–157
Mycobacterium tuberculosis, 26
Myocardial infarction
    acute, 316
        in elderly, 481

Myocardial infarction (*Continued*)
    silent, 317
        in elderly, 481

N

Narcotics, 372
Nasal bones, 178
Nasal cannula, 123
Nasal trumpet, 122
Nasopharynx, 120
    airway, 122
Near drowning, 394–395
Neck
    in children, 460
    physical examination of, 260
    trauma assessment, 140
    wounds, 204
Neglect, elderly, 483
Negligence, 37
Negligence per se, 37
Neisseria meningitidis, 27
Neonates. *See* Newborns
Nerve agents, 530
Nervous system, 51–52, 52f
    in children, 460
    in elderly, 479
Nervous tissue, 47
Neurogenic shock, 206, 230
Neurologic examination, 180
Neuropsychiatric disease in elderly, 482
Neurotoxins, 530
Newborns
    blood pressure of, 459t
    breathing rate, 121
    development of, 458
    pulse rates of, 459t
    respiratory rates of, 459t
    resuscitation of, 442
Nicotine, 372
Nitrogen mustard, 531
Nitrogen narcosis, 395
Non-English speaking patients, 502
Non-rebreather mask, 123
Nonurgent moves, 79–80
Normal blood volume, 204
Normal delivery, 441
Normal sinus rhythm, 318, 318f
Nose, 50, 120

O

Obese, 393
Obstetric and gynecologic emergencies, 438–456
Occupational Safety and Health Administration (OSHA),
    511

One-person cradle carry, 78f
One-rescuer assist, 75–78, 77f
One-rescuer carries, 75–78
Open extremity injury, 157
Opium, 372
Orbits, 178
Organ, 47
Organism, 47
Organophosphate pesticide, 530
Organ system, 47, 48–49
Oropharynx, 120
    airway, 122
OSHA. *See* Occupational Safety and Health
        Administration (OSHA)
Osteoporosis, 479, 483
Ovaries, 52, 439
Overdose, 372
Oxygen cylinders, 123

P

Pack-strap carry, 76, 78f
Palmar, 11
Pancreas, 51, 52
Panic attack, 422
Paramedic, 3
Paranoia, 423
Parathyroid glands, 52
Parietal pleura, 285
Patella, 157
Pathogens, 25
Patients
    assessment using acronyms, mnemonics, and
        abbreviations, 12–13
    carrying devices, 83–84
    moving and lifting, 74–95
    non-English speaking, 502
    refusal documentation, 504
    responsive medical, 260
    seated
        spinal motion restriction, 181
PCM, 372
PCP, 372
Pediatric. *See* Children
Pelvic girdle, 156
Pelvis, 48
    physical examination of, 261
    trauma assessment, 140
Penetrating chest injuries, 203
Perineum, 439
Periosteum, 156
Peripheral nervous system, 52
Pesticide, organophosphate, 530
Petit mal seizure, 352
Phalanges, 156, 157

Pharyngotracheal lumen airway (PTU), 548–549
Pharynx, 50, 120
Phenol, 399
Phobia, 422
Phosgene, 532
Phosgene oxime, 531, 532
Physical examination
    of children, 461
    of elderly, 481
    of respiratory disease, 286–387
    of unresponsive medical patient, 260–261
Physiology, 47–65
Pia mater, 178
Piggyback carry, 77, 79f
Pituitary gland, 52
Placenta, 439
Placental delivery, 441
Placenta previa, 440
Plague, 533–534
Plantar, 11
Pleura, 285
Pleural space, 285
Pneumatic antishock garment, 232
Pneumonia, 289
    in children, 462
    in elderly, 481
Pneumonic plague, 534
Pneumothorax, spontaneous, 290
Pocket mask, 123
Poisoning, 370–371
Poisons, 369–380
Polypharmacy, 480
Portable ambulance stretcher, 83
Portable receiver, 501
Portable transmitter, 501
Positions, 11
Posterior, 10
Potassium, 399
Power lines, 522
Pralidoxime, 530
Predelivery emergencies, 439–440
Preeclampsia, 440
Prefixes, 11–12
Pregnancy, ectopic, 440
Pregnancy-induced hypertension, 440
Premature infant, 443
Preschoolers, 459t
Presenting information, 501
Pressure-compensated (Thorpe) flowmeter,
        123
Pressure point, 205
Pressure regulators, 123
Prolapsed umbilical cord, 442
Pronation, 11

Protective clothing, 522
Protocols, 3
Proximal, 10
Psychiatric disorders, 422
PTU. *See* Pharyngotracheal lumen airway (PTU)
Pulmonary artery, 50
Pulmonary edema, acute, 289
Pulmonary embolism, 290
  in elderly, 481
Pulmonary irritants, 530, 532
Pulmonary veins, 51
Pulse, 99
  rates, 459t
Punctures, 203
Pupils, 100

Q

Quality improvement, 3

R

Rabbit fever, 534–535
Radio communications, 500
Radius, 156
Railroads, 512
Reactive airway disease in children, 461
Records, medical, 503–504
Reeves stretcher, 84
Removal preparation, 524
Renal system in elderly, 479
Repeaters, 501
Reproductive system, 55, 55f
Rescue, 520–528
  hazard control, 521–522
  size-up, 521
Res ipsa loquitur, 37
Respiration, 99
Respiratory disease, 284–313
  in elderly, 481
Respiratory rates, 459t
Respiratory system, 49–50, 49f
  anatomy of, 120
  in elderly, 479
Responsive medical patient, 260
Restraints, 426
Resuscitation of newborn, 442
Rhythm, 121
Rib cage, 48
Ribs, 156
Ricin, 536
Ricinus communis, 536
Right lateral recumbent, 11
Right ventricular failure, 317
Road rash, 203
Road surface, 512

S

Sacral spine, 156, 178
Safety, 97
Salmonella, 535
Sample history, 100, 260
Sarin, 530
Scapula, 156
Scene size-up, 97
Schizophrenia, 423
School age children, 458, 459t
School buses, 512
Scoop stretcher, 83
Scuba emergencies, 395–396
Sedatives, 372
Seizures, 351–352
  in elderly, 482
Septic shock, 206, 230
Shin, 157
Shock, 11, 206
  anaphylactic, 206, 230
  cardiogenic, 206, 230
  compensated, 231
  decompensated, 231
  elderly, 483
  in elderly, 483
  hemorrhagic, 206, 230–231
  hypovolemic, 206, 230
  irreversible, 231
  management, 229–257
  neurogenic, 206, 230
  septic, 206, 230
  stages, 231
Short spine board, 83
Shoulder blade, 156
Shoulder drag, 74, 75f
Shoulder girdle, 156
Silent chest, 288
Silent myocardial infarction, 317
  in elderly, 481
Simplex frequency, 500
Sinus rhythm, normal, 318
Siren, 513
Skeletal muscle, 156
Skeletal system, 48, 48f, 156
Skin, 53, 202
  color, 99
  irritants, 530
Skip, 500
Skull, 48, 156, 178
  fractures, 178–179
Slander, 37
Small intestine, 51
Smallpox, 535
Smooth muscle, 156

Sodium, 399
Sodium thiosulfate, 531
Soft tissue injury, 202–228
Somni, 530
Spinal column, 156
   injuries, 178–181
Spinal cord, 52, 178
   injuries, 180
Spine, 48, 156, 178
   motion restriction, 181
Splints, 157
Spontaneous abortion, 439
Spontaneous pneumothorax, 290
Sprain, 157
Squeeze, 395
Stable angina pectoris, 316
Stair chair, 83
Standard of care, 38
Standing orders, 3
Staphylococcal enterotoxin B, 537
Staphylococcus aureus, 537
Status epilepticus, 352
Sternum, 156
Stimulants, 372
Stokes basket, 84
Stomach, 51
Strain, 157
Stress, 23, 24
Stretchers, 83–84
Stroke, 352–353
   in elderly, 481
Stroke volume, 315
Stylette, 546
Subarachnoid space, 178
Subcutaneous layer, 54, 202
Subdural hematoma, 180
Subdural space, 178
Substance abuse, 372
Suctioning, 122–123
Sudden cardiac death, 317–318
Suffixes, 11–12
Suicides, 422, 423
   assessment of, 425
Sulfur dioxide, 530
Sulfuric acid, 530
Sulfur mustard, 531
SuperChar, 371
Superficial, 11
Superior, 10
Supination, 11
Supine, 11
Supine hypotension, 440
Supine patient, spinal motion restriction, 181
Supplemental oxygen, 123

Syncope in elderly, 482
Systole, 315

T

Tabun, 530
Tachypnea, 121
Tail bone, 178
Talus, 157
Tar, 399
Tarsals, 157
Teenagers. *See* Adolescents
Tendons, 156
Terminology, medical, 10–21
Terrorism, biological and chemical, 529–544
Testes, 52
Tetrahydrocannabinol, 373
Thigh, 157
Thoracic cage, 156
Thoracic spine, 156, 178
Throat, 120
Thyroid gland, 52
TIA. *See* Transient ischemic attack (TIA)
Tibia, 157
Tidal volume, 120
Tissue, 47
Toddlers
   blood pressure of, 459t
   breathing rate, 121
   development of, 458
   pulse rates of, 459t
   respiratory rates of, 459t
Toes, 157
Tort, 38
Tourniquet, 205
Trachea, 50, 120
Traffic laws, 511, 521–522
Traffic patterns, 512
Tranquilizers, 372
Transient ischemic attack (TIA), 481
Transmitting information, 501
Trauma
   assessment, 138–140, 139f
      body substance isolation, 138
      mechanism of injury, 138–140
      scene size-up, 138
   in elderly, 483
Trendelenburg, 11
Trunking, 500
Tuberculosis, 26
Tularemia, 534–535
Tunnels, 512
Two-rescuer assists, 78–79, 80f
Two-rescuer carries, 78–79
Type I diabetes mellitus, 350

Type II diabetes mellitus, 350
Typhoidal tularemia, 535

U

UHF. *See* Ultrahigh frequency (UHF)
Ulceroglandular tularemia, 534
Ulna, 156
Ultrahigh frequency (UHF), 500
Umbilical cord, 439
  prolapsed, 442
Unconscious with foreign body airway obstruction, 287
Unresponsive medical patient, 260–261
Unstable angina pectoris, 316
Unstable vehicles, 522
Upper airway, 120, 285
Upper airway burns, 399
Upper extremities, 48, 156
Ureters, 54
Urethra, 54
Urinary bladder, 54
Urinary system, 54, 54f
Uterus, 439
  rupture, 440

V

Vagina, 439
Valium (diazepam), 530
Vehicle windows, 523
Veins, 315
Venae cavae, 50

Venezuelan equine encephalitis, 535–536
Venous bleeding, 204
Ventilation, 120
Ventral, 10
Ventricular fibrillation, 318, 319f
Very high frequency (VHF), 500
Vest-type extrication device, 84
VHF. *See* Very high frequency (VHF)
Vibrio cholerae, 534
Violence, 423
Viral hepatitis, 26–27
Visceral pleura, 285
Vital signs, 99–100
Voluntary muscle, 48

W

Walkie-talkie, 501
Warning lights, 513
Wet lung, 394–395
Wheeled ambulance stretcher, 83
Windpipe, 120
Withdrawal, 372
Womb, 439
Writs, 156

Y

Yersinia pestis, 533

Z

Zygoma, 178